THE FRAGRANT MIND

Aromatherapy for Personality,
Mind, Mood and Emotion

Valerie Ann Worwood

BANTAM BOOKS

London • New York • Toronto • Sydney • Auckland

THE FRAGRANT MIND
A BANTAM BOOK : 9780553407990

Originally published in Great Britain by
Doubleday, a division of Transworld Publishers

PRINTING HISTORY
Doubleday edition published 1995
Bantam edition published 1997

13 15 17 19 20 18 16 14

Set in 11 on 12 point Times by
Falcon Oast Graphic Art.

Bantam Books are published by Transworld Publishers,
61–63 Uxbridge Road, London W5 5SA,
A Random House Group Company.

Addresses for Random House Group Ltd companies outside the UK
can be found at: www.randomhouse.co.uk
The Random House Group Ltd Reg. No. 954009.

Printed and bound in Great Britain by
Cox & Wyman Ltd, Reading, Berkshire.

The Random House Group Limited supports The Forest Stewardship
Council (FSC), the leading international forest certification organisation.
All our titles that are printed on Greenpeace approved FSC certified paper
carry the FSC logo. Our paper procurement policy can be found at:
www.rbooks.co.uk/environment.

DEDICATION

For my Dad who read me Omar Khayyám, told me stories about his
Fairy and the Tiger, and gave me gifts of dreams and imagination.

ACKNOWLEDGEMENTS

A sincere thank you to Julia Stonehouse for her invaluable
assistance, encouragement and humour, and to my daughter,
Emma, for giving me precious space and the time to write.

Thanks also go to the following tutors and practitioners who
gave up precious personal time to send me their thoughts on
favourite essential oils for Part Three: Susan Worwood, Vivian
Lunny, Norma Gilbert, Elizabeth Jones, Teddy Fearnhamm,
Nicole Perez, Maureen Farrell, Anne Marie Joyeux, Olive
Beachamp, Shirley Price, Rodolphe Balz, Dietrich Gumbel,
Jan Kusmirek.

Over the last two decades many people have contributed
directly and indirectly to the concept of *The Fragrant Mind*,
including my patients and students, fellow practitioners and
lecturers, as well as researchers and scientists exploring the
universal mind. To these, and the unseen hands that guide me,
I give thanks.

PLEASE NOTE:

The material in this book is not meant to take the place of diagnosis and treatment by a qualified medical practitioner. Since the actual use of essential oils by others is beyond the author's control, no expressed or implied guarantee as to the effects of their use can be given, nor liability taken. Essential oils are to be used at the user's own discretion.

Any application of the recommendations set forth in the following pages is at the reader's sole risk. The author and publishers disclaim any liability arising directly or indirectly from the use of this book.

CONTENTS

INTRODUCTION

'I planted the seed, Apollos watered it.
But God made it grow.'

1 Corinthians, 3:6

The Alternative Service Book

WELCOME TO *THE FRAGRANT MIND* — A NEW APPROACH TO emotional well-being. The subject of this book is essential oils – highly concentrated aromatic plant essences that are used in aromatherapy – and their application to enhance mind, mood and emotion. This is not a new subject, of course, and plant essences have in various ways been used for thousands of years to cheer people up, calm them down, and make them feel good about themselves. This book, for the first time, presents a comprehensive guide to this subject of natural mind enhancement with essential oils.

Over recent years there has been a significant growth of interest in aromatherapy and what has made it so successful is the fact that people gain tremendous benefit from essential oils in terms of emotional well-being. Indeed, when most people think about aromatherapy, they think about it being able to alleviate stress and tension. However, this is just the tip of the iceberg, so to speak, because in fact essential oils provide a complete *materia medica* for mind, mood and emotion.

You do not have to be ill to use essential oils for the mind. Indeed, essential oils are all about potential – not only the potential of the body to be healed, a medical system, but about the potential of the mind to work at optimum emotional harmony, a system of aromatology – well-being of the mind – and a huge spectrum of possibility presents itself.

The Fragrant Mind is presented in three parts. The first, *Pathways to the Mind*, explains how essential oils appear to work on the brain, and the many diverse ways in which they can be used, both by the lay person and the professional. Part Two, *Emotional Healing and Aromatherapy*, gives detailed suggestions relevant to a very wide variety of emotional conditions. This includes blends for happiness and other positive states, as well as an essential oil guide for an A–Z of negative emotional problems. Part Three, *Aroma-Genera: Human Characteristics and Personalities of Essential Oils*, explains the typology of essential oils, and acts as a guide for choosing the right oils for your personality.

This last section, *Aroma-Genera*, is used in the field of aroma-psychology – a brand new branch of aromatherapy. It is about using essential oils in a positive way to enhance personality. The groups into which essential oils fall are known as the typology, and these are described here for the first time as *Florals, Fruities, Herbies, Leafies, Resinies, Rooties, Seedies, Spicies* and *Woodies*. These classifications act as a guide to positive and negative personality traits, and help indicate which particular essential oils would suit a particular person. In addition to this, each essential oil has its own unique personality, and forty-five essential oils are described here.

Not only can essential oils be used for anxiety, doubt or fear, they can also be used to make a person more assertive, confident or creative. Aromatherapy is not just about 'stress and tension', although of course it is tremendously beneficial in these areas, it goes very deeply into the psyche on all levels of human experience. Essential oils are nature's pharmacopoeia, fully able to deal with the mind in all its aspects, a fabulous gift for us all.

This book has been many years in the making and the material on these pages is a synthesis of practical application and knowledge, experienced by real-life people who have benefited from essential oil use. The information presented here is not based on some ancient texts which may have had relevance many hundreds of years ago but on many years experience as a clinical aromatherapist, in contact with others in my profession.

Today, all over the world, for different reasons, researchers are increasingly becoming interested in the fact that these precious concentrated substances actually work, and are more than the sum of their component parts. Pictures produced by sophisticated technology can now be taken showing aroma molecules working on the brain. We are talking here about powerful aromatic substances which, through the olfactory bulb, gain an immediate access to our mind, mood and emotions. Aromatherapy may be an ancient art but it is also, and increasingly so, being seen as a hugely interesting field of future research and development.

Essential oils allow you to take control of your emotional well-being. These are not unknown quantities but substances that have been used by millions of people over thousands of years and continue to be used today in a wide variety of ways – some of which you will be familiar with. For example, some of the essential oils mentioned in this book are used in perfumery and cosmetics, others are ingredients in food and drink products and, of course, essential oils are used as medicines.

Essential oils are distilled from certain varieties of certain species of plants, some coming from petals, others from stems, twigs, leaves, roots, trees, grasses or fruits. These exquisite aromatic substances provide a rich treasury for human beings, in all their aspects of mind, body and spirit. Well-being is a difficult thing to quantify, but essential oils can certainly help us discover it. My aim with *The Fragrant Mind* is to pass on some of the information I have acquired in an easy-to-use form, so that others can walk on Mother Nature's pathway to a fragrant mind.

Part One

PATHWAYS TO THE MIND

'The most beautiful and deepest experience a man can have is the sense of the mysterious. It is the underlying principle of religion as well as all serious endeavour in art and science.'

ALBERT EINSTEIN
*In a speech delivered at the
German League of Human Rights, 1932*

Chapter One

THE HISTORY OF DRUGS

I wonder what's around the bend? said the explorer
I wonder what that plant is? said the collector
I wonder what's in it? said the chemist
I wonder what activity it has? said the pharmacologist
I wonder if it'll work in this case? said the physician
I hope she lives! said the father
Please God! said the mother
I think she'll be all right in the morning, said the nurse

MARGARET KREIG
Green Medicine

EVER SINCE HUMAN BEINGS FIRST WALKED ON THIS EARTH THEY
have searched for materials which would ease their suffering.
As time went on they came to know which plants would feed
their hunger, which would poison, and which would heal. In
the ancient Sumerian town of Nippur, prescriptions were
written out on clay tablets and from these we know that over
4,000 years ago people used flowers, seeds, leaves, fruits,
roots and barks in their medicines. Among the plants they used

were thyme, myrrh and pine – which are still used today in the form of essential oils – and willow, the source of aspirin.

Aspirin is another name for acetylsalicylic acid, a synthetic first produced in 1899 and derived from salicin, the active ingredient, named after salix – a family of willow tree. For thousands of years resins and juices from the bark and leaves of the willow have been used to treat rheumatism, neuralgia and other ailments, but the scientific history of the willow is traced to an eighteenth-century clergyman, Edmund Stone, who had by recommendation or accident acquired the habit of chewing the bark. Interestingly, salicin is also a drug for the tree itself – conferring 'systematic acquired resistance' on it, according to scientists at the Agricultural Biotechnology Research Unit of Ciba-Geigy Ltd, the multinational chemical company. Apparently, the willow trees use it to ward off infections, which they are prone to because they often grow by stagnant water.

Malaria has killed more people in this world than any other disease. The first drug treatment was quinine, which continues to be used against strains of the disease which are resistant to newer antimalarials, and is more commonly prescribed to prevent painful leg cramps at night. The source of this drug is the bark of a flowering evergreen, *Cinchona*, which grows on the Andean slopes of South America. The bark was first imported to Europe in 1645 and widely used as an antimalarial although its mysteries were not uncovered until 1819 when pharmaceutical chemists extracted one of the alkaloids and named it quinine after the Peruvian Indian word *quina-quina*, the 'bark of barks'.

As they explored their natural environment, people inevitably came across those plants which have an effect on the mind. So it was in India and Africa where for hundreds and perhaps thousands of years people used the root of related species of rauwolfia as a tranquillizer and treatment for 'moon madness' – lunacy. In 1925 an eminent Nigerian living in London became psychotic but the doctors treating him couldn't help. The witch doctor was summoned and arrived with his rauwolfia root – which did the trick. The active substances in rauwolfia (named after Leonhard Rauwolf, the sixteenth-century physician and plant explorer) were isolated in the late 1940s by Indian scientists and after more work by the Swiss drug company, Ciba-Geigy Ltd, the first mind or mood altering drug based on rauwolfia alkaloids, reserpine, hit the market. And what a market it was – $80 million by the mid 1970s.

Not all alkaloids are so easy to reproduce chemically because they have large compounds which are difficult to synthesize. An example of this is the Madagascan Periwinkle, the source of vincristine sulphate, an essential drug in any pharmacy dealing with childhood leukaemia and certain lymphomas. It still takes twelve tons of crushed leaves to produce one ounce of the drug – also the source of Vinblastine, used to treat Hodgkin's disease. Over the years untold suffering has been alleviated by this innocent-looking pink and white ornamental, *Catharanthus roseus*, which gardeners appropriately call 'bright eyes'. Cancer treatment would be a harder task today without the 70 per cent of antitumor drugs derived from native medicines.

Originally, all drugs were natural. The Ayurvedic system of medicine, thought to be at least 5,000 years old, is still extensively used in the Indian subcontinent and is studied by many western medics as well. The textbooks mention 8,000 different natural medicines, using plant, animal and mineral materials. Chinese herbal medicine is also becoming popular in the West, and of course continues to be of central importance in the *materia medica* of China. The first drug directory that we know of is the 2800 BC *Pen Ts'ao*, written by herbalist Shen Nung. In the western tradition, credit for establishing medical botany as an applied science is given to the Greek physician Pedanios Dioscorides who in AD 78 published his *Materia Medica* which detailed the properties of about 600 medicinal plants, as well as the medicinal value of certain animal products. Books such as these, recording the properties of natural products, were the mainstay of western medicine for about 1,400 years. The concept of medicinal chemistry was introduced in the 1520s by Paracelsus, a Swiss pharmacist-physician whose 'real' name was Theophrastus Bombastus von Hohenheim. Paracelsus advocated the use of mineral salts and acids, and experimented with various chemical processes including distillation. It would be another three hundred years before medical chemistry really took off, however, inspired by the German apothecary's assistant, Friedrich Serturner, who in 1806 isolated the first active alkaloid of a natural drug – raw opium from the poppy *Papaver somniferum*. Serturner named it morphine after Morpheus, the Greek god of Dreams. Codeine is a derivative of morphine.

The history of drugs clearly shows the source of inspiration – nature. However, nature has its disadvantages. Imagine yourself the manager of a drug company looking at your storehouse full of bags of herbs, barks, roots, leaves and flowers imported from all over the world. You start thinking about what could go wrong with your supplies. Natural products are vulnerable to adverse weather conditions, including flood and drought, as well as to pest catastrophes. But if just one of these raw materials fails to make it to the factory, drugs cannot be made and people die. Also, natural raw materials are unpredictable in terms of the quantity of active ingredient they contain, and huge quantities of the stuff have to be processed to produce small quantities of the required drug. On top of that, the raw material has to be purified and quantified – all of which is more effort. You can see why chemists tried to find a way of creating the active ingredients of medicinal plants by more easily controlled, chemical means.

Over the years we have seen a major shift of emphasis. To begin with, natural products were either the raw material of drugs, or the inspiration for man-made copies. As chemists became more confident, they made cocktails using more and more compounds – some natural, some not. Nowadays, scientists create chemical cocktails which have little to do with nature as we know it. What effect these will have on the population is still little understood because long-term studies cannot yet be made. Unlike natural drugs, these chemical cocktails have new molecular arrangements which haven't been on trial for thousands of years. Indeed, their trials are of necessity rather short because a company has to register the thirty-year patent for the new drug before it can carry out trials. The patent is liable to run out if the company doesn't get

Clove

its act together quickly, and produce the evidence of efficacy and safety required to get a product licence. The quicker a trial can be done, the more time there is left on the patent in which the company can exclusively exploit its invention.

Chemical companies are still interested in nature. In the deepest jungles and the most far-flung corners of the earth, representatives from drug companies continue to scour the landscape looking for new varieties of nature to exploit. They are not intending, however, to manage huge fields of these natural products, and extract from them the drug required. They are simply going to try to isolate the active substances and replicate them in the laboratory. In their dreams, scientists imagine a future biotechnology when the physiological and psychoactive substances in plants can be produced cheaply and easily, using microbes or whatever.

Biotechnology is here, however. Take Hirudin, for example, the latest potential drug from Ciba-Geigy Ltd, which is at the

human trials stage. The leech *Hirudo medicinalis* was used for
centuries to draw blood from patients. The saliva of the leech
is now known to contain substances which act as a powerful
and highly predictable anticoagulant, which may be very useful in the prevention of thrombosis, stroke and heart attack –
the western world's largest killer disease. The problem is, it
takes the saliva from 10,000 leeches to make a single human
treatment and, I imagine, extracting it is quite a job! Bio-
technology, however, gets around the problem by taking the
appropriate gene from the leech and putting it in yeast cells,
which produce Hirudin molecules.

New discoveries continue to be made. In a recent article in
the *Lancet*, co-authored by Nobel Laureate B. S. Blumberg,
clinical research was presented which proved that the hepatitis
B virus was eliminated from the bodies of 59 per cent of
people treated for thirty days with dried and powdered
Phyllanthus amarus, a plant used for over 2,000 years in
Ayurvedic medicine to treat liver disease, including jaundice.
The plant has also been used in China, the Philippines, Cuba,
Nigeria, Guam, East and West Africa, the Caribbean, and
Central and South America. Despite the fact that the plant is
used so extensively, and the fact that it has now been studied
for over ten years, and has shown no toxic or side effects in
animals or humans, it will probably never reach the market
place in Britain or America. *Phyllanthus* needs more than the
keen advocacy of the eminent Blumberg, who got his Nobel
prize for discovering the hepatitis B virus and developing the
blood test to detect it. *Phyllanthus* needs tens of millions of
pounds to go through clinical testing, and chemical companies
aren't going to support that work because to date they have
had no intention of selling herbs. They may well look at
Phyllanthus, and try to copy its active constituents, but that is
another matter.

In the land of the BMW, Germany, things are different. The
laws allow natural medicines to be sold, but as food supplements without any indication of use on the label. Even so,
everyone knows what they are for and so, for example, we see
Gingko biloba extract taken from the tree much used in herbalism, becoming the best-selling prescription drug in Germany –

Vanilla

where it is used to stimulate cerebral circulation in the elderly.[1]

Chemical companies are not keen to switch their attention to producing extracts or essential oils from natural plants and it may have something to do with the difficulty in patenting remedies that have been known for centuries. But it is possible to extract the active constituents of plants quite easily, and it's much easier than trying to replicate their extraordinary complex powers in chemistry. Lavender essential oil is the classic case in point. It is the treatment *par excellence* for burns. Put on badly burnt skin, lavender, nothing short of miraculously, returns it to normal, and very, very quickly. But, for all the work on it, lavender will not easily give up her secrets. Chemists can make a liquid that *smells* like lavender, and they can even break it apart and label a certain number of its constituents, but they cannot make a substance that is like lavender in that it heals burns. As systems of analysis get better, more molecular and other secrets will be revealed.

Meanwhile, in burns departments in hospitals, people suffer.

Of course science has made great strides in the field of medicine, and we all have reason to be grateful for it, but let us not forget the relationship between science and nature. Science looks to nature in amazement, tries to break it apart and copy it. Nature makes cells and gets them to interact in unbelievably complex ways, while the whole of science and technology cannot between them make a single cell – plant, animal or human. Looking at nature and science, we must ask ourselves which is the more clever?

THE SHAMANS

Consciousness is at the core of humanity. Deprived of sight, hearing, touch, taste and smell, we still have consciousness. It is, if you like, the essence of being, but throughout time people have strived to enlarge their consciousness or to change it so that other dimensions of being are reached. Substances which alter perception are used to put people in touch with the spirits of dead ancestors; or to seek union with the godhead; or by traditional healers who want to gain a more profound insight into the nature of a patient's disease – often perceived as the result of outside, non-material, forces. Other people use them to get 'in tune' with the animals they want to hunt.

The Matse are a small, semi-nomadic tribe of hunter-gatherers who live in the rainforest on the Peru/Brazil border. Their pharmacopoeia includes a drug, *nu-nu*, which hunters use to induce visions of the future movements of animals. They see the animal situated in a particular place, and from clues in the vision, they estimate the time of day. Armed with this information, they lie in wait and make the kill. Peter Gorman may be the only westerner who has tried *nu-nu*, which is blown into the nostrils down a hollow reed tube, and this is his description of the experience:

> When the *nu-nu* hit, it seemed to explode inside my face.
> It burnt my nose and I began to choke up wretched green
> phlegm. But the pain quickly subsided and I closed my
> eyes. Out of the blackness I began to have visions of

animals – tapir, monkey and wild boar – that I saw more
clearly than my limited experience with them should have
allowed. Then suddenly the boars stampeded in front of
me.[2]

Gorman told the Matse what he had seen, and from the clues
in his vision, the time and place of the stampede was determined. The next morning Gorman and several Indians set off
for the place seen in the vision. He writes: 'As we neared it, I
was astounded to hear the thunderous roar of dozens of boars
charging across the river in front of us. We jumped out of the
boat and chased them.' They returned to the village with seven
boars – 'enough meat for the entire village for four days'.

Gorman also took another Matse drug, *sapo*, which is made
from the secretions of a frog, *dow-kiet!* or *phyllomedusa
bicolor*. The immediate physical effects of ingesting this drug
were horrendous, according to Gorman's account, but the
results were worth it. His hearing was greatly improved, and
more besides:

> My vision, my sense of smell, everything about me felt
> larger than life, and my body felt immensely strong . . .
> During the next few days, my feeling of strength didn't
> diminish; I could go whole days without being hungry or
> thirsty and move through the jungle for hours without
> tiring. Every sense I possessed was heightened and in tune
> with the environment, as though the *sapo* put the rhythm
> of the jungle into my blood.[3]

The Matse use huge quantities of the drug *sapo* to do nothing
less than project their anima, their spirit, into the form of an
animal – which they use as a lure for real animals. Gorman's
informant, Pablo, set a trap in the forest then returned to the
village where he took the *sapo* for two days. The next morning he woke Gorman up before dawn and, with the rest of the
village, rushed to the place where the trap had been set. Just as
the people arrived, a tapir was approaching the trap – and was
duly caught. On analysis, it turns out that *sapo* contains seven
bioactive peptides – triggers which cause chemical reactions
in the body. However, why *sapo* should give a person the

ability to project their anima remains a mystery!

People living in the depths of nature seem to have an extra-ordinary sensitivity. One thinks about the reports of people back at camp whooping and shouting at the precise moment the hunting party, many miles away, makes a kill. How did they know? These are mysteries of communication we can only guess at but, on top of this degree of 'extra-sensory' perception, native peoples seek to go further. With a little help from nature, they project themselves into the very form of animals, they see the future, they communicate with dead relatives, they speak to nature spirits, they get outside their conscious selves and into another, equally real, dimension.

In our culture, such concepts are difficult to grasp but we too experiment with consciousness-raising drugs, seeking our own understanding of the universe. Over the past three decades, LSD, mescaline and psilocybin have been widely used in this way and, interestingly, all these drugs resemble human brain chemicals in their chemical structure. The alkaloid mescaline comes from the peyote cactus and is closely related to noradrenaline, a neurotransmitter (which acts in the chemical transmission of impulses between nerves in the brain). Mescaline and the neurotransmitter noradrenaline (norepinephrine) have the same basic chemical structure and both are derived from phenylethylamine, another derivative of which is phenylalanine, an essential amino acid found extensively in humans. Psilocybin and psilocine are the active principles of the Mexican mushroom, *Teonanacatl*, and, like the brain hormone serotonin, are derived from tryptamine – as are the hallucinogenic properties of Morning Glory, *Ololuiqui*, the inspiration of the semi-synthetic LSD. Chemically, LSD is extremely close to lysergic acid amide and lysergic acid hydroxyethylamide, the hallucinogenic principles of *Ololuiqui*.

In the very excellent *Plants of the Gods*, Richard Schultes MD and Albert Hofmann MD (the man who discovered LSD) explain the psychotropic potency of these hallucinogens:

> Having the same basic structure, these hallucinogens may
> act at the same sites in the nervous system as the ... brain

hormones, like similar keys fitting the same lock. As a result, the psychophysiological functions associated with those brain sites are altered, suppressed, stimulated, or otherwise modified.[4]

But it isn't just about chemistry. According to Schultes and Hofmann:

> The ability of hallucinogens to provide changes in brain function is due not only to their having a particular chemical composition, but also to the peculiar spacial arrangement of the atoms in their molecules.[5]

LSD is a case in point. The semi-synthetic hallucinogen LSD differs from the semi-synthetic compound iso-LSD only in the spacial arrangement of the diethylamide group, but the iso-LSD has practically no hallucinogenic effect.

Life teaches us that the mind is a very strange thing. Speed alters in an emergency. It goes in slow motion as we helplessly watch our car smash into another. For one friend, time stood still when, walking in the wilderness, she inadvertently stepped into a mud pool – like quicksand – in which she could quite easily have disappeared without trace. With the mud more liquid below her feet, and her companions walking on ahead, she knew she was on the fence between life and death. Time stood still, she tells me, and to this day she doesn't know whether she was there for five minutes, five hours or five centuries!

The mind is clearly capable of playing tricks on us, and there is probably some self-preservation reason at root. The point, however, is that this Pandora's box of perceptual tricks can be stimulated by outside means – life experiences which provoke exceptional chemical phenomena, synthetic hallucinogens, and natural plant and animal materials.

There are essential oils that have narcotic or mind-altering principles, but I shall not list them here, you won't find them in other aromatherapy books, and they are not discussed in aromatherapy schools. Indeed, it is a matter of professional responsibility to ensure that no potentially harmful substances are used. In *The Fragrant Mind* I promote the use of subtle and gentle substances which allow you to seek your own visions or understandings – a vision quest in which you have the control. Essential oils are the non-toxic and harmless way to allow your mind free will to explore its untapped potential.

Chapter Two

ESSENTIAL OILS AND THE MIND

ESSENTIAL OILS AND HUMAN BEINGS HAVE A GREAT DEAL IN common. We are both alive – chemically, electrically, and in terms of infrared radiation. Essential oils come from plants, while we ourselves rely totally on plants for our sustenance – we eat plants, and animals which eat plants, and breathe air made possible by plants. Human beings and plants are related because all living organisms are descended from the same single-cell line.[1] The chemical composition of DNA in plants and people is virtually the same.[2] Neurobiologist Donald Kennedy has done a detailed study of the difference between plants and animals and come to the conclusion that there is very little difference! He took tissue from a spruce tree and compared it with that from a moose, the animal. Cells from both the spruce and moose have walls, both contain little organs called *organelles*, and both have a nucleus, with its own membrane, and genetic material – DNA – the chemical composition of which is identical between spruce and moose.[3]

Plants and humans both depend on a chelating chemical, which in humans is red *heme* – which transports the oxygen released from plants in the blood – and in plants it is *chlorophyll*. Chemically, the only difference between these two is that a magnesium atom replaces an iron one.[4] The similar chemical composition of plants and humans may explain why essential oils, which are distillations of certain parts of certain plants, seem to act like keys to our physical and mental mechanisms.

It's becoming increasingly clear that there is still much to learn about plants. Trees might look helpless, locked to one spot in the ground, but we now know that, using chemistry, they talk to each other, defend themselves against animal invaders, and attack plant species to protect resources. Genetically, trees are very resourceful, adapting over one generation to deal with many generations of short-lived but highly adaptive insects. An old oak tree, for example, could have ten branches carrying ten different genetic messages. This evolutionary advantage may help explain why some trees, like *Pinus aristata*, can live for over 2,000 years!

Chemically, trees are very active. When under attack from a predator they can produce extra chemicals called tannins – which deter and even kill the predator – and then distribute them to the leaves. In Africa, Professor Wouter van Hoven set about testing a variety of trees to see how *much* extra tannin the trees produced. He got his students to thrash the trees with sticks and belts, replicating the harsh treatment trees get from browsing deer and the like, and then he tested the increase. After fifteen minutes, *Acacia caffra* had increased its tannin production by 94 per cent while *Rhus leptodictya*'s went up by 76 per cent. After an hour, the off-putting tannins had increased in the leaves of wattle by 256 per cent and in the acacia by 282 per cent. Other species show similar reactions. It took the trees between 24 and 100 hours after the attack to return to their normal chemical state. Somehow too, the trees had transmitted the news of 'predators about' to nearby trees, which also started to produce extra tannins. Because the message was relayed to trees not connected by their root systems, as Dr David Rhoads of the University of Washington has suggested with red alder and sitka willow, what we may have at work here are 'airborne pheromonal substances' – chemical messengers . . . hormones. As another piece of chemical wizardry, to protect their personal space, trees produce allelochemicals which insects ingest and, through their droppings, deposit on the ground around the tree. These allelochemicals prevent other plants from growing nearby, thus conserving resources for the tree.

There is a whole chemical way of life for plants which we are only just beginning to discover – speaking from a laboratory perspective, at least. People have for countless millennia been interacting with plants and a knowledge has built up about the chemical movements within plants – so they can be harvested at their peak. An essential oil could be distilled from a jasmine flower that is not one day old, or a sandalwood tree that is not less than thirty years old. Some plants are harvested in the morning, some at night. And, of course, there are seasons. People have learnt to pick the plants at the optimum moment, even though they haven't understood why the particular required chemicals should be in that particular part of the plant, at that particular time. But there is more to life than chemistry, as we shall see later, and the beauty of essential oils is that whichever way you look at them, they seem to be in perfect harmony with the human organism.

WHAT ARE ESSENTIAL OILS?

For as long as we know, people have been distilling and otherwise processing certain plant materials to extract their powerful healing essences. The word *chemistry* comes from the Greek word *chemia*, meaning plant juice. In turn, according to some scholars, *chemia* may derive from the Persian word *kimiya*, which referred to a group of Chinese tonic herbs. In medieval Latin, Paracelsus referred to the oils he distilled from medicinal plants as the *quinta essentia* – the quintessence of the plant – and that is where the term 'essential oil' comes from.

Essential oils are distilled or otherwise processed from very specific parts of particular species of plants. Vascular plants such as flowering species and conifers contain special tissues or vessels for the circulation of fluids. In the case of lavender, the oil is distilled from the flowers, in the case of ginger it's the root, and in patchouli it's the leaves. Essential oils are made from flowers, leaves, barks, roots, fruits, seeds, grasses and resins. They're produced in practically every country of the world. Oil of spearmint comes from America, oil of chamomile from England, bergamot from Italy, rose from Bulgaria, frankincense from Somalia, pine and cypress from Bhutan and so on. Oils come from *specific* species of plant groups. For example, there are over three hundred varieties of tea tree in Australia, but only a few produce oil with medicinal properties.

There are an estimated half-million species of flora in the world, of which about three hundred produce an essential oil which is used in modern aromatherapy although, of course, traditional medicine and shamanism throughout the world utilizes many more, whose properties we do not yet know. Essential oils are examined in various ways, particularly in terms of chemistry by gas chromatography and the mass spectrograph. Although over 1,000 compounds have been found in essential oils, there are many other compounds which have yet to be isolated, named and understood. These unknown compounds tend to be 'disappeared' by the literature, which concentrates on what we *do* know. Long lists of components in oils may look very impressive but what science doesn't tell us is that if all the known chemicals were mixed together in a pot, they would not make the essential oil they were trying to copy. Something vital is missing, the question is, 'what?'

Reductionism, with essential oils, doesn't work. Tea tree oil is powerfully antimicrobial, but its two main components – terpinen-4-ol (40 per cent volume) and gamma terpinene (28 per cent) are much less so. It is the *synergistic* effect of *all* the components that makes an essential oil what it is. This is why there isn't a chemist in the world who can tell you *how* essential oils work. In a rose oil, for example, there may be over 100 compounds, some known and some not, and figuring out how they all work as an integrated unit is not at all easy. Essential oils are complex chemical structures, still beyond the powers of scientific analysis.

As individual oils are so mysterious, imagine the difficulty in analysing *mixtures* of oils. But blends of different oils are used every day by millions of people all over the world. Indeed, complex blending has been a feature of herbal life for as long as we know, and as the medicine men and women and shamans working to help the people around them know, it is not only individual plants that are interesting, but the synergistic effect of them when combined.

ABSOLUTES

In the general term 'essential oils', there are some which are more accurately called 'absolutes' because they have been through a particular form of extraction which brings into the 'oil' more components than essential oils produced by steam distillation. The process of distillation releases only the lighter aromatic molecules, which are subsequently separated and packaged, while the absolutes contain both the lighter and the heavier molecules. The absolutes include jasmine, tuberose, rose maroc, narcissus, cistus and hyacinth, amongst others, and are made from the most fragrant and delicate of flowers.

It is an ironic yet poetic fact of nature that the most fragrant flowers are the most difficult from which to extract the fragrance. You might simply pass a rose in the garden but the aroma wafts towards you and stays with you for half a day. One jasmine plant can perfume an entire garden. Capturing this power is phenomenally difficult with many millions of petals being required to fill one small bottle of, for example, jasmine oil.

It is not an easy job to coax the powerful aroma from the delicate flowers from which absolutes are made. Distillation is too harsh, so over the years other methods have been employed. The ancients used fat-extraction, a method which has been continued during the following many centuries in the form of maceration or enfleurage, but today we have CO_2 (carbon dioxide) extraction to obtain the aromatic material. This produces an 'essential oil' or, if you want to be exact, 'an absolute', which smells exactly like the flower from which it came. The same cannot be said for steam-distilled essential oils, which often differ somewhat in aroma from the plant itself.

Absolutes contain in them more components of the plant from which they came, including waxes, colour pigments, fatty acids, vitamins and minerals. These tend to give the absolute a more three-dimensional aroma, much appreciated by the perfume industry. The very name 'absolute' does, in fact, describe this class of oils very well because they are absolutely complete in their aromatic complexity.

In the aromatherapy field there has been a long debate about these absolutes, with some people saying that the extraction methods bring into the 'oil' residues of solvents and particles of the plant which are not therapeutic. It has now been shown that absolutes do not necessarily contain residues of solvents which, in any case, can be organic substances. Also, the newer method of CO_2 extraction eliminates the question of solvents.

The growing appreciation of absolutes has generated the new practice of extracting absolutes from plants usually distilled by steam distillation. We are discovering that chamomile absolute, as distinct from chamomile essential oil, smells different to it, and may have properties different to it too. The difference between essential oils and absolutes could be said to be a degree of dimension. The absolutes are as their name implies – more absolute, i.e. whole or entire. In essential oil terms, this means they extend, perhaps more than some essential oils, from their medicinal therapeutic value into aroma-psychology and the dimension of emotional and even spiritual value.

CHEMISTRY

On average, an essential oil is made up of over a hundred components. Some are ten times more complex than this. The main categories of compounds are terpenes, alcohols, esters, aldehydes, ketones and phenols. At the present time it is known that up to 50 per cent of the essential oil of *Lavendula officinalis* is made up of alcohols including lavandulol, borneol, terpineol, geraniol and linalol – in esterified form, linalyl acetate. Between 48–52 per cent is comprised of esters derived from the alcohols: lavandylyl acetate, linalyl acetate, bornyl acetate.

Oxides account for between 2–3 per cent, like 1,8 cineole, linalyl oxide and caryophyllene oxide. There are also minuscule but vital other components such as coumarin, herniarine, umbelliferone, santonine. Terpenes such as myrcene, limonene and ocimene can account for up to 5 per cent, while the sesquiterpene, caryophyllene, is about 3 per cent. There is also ketone camphor, methyl heptyl ketone, lactones and aldehydes. The trouble is, if you were to put together a stew of chemical ingredients, following the above formula, you would not get a lavender oil capable of healing burns. There are still as yet undiscovered compounds in essential oils, or perhaps other forces, which may one day explain their extraordinary healing powers.

It should also be said that current methods of analysis depend very much upon the sensitivity of the machine and the operator. Different chromatography machines give different readings so an operator needs to be familiar with his or her machine. The operator doesn't exactly *read* the data so much as *interpret* it. For this reason, accurate analysis of essential oils may have to wait until technology has built the tools which can interpret nature.

ELECTROMAGNETISM

The word electron was adopted from the Greek by William Gilbert, physician to Queen Elizabeth I in the sixteenth century. Gilbert demonstrated the electron factor by applying friction to amber (which is of course a plant resin), which makes light objects like feathers attract to it. But electricity and magnetism are more impressive than this. In the 1960s Wilderanck showed that if an electric field was applied to cells in a fluid suspension they would join up to make strings or chains which would orientate along the lines of magnetic force. When the field was turned off, the cells returned to their individual unconnected state.

All life has electric properties. The ion channels in cell membranes cause a voltage difference across the membrane of nearly one tenth of a volt. If you put twenty neurons together

in the correct way you could get a charge of 1.5 volts – enough
to run a small torch. Chains of molecules (polymers) are polar-
ized like the DNA helix, which has a positively charged end
and a negatively charged end – just like a magnet. Human
beings react to sunspots happening 93,000 miles away like
receivers of energy. Doctors apply electrical impulses to
broken limbs, which have proved difficult to mend, and hey
presto, they heal! Electrical osteogenesis is just one aspect of
the new branch of science, electrical medicine, which is
developing all the time.

Essential oils have electrical properties, which are defined in
terms of positive-negative and polarity. Thus an aroma molecule
might be negative and polar, negative and non polar, positive
and polar, or positive and non polar. Even the electrical properties of individual components in essential oils can be measured
and we know, for example, that aldehydes have an electro-
negative character, while monoterpene hydrocarbons have
moderately electro-positive molecules. Phenols are electro-
positive while turpenic alcohols are for the most part mildly
electro-positive. Esters are electrically neutral, aldehydes have a
distinct electro-negative character and phenols have an electron
deficiency.[5] The electrical cocktail going on in essential oils is
similar to the electrical cocktail going on in the human body –
positives and negatives all firing at different times, yet in syn-
chronicity. According to essential oil researchers Franchomme
and Pénoël, they are carriers of negative or positive energy
depending on whether they have an excess or lack of electrons,
whether donors or acceptors of electrons. This makes essential
oils very dynamic, and a good set of therapeutic tools to work
with.

INFRARED RADIATION

The aroma molecules which rise up from a corn field can be
detected by moths flying between 500 and 2,000 feet above.
This remarkable perception was once attributed entirely to the
moth's sense of smell, but it's now thought moths also recognize the infrared radiation produced by the aroma molecules.

The scientific field of infrared spectrophotometry was discovered by the nineteenth-century Irish genius, John Tyndall, who, aside from discovering why the sky is blue, found that infrared radiation is absorbed by the essential oils of patchouli, sandalwood, cloves, lavender, rose, lemon, thyme, rosemary, spikenard and aniseed, among others.

What significance this infrared factor has *vis-à-vis* humans is not known, but humans are themselves surrounded by an aura of infrared emanation.[6] According to Tompkins and Bird in *Secrets of The Soil*, 'the subtle molecular odors that surround human bodies are stimulated to radiation by this infrared emission'.

When I was working in Europe over twenty years ago it was usual for therapists to leave the client under an infrared lamp for five minutes before starting an aromatherapy treatment because it was thought this helped the absorption of essential oils. This may well be so because infrared improves circulation, opens blood vessels, brings blood to the surface, so it can absorb better. On the infrared question then, we have several factors to consider: aroma molecules may produce infrared radiation; they also absorb it; human beings are surrounded by infrared emissions; and circulation is helped when they are exposed to more of it. Clearly, there are interactions between essential oils and human beings on the infrared level, interactions that need further investigation which may one day help to explain their efficacy.

HOW DO ESSENTIAL OILS GET INTO THE BODY?

There are several ways of taking essential oils into the body. One of the most effective ways is through percutaneous absorption – through the skin. As aroma molecules, essential oils set off reactions in receptor cells in the nose, leading to enzyme activity and electrical impulses to the olfaction bulb – which is actually an extension of the brain. Some people, under some very particular circumstances, also take essential oils orally, but generally, this is their least effective means of absorption because they end up in the digestive tract with all sorts of other materials with which they will react (which is also the case with chemical drugs). Because of the high absorption of essential oils by the mucous membranes of the respiratory tract, they can be inhaled as airborne particles. In France, essential oils are delivered in suppositories and pessaries. The state of acidity in the delicate mucous membranes allows them to absorb materials into the body very effectively. There is a particularly absorbent area under the tongue, which is now being utilized in the delivery of 'sublinguals', usually vitamin supplements – the latest medicinal delivery system. But also the nose has many surface capillaries, through which molecules can go straight into the bloodstream. For this reason, you can now buy vitamin supplements like B12, for example, which are packaged in gels which you squirt up the nose. Cocaine and the South American drug *nu-nu* are other substances which may enter the bloodstream via this route.

When you have essential oils in your environment, then, they could have an effect on you via many routes. As airborne particles in a diffuser, say, their effect would be very subtle – affecting the mind via receptor cells in the nose and the olfaction bulb, and getting into the bloodstream when absorbed through mucous membranes – of the nose, mouth and respiratory tract. In the bath, essential oils work both percutaneously and through airborne manners, as they do during massage – which generally gives much higher concentrations. With essential oils more is not always best. Sometimes, less is better. The different methods of use all have their advantages, depending on the circumstances.

In a later section I discuss how essential oils work on the brain, but here it is just worth noting that essential oils manage to do what no other known substance can do – seemingly they move through the body with great ease, passing through the interstitial fluid with no problem. The ease with which essential oils pass through the body makes them a perfect drug delivery system, a fact fully appreciated by manufacturers looking to develop 'the magic bullet' – a drug which will go directly to the place in the body where it's required.

The Sense of Smell

According to Dr Alan Hirsch of the Smell and Taste Treatment and Research Foundation in Chicago, by the year 2000 many of us will be living in houses that have aroma-air-conditioning systems. Ten minutes before we want to wake up they'll start to pump a stimulating aroma into the air. Our eyes will open. When we go into a café for breakfast we're induced by pre-packaged aromas to eat more (or less). At work, aromas will be designed to cut the error rate, while in the gym they'll be designed to invigorate. When you come home, there will be a relaxing aroma in the house, and when you go to bed, a soporific or amorous one, depending on your choice. Dr Hirsch and his team have carried out forty-six research studies including one involving 12,000 people which looked at the effect of olfaction on learning. Among other things, Dr Hirsch has discovered that people will judge a product better value when bought from a shop where there is a pleasant aroma, and in another trial he found that when a mixed floral aroma was suffused throughout a room of calculus students, they increased their speed of learning by 230 per cent. When gambling machines in Las Vegas were 'aromatized' with a certain aroma number 1, Dr Hirsch discovered that the punters spent 45 per cent more cash! These and other recent dis-coveries are leading us into an aromatic future – whether we know it or not. Next time you go into an office to make a furious complaint, and come out unplacated but subdued, con-sider the possibility that the waiting room was suffused with an aroma to make clients calm down. It is possible, and it gets more probable every day.

Science is catching up with what aromatherapists have been saying for years: aromas can improve performance and capacity to remember, and they can make you alert or relaxed and change your mood. Aromatherapy uses natural aromas which have, of course, been used for similar purposes through-out the centuries. But, while it is nice to have one's work confirmed, we now have the situation where even more man-made, synthetic, non biodegradable chemicals will be pumped into the atmosphere. Do we really need them when

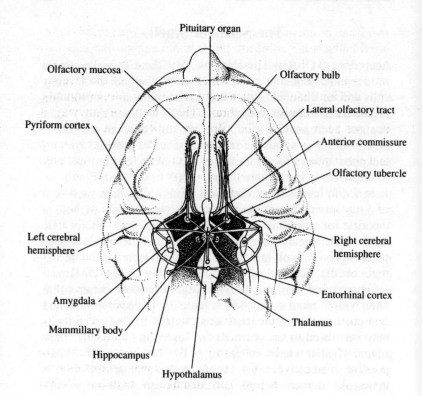

Pituitary organ

Olfactory mucosa

Olfactory bulb

Lateral olfactory tract

Pyriform cortex

Anterior commissure

Olfactory tubercle

Left cerebral
hemisphere

Right cerebral
hemisphere

Entorhinal cortex

Amygdala

Thalamus

Mammillary body

Hippocampus

Hypothalamus

Olfactory nervous pathways

naturals will do as well, if not better?

The reason aroma has such a direct action on the brain is that aroma molecules connect with receptor cells in the cilia extending from the two olfaction bulbs – which are themselves actually an extension of and part of the brain. Olfaction is thus the most direct interface between the brain and the outside world. Through our sense of smell, aroma molecules set off a cascade of reactions involving proteins, enzymes, cell depolarization and second messengers – all leading to an electrical impulse being sent to the brain. The part of the brain most directly involved is the limbic system, evolutionarily the oldest part of the brain, and home of our emotions.

The olfaction bulbs are extraordinary organs, looking like

two small upside-down spoons. Directly under the match-head-sized bulbs is the cribiform plate, thin bone, but the olfactory neurones pass through perforations in this and end – inside the nose – in protein-rich cilia, which are the site of the receptor cells and ion channels which convert an odour into, eventually, an electrical impulse to the brain. That's the theory anyway; it has not been proved. The cilia are embedded in a layer of mucus which is about the size of two shirt buttons on the top and either side of the nasal cavity. Aroma molecules must pass through this before reaching the receptor cells on the cilia.

In 1991, Linda Buck and Richard Axel identified a family of 7-transmembrane domain receptors, which are thought to be the first known olfaction receptors. They look likely candidates because they are found only in the nose and resemble other neurotransmitters in structure. However, attempts to replicate the function of the receptors have so far failed.

Because we have not yet definitely identified the receptors with which odour molecules interact, it is impossible to say *how* an aroma molecule translates into smell. The crucial factor may be related to the chemistry of the aroma molecule, or its shape, whether it is laevorotatory or dextrorotatory, electrically positive or negative, polar or apolar, or some combination of these. As human beings can distinguish between 10,000 aromas, it is thought by some that there are, among the 50 million receptors on the cilia, 10,000 types of receptor. Others think there are just a thousand or even a mere hundred types of receptor, which in some way adapt or amplify (or both) the aroma molecule, thus giving the system its extreme subtlety. For example, the same aroma molecule might smell like one thing if the connection with the receptor is strong, but like another thing if it is weak.

Olfaction is a very complex business. For example, the compound carvone is molecularly identical whether L-carvone or D-carvone but the L-type smells like spearmint and the D-type smells like caraway. These two are stereo-isomers – which means they are copies of each other except that a hydrogen atom sits either to the left or to the right. This difference causes the plane of polarization of light to rotate either to the left or right, giving the definitions 'L' for laevorotatory (to the left) and 'D' for dextrorotatory (to the right). When identical aroma molecules, differing only in their laevorotatory or dextrorotatory characteristics, are perceived as two completely different smells – spearmint and caraway – you can begin to see how complex the problem of olfaction is.

Discoveries are being made all the time, however. Researchers are currently working on a group of enzymes known as the P450s. These have been found in the nasal mucus and are thought to chemically change odorants, perhaps disintegrating them and facilitating their expulsion from the body. It has been suggested that an absence of these enzymes may be the reason some people have lost their smell sensitivity and as there are about 2 million anosmic people in America alone, any further research in this area would be welcome.

Nasal passage

The machinery used to analyse odours by gas-liquid chromatography and mass spectrometry is less sensitive than a healthy human nose. Olfactory neurones are physiologically remarkable in that they are in a state of continuous regeneration. This seems to indicate their importance for our survival, perhaps not so much now as a few thousand years ago. The system remains, however, and it connects directly with the oldest part of the brain, the limbic system. In the old days, aromas would come to us and depending on them, we would approach, attack, make love or run, and although today we may be less aware of it, aroma still plays a crucial role in our emotions and reactions. The limbic system is made up of the hippocampus, amygdala, the septal area and several regions of the cerebral cortex. The hippocampus is believed to be involved in memory and learning. The connection between aroma and memory is well known, of course, but the connection between aroma and learning is only now being scientifically appreciated.

Olfaction research involves chemistry, stereochemistry (the shape of the molecule), vibrational frequency, electrochemical factors, enzymes and proteins and a whole lot more besides. It is multi-dimensional in a way sight and hearing are not. This will make the sense of smell a very difficult mystery to unlock but, in the meantime, olfaction research is becoming more interesting to biologists, psychologists, teachers, sales managers, people managers and even defence departments. Olfaction is no longer the forgotten sense.

Most of the research currently being carried out on smell is by people who want to bombard you with it for commercial reasons, as we shall see later. In the labs, subjects are exposed to fragrance and wired up to equipment which measures electrical skin response, skin temperature, muscle tension, heart rate, respiration and blood pressure. Pictures of the brain can be seen changing under the influence of aroma. According to Drs Craig Warren and Stephen Warrenburg at International Flavours and Fragrances, New Jersey, 'pleasant odours tended to enhance creative performance, generate more positive evaluations of words and pictures of people, and elicit more happy memories'.[7] It is this aspect of olfaction big business wants to harness, but we can harness it too – the natural way.

Percutaneous Absorption

Applying essential oils, in a base oil, directly onto the skin is central to aromatherapy and many trials have shown that essential oils, or components of them, show up in the blood or urine shortly after being applied through massage. Meanwhile, their absorption through the skin during bathing is less of a mystery since Dr Peter Slynko at the Kiev Institute of Physiology (Ukrainian Academy of Science) proved that for several minutes after sweating, the pores remain open and suck in whatever happens to be on the surface of the skin, which later shows up in blood and the lymph.

Clearly the essential oils pass through the skin, the questions are how many of the components in essential oils pass through, and how do they do it? The first question is raised by the fact that the skin, the largest organ of the human body, is a site of metabolism – a place where chemicals in the body alter molecules, either to incorporate them into the body, to use them as fuel, or to expel them more easily. Esterase enzymes, for example, are involved in these functions. The skin is also a place where one of the body's most efficient metabolic alterants are at work in the form of P_{450} enzymes. These enzymes are found in high concentrations in the liver – the ultimate detoxification machine – and, as we have seen, in the olfactory mucus. As the purpose of the P_{450}s is to prevent toxins damaging the body, this may help to explain the remarkably safe history of percutaneous essential oil use. It could be that the P_{450}s either alter any harmful molecules or immobilize them, leaving them in the upper, dead layer of skin, ready to be expelled.

The excellent skin permeability of essential oils is usually attributed to their high lipophilicity. Once through the epidermal (outer) layer of skin, the molecules are transported by the capillary blood and by interstitial fluid. Heat tends to favour their absorption – by having the room warm, the massaging hands warm, and by warming the oil in the hands before applying to the skin. Absorption is also helped by covering the areas of skin to which oil has just been applied, with a towel for example, thus preventing evaporation. The great advantage of percutaneous absorption is that essential oils can be applied directly to the area where they are required – to treat pain or inflammation, for example – and it is also an excellent way to get essential oils into the bloodstream and from there into all areas of the human body, including the brain.

Their Exit

Essential oils have different routes of exit, depending on their variety. It's thought that eucalyptus is exhaled through breath, sandalwood leaves in the urine, patchouli in the faeces and rose oil via perspiration through the whole skin. After a massage with 2 per cent lavender oil, the main constituents – linalol and linalyl acetate – can be detected in the blood after just five minutes, with a maximum concentration after twenty minutes, while after ninety minutes most of the linalol and linalyl acetate has been eliminated from the blood.[8] This isn't to say that the effect of the lavender doesn't linger on – lavender and the other oils set off all kinds of chemical reactions in the body. The keys are turned in the locks, their jobs are done, and they can leave. It should also be said that while some of the more detectable components exit the body, the smaller compounds may be left behind in the body for a longer time, to finish their job perhaps and, as we shall see later, there may be other factors at work.

THE MIND

Philosophers throughout the millennia have spent much effort in trying to define 'the mind' and even today, it's not at all clear what exactly it is. Some would say the mind is the seat of the soul and others that it is nothing more that the sum total of one's experiences, which could also be called 'consciousness'. For the sake of simplicity, I am calling 'mind' here all that which can be said to be primarily experienced in the head – personality, thinking process, intellectual capacity, moods as in feeling 'up' or 'down', and emotions such as love and fear.

Ironically perhaps for the 'seat of feeling', the brain has no pain receptors, so after cutting through the skull with local anaesthetic, brain surgery can be done without anaesthetic and with the patient conscious. The brain seems a well-defined organ but some of the nerves within it are over a metre long . . . so where does the brain end and the body begin? One could say the brain ends at our fingertips because, working on a computer terminal, for example, that's how far the brain's messages go (biologically, at least). Technically, the brain is about three pounds of pink and grey wet matter, 90 per cent water. From an engineering and computational point of view, the brain is the most complex structure known as it is thought to have 100 billion cells and 100,000 billion possible connections.

With training, people with a certain aptitude can perform remarkable mathematical feats, as in the case quoted in Lyall Watson's *Supernature II*, of A.C. Aitken who, when asked to turn 4/47 into a decimal he replied in four seconds with 'Point 0851063829787234042553191 4', then he paused for breath and continued, '89361702127659574468 – and that's the repeating point. It starts again then at 085.' Aitken, who was professor of mathematics at the University of Edinburgh, is obviously a smart guy, but to accomplish these feats he had to train his memory, which everyone can do. As far as can be guessed, good memory was evolutionarily advantageous in the days when we needed to communicate survival information, history and custom from generation to generation, but had no writing with which to do it. The memorizers were the libraries. Then, as now, the brain constantly modifies itself, learning more each day, using and re-using connections, finding new ways to do things. As we know, if children are started early enough with intense teaching, they can absorb a phenomenal amount of information by their teens. Why we have this huge mental capacity and whatever its evolutionary past may be, it is a delight for humans to exercise and test our brains. We take pride in being able to fix the car, finish the crossword, win an argument, put across our political point, pass an exam and so on. But the brain is more than our most valued tool, it is our friend, our confidant, our security and our home.

We more than remember and compute, we *feel*. Tears pop out of our eyes; rage turns our face red. All this may be an evolutionary advantage – if we didn't feel angry when someone stole our last fish, we wouldn't fight to get it back and maybe we would have starved; and if we didn't feel love, who would take care of the babies? Emotions may not seem so great when you're sitting on the sofa, tears rolling down the cheeks because your partner has just moved out, but it's a mechanism, feeling loss, which accentuates its other side – feeling great together, which is the glue that keeps us in evolutionarily favourable pair-bonding and social groups. Working in small or large teams, whether specialist or not, means we can get more done more easily. That's one reason why we are where we are – in control of the world.

These days the brain is under tremendous pressure. Was it designed, I wonder, to do what a typical day in a modern city requires of it? We all wake up to the news – which is usually bad, if not horrifying (and depressing), then the post arrives, with more bills we can't pay. The drive to work is a nightmare of split-second life-or-death decisions, or a torture of being packed with too many people in an underground train. Breathing in the polluted air, commands come at us: 'walk' or 'don't walk' the signals say. The commands continue when we get to the workplace, in which we have to watch our mouths and our moves or we might get made redundant. Whatever politics and unpleasantness is thrown at us, we have to get on with it, or there's no money on payday. Flicking through magazines during our ten-minute tea break, we read articles telling us to be better mothers, fathers, lovers, slimmers, dressers, lookers and achievers. We start feeling guilty. On the way home from work we stop at the supermarket. More decisions. We pick up an apple – is it fresh enough? Has it been waxed, irradiated, or sprayed with chemicals? We pick up a yoghurt – has the out-of-date ticket expired, what's in it? We look in the freezer – will one of these products be acceptable to all members of the family or is someone going to say, 'I don't eat that'? Temptation looms at the checkout, then the bill arrives. We go home and watch TV. We cry at a sad old movie, then watch horrified at the news pictures of a plane crash. Half an hour later we're sitting on the edge of our seats, cheering our team on in football. Then the ads come on and scream 'Buy me! Buy me!' We think about tomorrow, put a load of washing in the machine and iron a couple of shirts. By the time we get into bed, we're exhausted – mentally as much as physically. Was the mind designed for all this, or was it meant to look out over a clear night sky and ponder the nature of the universe?

It would be convenient for scientists if all brains were the same because it would be much easier to establish a 'normal' brain from which others could be judged. But it's not that simple – every brain is different. Nevertheless, the measuring goes on. Not only do we have static computerized axial tomography (CAT) scan photos, we've got moving living images through positron-emission tomography (PET), magnetic resonance imaging (MRI), and superconducting quantum interference devices (SQUIDS).

A great deal has been heard this past couple of decades about neurotransmitters or brain chemicals. You hear the words serotonin, noradrenaline and so on bandied around as if they were everyday things we knew everything about, especially as many modern drugs are intended to mimic them in some way. In fact the only synapse in the mammalian central nervous system, where scientists are *certain* what the transmitter is, is in the case of the acetylcholine (ACh) synapses between the motor neuron axon collaterals and interneurons.[9] Except in this case, scientists have been unable to make pure cultures of other synapses and, although the action of ACh is understood at neuromuscular junctions, how the ACh circuits in the brain work is still not known. Books on the brain are full of words like presumably, probably and may, and expressions like 'one must be very careful about drawing conclusions'. This isn't out of misplaced lack of confidence, but actual fact – we don't know how the brain's chemicals work.

According to Richard Thompson in *The Brain*, 'we are only beginning to understand the functional circuitry of the brain'.[10] Apparently, 'the most is known about the least common transmitters in the brain'[11], dopamine and norepinephrine, and the neurons that contain them – but they account for only a few per cent of total neurotransmitters in the brain. Besides transmitters, many neuron terminals also contain peptides – which could act as transmitters, but not a great deal is known about their function.[12] Although human beings have been building up a library of information on opium for at least five thousand years, science discovered only relatively recently that the brain produces opiates in the neurons and the pituitary which, like morphine, alleviate pain and produce pleasurable sensations. We know there are several opiate receptors on neurons in the brain but Thompson admits 'little is really known about the possible differential functions of the different brain opioids and the different opioid receptors'.[13] What little we know about opiates has been highlighted by the very recent discovery, by Dr Goldstein at Stamford University, of dynorphin, which is over 200 times more potent than morphine. The mind boggles!

Scientifically, there's a world of difference between knowing *that* a certain chemical can effect a certain change, and knowing *how* it does it. Brain science is at the stage of recognizing that certain brain chemicals elicit a certain response, and mostly they seek to inhibit or encourage the flow of these chemicals. However, let us not overestimate what is known or how well understood modern drugs are. According to Thompson, on the drug used to treat manic depression, for example, 'the reasons for lithium's effectiveness are still largely obscure'.

HOW ESSENTIAL OILS WORK ON THE BRAIN

Essential oils have an effect on the brain via two routes: olfaction and essential oil absorption. The olfactory bulbs, which are just above the top of the nose and are actually a part of the brain, extend from the 'limbic system'. The name comes from Latin, *limbus*, meaning border because, comprising several structures, it forms a ringlike base to the cerebral cortex. It is the home of our emotions, sexual feelings, memory and learning, and with olfaction these can be evoked – even subconsciously. The limbic system is a link between the voluntary and involuntary nervous centres, and a link between left and right brain. Essential oils connect directly into this system through the olfactory bulbs. As for the science of olfaction, it's like a huge jigsaw made up of many pieces, a few of which we have. These tell us something, but not how olfaction works.

One thing we know is that benzodiazepene receptors are located all through the human brain, and it is on these that drugs such as Valium and Librium work. But these receptors were put in the brain long before chemists invented drugs, presumably because there are substances in nature that do the same thing. We also now know that benzodiazepene receptors are found in large quantity on the olfactory bulbs of rats and, it is thought, humans. Perhaps we were designed to receive tranquillizers through the nose – in the form of aroma molecules from plants.

The circulatory system has devised structures that prevent large molecules passing into the brain – this is 'the blood-brain barrier'. Presumably because of the small size of certain essential oil molecules and their lipophilic nature, they pass the blood-brain barrier and thus enter the brain. (As do many chemical drugs.) Essential oils get into the bloodstream in many different ways – through the capillary system at the top of the nose, through the delicate mucous membrane of the mouth and respiratory tract, through the vagina and anus if given in pessary or suppository form, through the digestive system if given orally, and through the skin if applied through massage. Although the brain only accounts for 2 per cent of our body weight, it gets 15 per cent of the blood supply.

The simple answer to the question 'how do essential oils work on the brain?' is 'we don't know'. Because human beings rely so totally on plants for their sustenance and well-being, and because the chemistry of plants and humans is so similar, they might be thought of as a set of keys for turning on the body's mechanisms – whether this is thought of in terms of chemistry or stereochemistry (the shape of the molecule). There are many different ways drugs can affect brain chemicals – they can block the synthesis of a naturally occurring chemical, or block its transport down an axion, its formation into vesicles, its release into the synapse, its attachment to the receptor and so on. Science does not often exactly understand which mechanisms are at work. It seems unreasonable, therefore, to expect us to know how essential oils work.

However, the science of brain chemistry has introduced a new element into the discussion as to why certain essential oils should be 'adaptogens'. For example, lavender oil taken in small quantity is sedative but when taken in larger quantity, becomes a stimulant. This apparent paradox has mystified students of essential oils but we now know that even within our own brain chemical system such adaptogenic processes are going on – as with dopamine, for example, or acetylcholine – which inhibits the activity of cardiac muscle cells, yet excites the activity of skeletal muscle cells. Dr Wagner and his team at the University of Munich, Germany, published a review of herbs used as 'adaptogens'. Their definition is: 'substances meant to put the organism into a state of nonspecific heightened resistance in order to better resist stresses and adapt to extraordinary challenges'.[14] That seems a pretty good definition to me!

Essential oils have many interesting features which may help explain how they work. They seem to affect the working of enzymes – a class of complex organic substances that cause chemical transformations in animals and plants. According to Dr Gerhard Buchbauer, '. . . some monoterpene derivatives, such as frenchone or carvacrol, inhibit enzymes like the acetylcholinesterase which inactivate the spasmogenic musculotropic inhibition mechanism'.[15] He also says:

> The constituents of essential oils, the aroma chemicals, accumulate in the nerve cell membrane, thus causing a sterical blocking of embedded function proteins, which are the ion channels. This blocking causes a change in the physical properties of the membrane, especially a modification of its ion permeability.[16]

If, as is thought, essential oils interact with certain membrane lipids causing a change in the calcium ion channel functions, we are talking here about effecting change in a fundamental physiological process. Also, as we have seen, essential oils affect enzymes. Neurotransmitters are often

made from substances which come from plant foods. For
example, serotonin is made (via 5-HTP) from tryptophan
(once sold as a natural antidepressant) – a naturally occurring
amino acid found in bananas and other vegetative materials.
Add to this the fact that essential oils have electrical properties, polarity, are dextrorotatory or laevorotatory, and emit
infrared radiation, and you have a cocktail of factors we are
nowhere near understanding. Whether essential oils are seen
as keys unlocking chemical reactions, as catalysts that cause
chemical transformation, or as electrical moderators, they are
basically *effectors* – bringing about a stimulation of the body's
healing mechanisms.

My feeling is that the energetic state and medicinal value of
most essential oils starts to diminish after two years. They still
smell good, but therapeutically they don't work nearly so well.
Some oils defy this rule and retain their antiseptic value for
many years – thyme, eucalyptus and oregano being examples.
Essential oils feel to different degrees 'alive'. That's not a very
scientific explanation, I know, but some oils just don't have a
vibrancy in them, a difficult thing to judge without experience
or very sophisticated equipment.

The fact that essential oils leave the body by different
routes – exhaled air, perspiration through the entire skin, via
urine or faeces, raises the question of why a particular oil
should take a particular direction. Aromatherapists sometimes
talk in terms of particular organs being 'in resonance' with a
particular oil while physicists might talk about it in terms of
'selective synchronous vibration' (the opposite of gravity)!
Another curious fact is that people are often strongly attracted
or repelled by certain aromas, and not simply because good or
bad memories are evoked. Spikenard is an oil people seldom
come across, for example, and when they first smell it, they
react in different ways. Aromas are very *personal*, for reasons
we do not know.

The Water Connection

There is a common misconception that essential oils and water
do not mix. In fact, as a by-product of essential oil distillation,

rose water and other hydrolats are routinely produced. The steam carrying the aromatic molecules of plants rises during the distillation process and, after cooling, separates into essential oil at the top and water, the hydrolat, at the bottom. Hydrolats are used most particularly in European phytotherapy, a form of herbal medicine, but rose water has been used for centuries in Europe for cooking. Although one might not see how, technically, any of the rose could be left in the water during the process of distillation, the fact is that the water is distinctly rose-scented, or scented with the particular plant being distilled. Even if you put, say, six drops of geranium essential oil in a bath, and can see that the essential oil floats on the top of the water, if you were to taste some of the water that seems untouched by it, the geranium is nevertheless evident. In some way, the aromatic molecule, or the vibration of the essential oil, has managed to become imprinted in the water.

I was, then, very interested to read in the scientific journal *Nature* (30 June 1988) a paper written by thirteen scientists which showed that, even when antibodies were not technologically detectable in a highly diluted aqueous solution, the memory of them lingered on, making the solution still biologically active. Commenting on the paper, the deputy editor of *Nature*, Peter Newmark, said that if the results were confirmed to be true, 'we will have to abandon two centuries of observation and rational thinking about biology because this can't be explained by ordinary physical laws.'[17] The man at the centre of this discovery, Dr Jacques Benveniste, later appeared with his detractors on Channel 4's three-hour discussion programme, *After Dark*,[18] in which his work was debated. As the argument heated up, the viewer was shown an example of how a totally new scientific pathway is very difficult for unimaginative people to grasp. Dr Benveniste was at the time of his discovery working for INSERM – the national medical research institution of France – and was one of France's leading biologists and immunologists, the author of four previous *Nature* articles and over 200 other scientific articles – two of which are called citation classics. Before he could publish this particular piece of work, however, Benveniste was forced by

Nature to have the work replicated by other labs – and this was successfully carried out in Israel, Canada and Italy. Nevertheless, the controversy continues.

The implications of Benveniste's discovery are far-reaching – for allopathic and homeopathic medicine, and for aromatherapy and essential oil use (not to mention public water management). When an aromatic molecule enters water, the function of the molecule becomes imprinted throughout that water-body. To understand how this may work, we need to look at water itself.

Water is ubiquitous in that it is everywhere, including our bodies (65 per cent) and brain (90 per cent). Yet, according to Patrick Flanagan, MD (MA), who was listed at age seventeen by *Life* magazine as one of America's top ten scientists, water is 'one of the world's most mysteriously anomalous substances.'[19] Flanagan became interested in water when he was a student of Dr Henry Coanda, who discovered in the 1920s that a fluid flowing over any surface tends to cling to that surface – the Coander effect. Coanda was interested in the profusion of colloidal (as opposed to ionic) minerals found in the water drunk by the Hunza people living on the western edge of the Himalayan range – who routinely live healthy lives to the age of a hundred and over. The word 'colloid' comes from the Greek word for glue and describes substances which are found throughout the human body, in plants, animals and elsewhere in nature. (One of their functions in plants is to prevent damage to the cell from freezing.) According to Flanagan, colloids in water take on the quality of tiny 'seeds' of energy. In the human body, they are known to be crucial in all body processes because of their impact on electrical flow.

Water is an excellent conductor of electricity, which is an important point to bear in mind considering that the brain is 90 per cent water. Water is fluid because the hydrogen atoms in it only have one electron to offer other atoms, so when it links with oxygen, the link is tenuous. Water could be described as one long molecule, which would explain why an input at one end – an essential oil for example – can be detected at the other end. Next time you see essential oil floating on water, bear in mind that the entire body of water is imprinted with the properties of that essential oil. What implications this has for the watery mucus at the top of the nasal cavity, which receives aroma molecules and translates them into messages for the olfaction bulbs, is yet to be discovered. However, it is known that substances put into water enter the body by osmosis, and this is how the benefits of essential oils are taken in while having baths, etc.

The Somatid Connection

One of the most interesting components of both living and non-living matter are things called *somatids*, named as such by Gaston Naessens. Somatids are described as ultramicroscopic, subcellular, living and reproducing entities. They are remarkable in that they cannot be destroyed by ultraviolet radiation (routinely used to sterilize), or by 50,000 rems of nuclear radiation, or temperatures of over 200 degrees centigrade, and they are impossible to cut by diamond, and do not respond to any of the strongest antibacterial or anti-fungal chemical agents.

Gaston Naessens was able to see somatids because working in the 1950s with artisans from the Lietz optical factory and the French military contractors Barbier-Bernard et Turenne, he constructed a microscope which can magnify *live* elements to enlargements of 30,000 X, with a resolution of 150 Angstroms (1 Angstrom = 100 millionth of a centimetre). The electron microscope can enlarge to the order of 400,000 X, with a resolution of 30–50 angstroms but, as Naessens explains it, it 'necessitates manipulations that alter the physical aspects of objects being observed'. To understand the somatids, or even identify them correctly, however, one has to be able to see the changes they go through. Consequently, when tiny bits and pieces were found in the blood they were called 'dross' or *crasse sanguine*. Naessens has discovered that these small particles are in fact polymorphous (which means they occur in many or various forms) living things.

In 1990 I had the opportunity to see a film showing somatids, which look like short, sparkling, aquamarine worms, tiny in comparison with red blood corpuscles and far more numerous. In a healthy person, somatids go through a three-stage cycle (somatids, spores, double spores), and produce, it is thought, trephone, a hormone indispensable to cellular division. However, when the immune system is weakened or destabilized through stress or trauma, the somatid goes through another thirteen evolving forms (including bacteria, mycobacterial forms, yeast-like forms, ascopores, asci and mycelial forms).

Somatids are found in all living organisms, including the sap in plants. According to Françoise Naessens, Gaston's late wife and assistant, '. . . the "tiny bodies". . . are fundamentally electrical in nature . . . Somatids are actually tiny living condensers of energy, the smallest ever found.'[20] To understand the significance of this discussion, consider the fact that if a cube of fresh meat is injected with an *in vitro* culture of somatids, placed in a vacuum-sealed vessel and put in the sun, the meat will not only remain fresh, but will grow!

Gaston Naessens says, '. . . we have observed, in all biological liquids and particularly in the blood, an elementary particle endowed with a movement of electronegative repulsion, possessing a polymorphic nature.'[21] Essential oils are a biological liquid and there is no reason to suppose that somatids are not present in them. It may well be that as further research is carried out, we will discover that essential oils in some way transfer somatids, the little condensers of energy, or influence the *trephone* factor – either chemically, electrically or energetically – and keep the somatids to a healthy (for us) three-stage cycle.

Not only has Naessens discovered an extraordinary and marvellous microscope, and discovered somatids, he has developed a product based on camphor and its derivative called 714-X which has arrested and reversed the progress of disease in over 1,000 cases of cancer as well as in several dozen cases of AIDS. Naessens writes, '. . . after having carried out numerous experiments on camphor and its derivative, we have discovered that this product is endowed with remarkable pharmaceutical properties . . . it carries to the tumour cells all the nitrogen that it needs, suppressing by the same action the secretion that would paralyse the immune system.'[22] Aromatherapists will find it interesting that he has chosen to work with camphor. Oil of Borneo

Camphor (*Dryobalanops camphora*) is used in aromatherapy for depressive bodily states, and acts as a tonic, among other things. Borneol is also found in small amounts in the essential oils of lavender, cinnamon, rosemary and certain types of hyssop.

Other Factors

Invisible forces are a fact of life. The air is full of invisible messages – from mobile phone conversations to satellite TV signals. No biologist discusses physiological processes without talking about electricity, which you or I don't see. Physicists tell us that all life is basically vibration, and there are even reputable scientists saying that life is just a big hologram![23] Compared with this, talk about etheric emanations seems positively old hat and perhaps it's not so surprising that university professors are proving the existence of auric bodies and chakras. Preliminary studies are proving what aromatherapists have long known – that essential oils have an effect far beyond the physical body.

SUMMARY

In the biological sciences there is still much to learn. To discuss essential oils solely in terms of chemical components is dismissive of other important factors in the nature of life. Aside from this, science has not yet identified all essential oil components. Life is *living*, that is the point! Nature has the capacity to retain life within it to a remarkable degree. In Denmark, *Spergula arvensis* seeds were germinated after 1,700 years and in China seeds of a Manchurian lotus were found to be fertile after 1,000 years. While recognizing and acknowledging the importance of the therapeutic value of the known chemical components of essential oils, they are probably working in tandem with other factors, and synergistically with each other. The fact is that certain essential oils work in therapy in certain conditions, yet chemically their effects cannot be explained. Sitting on the shelf in bottles, essential oils might be regarded as nothing more than a chemical cocktail, but they are powerful, energetic, dynamic liquids. Despite the criticism of being vague, aromatherapists continue to say that essential oils contain a 'life force', but it may be some time before science can prove them wrong!

WHICH MEDICINE?

Having worked in a clinical setting as an aromatherapist for many years, I find it immeasurably sad that there is a reluctance on the part of the medical professions to take advantage of the benefits offered by essential oils. A confrontational stance seems to have been adopted with 'them' (natural therapies) on one side and 'us' (doctors and chemical drugs manufacturers) on the other. Instead of scanning the various complementary therapies and asking 'what can you do for my patients?', doctors all too often dismiss complementary medicines, which they neither understand nor have experience of, as too weak, or too strong, just a placebo or unresearched.

There are historical reasons behind this divide, to do with the growth of the chemical drugs industry and the protection of market interests – financial profit, in other words. The drugs industry spends millions of pounds employing political lobbyists, public relations officers and sales representatives who influence the decision-makers, the public and doctors against natural alternatives. In this market protectionism, however, the patient suffers.

One can forgive general practitioners who have little enough time to talk to their patients, yet alone read the actual research behind many of the drugs they are prescribing. But hospital specialists, who have a limited number of conditions to treat, should most certainly look into complementary therapies and see what is on offer. It is a great shame that essential oils are not further researched for use in mind-related conditions and nor are the antiviral essential oils investigated for the alleviation of earache, colds and flu, and other more serious viral conditions. One can understand that chemical drugs are used when they are available, but there are many conditions for which nothing is available in the 'chemical medicine chest', but where natural options exist.

One criticism levelled against aromatherapy is that it is unscientifically tested – that we don't know how it works. On the face of it this might seem like a valid complaint until one realizes that the chemical drugs industry, who orchestrate the opposition to natural therapies for financial reasons, very often has little idea how its drugs work. For example, for many years doctors have been told that tricyclic drugs used to treat depression are effective because they work to change the natural levels of the neurotransmitters norepinephrine and serotonin. But, because of our limited knowledge about how neurotransmitters actually work in the brain, and the pathways they take, this is all just theory. The first problem with the theory is that testing urine for the level of these substances is an unreliable measure of how much is actually in the brain and there is, moreover, no convincing evidence that depressed individuals actually have lower levels of these naturally occurring chemicals. Also, and mysteriously, tricyclics act on norepinephrine and serotonin synapses within minutes but it takes weeks for their beneficial effects on depression to develop. This time gap cannot be explained (as it cannot for the dopamine/schizophrenia theory). Drug experts are aware in a way the general public (and even doctors) are not, that in chemical-medical practice it is routine for drugs to be prescribed although the treatment is more effective than the theory.

Doctors reluctant to use natural medicines, but happy to prescribe chemical drugs, should take a long hard look into the back-up research of those drugs and ask themselves – does anybody really know how these work? The fact is that chemical drugs are regularly given product licences although the exact mechanisms for them are not understood and, according to the American federal *Office of Technology Assessment*, 75 per cent of all currently available treatments have not had sufficient scientific scrutiny.[24]

Another criticism levelled against natural therapies is that they are potentially toxic. The argument is 'just because it's natural doesn't mean it's safe'. Of course nature is full of dangers, as we tell our children every time they reach out to pluck unknown berries from a bush. But it is also true that nature is full of natural remedies. Natural medicines have evolved over thousands of years, time enough for people to come to know which natural products are good to eat, which are poisonous, which heal and which do not. It is upon this wealth of experience that aromatherapy draws and, indeed, upon which chemical companies draw as they search for medications to synthesize chemically in the lab. Indeed, without certain plants, the pharmacies in cancer hospitals would have little to offer. With my hand on my heart I can tell you that in my long experience I have rarely heard of an adverse reaction to pure essential oils used correctly by registered practitioners in aromatherapy treatments in Britain, other than passing skin irritation in some people who have sensitive reactions to certain plants or plant products. According to Dietrich Wabner, professor of chemistry at the Technical University in Munich, skin irritation could be caused by biocide residues in particular essential oils, rather than being a reaction to that oil in general. The adverse 'side effects' of chemical drugs are becoming more well known due to the efforts of the media, and there are now several good books available to the public on that subject. It is ludicrous to criticize natural therapies on the basis of their potential toxicity when so very few toxic effects have been observed or reported, not only by me but by generations of serious medical researchers and government regulatory bodies.

Meanwhile, the toxic potential of chemical drugs is well documented. In the *Journal of the American Medical Association* (27 November 1987, p2891), we are told that one patient in every thousand admitted to hospital will be killed by the medicine they receive there. And according to the *Chemical Marketing Reporter* (2 January 1989), as a result of the 68 million prescriptions for non-steroidal anti-inflammatory drugs (NSAIDS) given to American sufferers of arthritis, 10,000–20,000 deaths occur each year. It is unfair to criticize essential oils for possible (unknown) side effects when chemical drugs are well known for their adverse side effects. For example, the data sheet for Eli Lilly's anti-depression drug Prozac contains not only a warning that rashes and other allergic reactions might be experienced, but a long list of 'adverse effects', far too long to go into here, which includes fever, nausea, diarrhoea, vomiting, insomnia, anxiety, dizziness, fatigue, seizures, pulmonary events, hair loss, sexual dysfunction and so on. Apparently, 'hypomania or mania occurred in approximately one per cent of fluoxetine (Prozac) treated trial patients'.[25] And this, supposedly, is a safe drug!

In America, drug safety is regulated by the Federal Drugs Administration but according to the Democratic representative Ted Weiss (NY), 102 out of 198 prescription drugs approved by them from 1976 to 1985 caused serious reactions which necessitated their either being relabelled or removed from the market.[26] How many of the chemical drugs currently being prescribed for the mind are destined, as time reveals their drawbacks, for the bin?

Natural medicines are often dismissed as being mere 'placebos' – chemically inactive substances that work only by the power of suggestion. The irony of this argument is that within the chemical-medical field the placebo effect is well known – after much worldwide research, 'the placebo effect' is said to cause wellness in 30–35 per cent of patients given nothing more than sugar pills. We are not here just talking about minor conditions. One group of doctors specializing in the treatment of angina pectoris (pain due to reduced blood flow to the heart) discovered that *pretending* to operate, by cutting the patients open and sewing them back up again, produced a cure rate equal to that produced by actual surgery (tying off the mammary artery);[27] while in a study to assess the effects of a new type of chemotherapy, doctors were surprised to find that 30 per cent of the *control* group, who had placebos and no drugs, lost their hair![28] Placebos have even been found to be as effective as morphine in relieving pain.[29] Clearly, placebos play a part in medicine, but the placebo effect involves all branches of medicine, not just the natural ones.

Indeed, placebos cost the National Health Service at least £77 million in the year 1992–3 because that's the value of the antibiotic prescriptions doctors wrote out for viral-induced colds and sore throats, which they knew full well they could not possibly cure. On this subject a recent *Audit Commission* report stated: 'Many doctors say that they often cannot afford the time to explain to patients the reasons why they do not need any medicine'.[30] In other words, the antibiotics were placebos. The report also states: 'Over-prescribing builds up resistance and disturbs the balance of micro-organisms in the body, permitting more severe infections to develop'.[31]

When I lecture on aromatherapy, I make it quite clear that essential oils are not cure-alls. Clearly, we all have reason to be grateful to the surgeons and other medical professionals, and many people are alive today only because of the chemical drugs they take. All this, however, does not negate the fact that essential oils have their benefits too. In some cases, as in chemical medicine, essential oils may act as placebos – and why not, if that makes the patient better? But essential oils are not just placebos, and there are hundreds of scientific papers to prove that point. As a complementary therapy, used correctly, aromatherapy is a very safe method of restoring well-being and one that, if made more widely available, would bring tremendous benefits to humankind.

Chapter Three

THE MODERN MIND

WHAT A CRAZY WORLD! WE'VE GOT PEOPLE KILLING THEIR neighbours on a vast scale and calling it war, children being abducted and killed, drugs being sold in the schools, workers being thrown out of their jobs, homes being repossessed, and countless pressures from all sides. I shake my head in wonder that any of us are sane. But, as our grannies used to say, 'we've just got to carry on'. The world isn't going to stop being the pressurized whirlpool it is, and unless we buy the lucky lottery ticket, we'll still have to carry on dealing with our daily problems much the way we always have. Will we ever get through?

Oh dear, no wonder half the population are strung out on drugs, or down at the pub, or smoking themselves into a grave! What is to be done? If you feel rotten you can go to your general practitioner where, in the waiting room, you might pick up a copy of an old magazine and see an article entitled, 'The Day I Went Insane' – about tranquillizer addiction. The doctor calls you in just as you get to the bit where the lady says: '. . . as the years went by I began to realize that my whole character was changing. My four children were young then and I started to get aggressive, and hit them – which is something I'd never done – I'd shout and scream at them about the most minor things. I'm not an aggressive person . . . so I knew there was a change taking place.'[1] Hoping nobody will notice, you take the magazine in with you. After you've told the doctor (in five minutes) what the problem is – your life is caving in – he pulls his prescription pad over and starts to scribble. 'What's that for?' you ask. 'Tranquillizers,' he says. 'But, eh, I was reading this . . .' – you show him the article. He sighs. 'Oh, yes,' he says, 'let's hope it doesn't come to that, we'll get you off them as soon as you feel better.' You ask if there are any alternatives. You're told your depression can be treated with a new family of seratonin re-uptake inhibitors but there have been reported side effects. 'Like what?' you ask. Like changes in personality. 'Any other alternatives?' you ask. 'Therapy, but the waiting list is at least six months.' You say 'thank you', and leave with your prescription.

If you live in America, like many other people you might decide to go into psychoanalysis. Then you work out how much it's going to cost you – $150 each 50-minute session, four times a week for four years equals $124,800. You decide you can't afford it, so pick up a local paper and scan the small ads – looking for help with your stressed-out life. On both sides of the Atlantic there are dozens of talk-therapists of various sorts; and people who'll hypnotize you so you can discover the *true* reason for your dissatisfaction with life – probably rooted in some previous incarnation, you're informed; then there are the astrologers and card readers and chanellers who say they can show you the way forward. You find adverts for pre-recorded tapes which will subliminally teach you to have confidence, or wealth, or make you feel younger, or more assertive, less aggressive, more relaxed, or in tune with the whales. You develop a headache trying to figure out which tape to buy and with which therapist to make an appointment, then remember you've got a health magazine somewhere. You find it and flick to the ads at the back. 'We can sort out your problems', they say, through re-birthing, or rolfing, bodywork, meditation, yoga, visualization and the list goes on and on. But which one do you choose? By now you've become so confused, you feel more depressed than you did to start with – are you the *only* person in the world who hasn't sorted themselves out yet? You pour yourself a drink and pull out the old packet of cigarettes you stashed away when you gave up smoking two years ago.

The expression 'modern-day stress' might seem like a cliché, but, boy-oh-boy, it is true. Look around you and try to think of one person you know who isn't weighed down with family responsibilities or financial obligations, or stuck in a relationship they want to get out of, or desperately looking for the relationship they'd like to have, or anguished by their dysfunctional family, or sick, or worried about a sick relative, or just plain overworked. It makes you wonder – is there anyone out there who is totally, truly happy?

I remember once seeing a TV film about people working in a factory where the interviewer went down the production line asking each person in turn what they were thinking about. About 90 per cent said they were working out what they were going to do when they won a million pounds on the football pools – this is escapism on a massive scale. Indeed, given the amount of stress we have to deal in, escapism seems to be a functional necessity. Without it, how many more of us would go mad?

I'm not going to say a word about the depleting ozone layer, or mention the scientists at the Naval Research Laboratory in Washington who have discovered a way of attaching living embryonic brain cells to computer silicon chips – the first step, apparently, in making a 'bioelectronic' artificial brain.[2] We can all read the papers – and scare ourselves rigid!

What I do want to do in this section is spend a little time discussing some of the issues that immediately face the modern mind. In *The Mind-Body Connection* we see that science is making us face up to the fact that mind and body are one. The implication is that, for physical as well as mental health, we have to address our psychological problems and deal with them. In *Drug Culture* we discuss the fact that some so-called 'recreational drugs' are causing new problems, with cocaine stripping people of their character for example, while in *Addiction* we see that a simple cup of tea can catapult a person into a vicious cycle of tranquilliser addiction, while heavy drugs turn normal people into monsters prepared to rob and murder for a fix. *Consciousness and Control* explores the difficulty of finding, through the jungle of media interference, who we truly are, while *Spirituality* addresses the problem of religious scepticism and spiritual void. *The Untapped Mind* reminds us that there is more to heaven and earth than we yet understand. *Psychotherapy, Counselling and Other Therapies* discusses ways forward for some, while *Meditation and Visualization* could be a way forward for others.

I have a friend who spent time in Ethiopia working with orphans who had literally nothing – no family, no home, no possessions. If they had a pencil, they considered themselves lucky. But, they were happy, she tells me, and on returning to London after a couple of years she was shocked to see the misery in the faces of people who, materially, seemed to have it all. Somehow we have lost our capacity for happiness. Not just the happiness we feel at particularly good times – a night out with friends, evening in with our lover, but the joyful openness and positivity we, surely, were meant to feel each new day. Life is a blessing, an adventure, a lesson with inevitable ups and downs. OK, it's hard and rocky in places, and like sailors in a storm we have to hold on tight sometimes. But life was meant to be enjoyed and happiness is our birthright. There is much out there to help us find a way through to the light, including, as we shall later see, nature's essential oils – our little helpmates.

THE MIND-BODY CONNECTION

Imagine one of the swords used in fencing, a foil, and then think of it being thrust straight through a body, but that body doesn't bleed or appear to feel pain. This was the highlight of a stage act performed at the Corsco Theatre in Zurich in 1947 by a Dutchman, Mirin Dajo. One of the audience had a heart attack and died and the show was banned, but a doctor heard about the strange goings-on and asked Dajo to undergo scientific enquiry. At a Zurich hospital, in front of a large crowd including doctors and journalists, Dajo's assistant again thrust the foil through his body and again there was no bleeding and the vital organs seemed undamaged. With the foil through his body Dajo, and everyone else, trooped up the stairs to the X-ray room where it was proved that the foil was indeed going straight through his body. It was removed after a total of twenty minutes, and there were just two faint scars showing. Dajo later obligingly undertook examination by more doctors in Basel, one of whom run him through with a foil. Thanks to Dajo's mind over matter, the doctor didn't have to be charged with murder.

In Valencia, Spain, today, there is a Dr Angel Escudero who has performed surgery on over 700 patients without using anaesthetic. Instead he uses psycho-anaesthesia – simply telling his patients that during surgery they will feel nothing. Observers of the procedure confirm that no hypnosis is involved. This is a different type of thought transference. The doctor says 'you will feel no pain' and the patient thinks 'I will feel no pain' – and they don't. According to Dr Escudero, the patient having liquid saliva in the mouth is a vital adjunct of therapy. He points out that having a dry mouth is a characteristic of stress, fear or panic. Unbelievably for more conventional doctors, Dr Escudero uses no antibiotics yet his patients have never once developed an infection.

Dr Escudero calls his method *noesitherapy* after *noesis* – action of thinking, and *noesiology* – the effects produced in human life by one's own thoughts. Thoughts produce changes in our arteries and in every organ, says Dr Escudero, and he advises we think positive thoughts, not negative ones, and learn to live happier lives. Dr Escudero takes his own advice and plays tennis regularly on the court in the lovely garden surrounding his home, which also houses the surgery and operating room. No commuting for him. In an operating room looking much like any other, Dr Escudero is assisted by the family he loves: his son – a doctor, his daughter – surgical nurse, and his wife, Marie-Jesus, who talks to the patient, holds their hand and generally keeps them company. The knife cuts deep into the flesh, metal rods are sometimes hammered through the limbs but the patient looks around happily, as if they were at a nice social gathering! The patient can feel heat and normal sensation – but no pain. All this is possible, apparently, because every thought is a programme in the biological computer of our brain. 'Think positive' is Dr Escudero's advice.

We've all read reports in newspapers about people being able to do extraordinary things in extraordinary situations. The mother, for example, who lifted a car to release her son, trapped beneath it, or the man who jumped a ten foot wall to escape a rabid dog. I heard about a woman caught in a war zone who pulled apart the iron bars across a window, to escape the enemy. Perhaps you or I could do the same.

In an emergency situation the brain tells the body to go on alert, and produces hormones which jolt us into action – the 'flight/fight reaction'. Fear also stops the instinctive sexual process. We can not only lose interest, but the penis can refuse to work and the vaginal muscles can contract sharply, preventing penetration. On the other hand, meditation can slow the body rhythms down, and correct breathing can control blood pressure. People on biofeedback machines watch the dials and control their brain rhythms. The mind-body connection is an observable fact.

The mind-body connection is also now a proven scientific fact. Indeed, one leading researcher in the field of brain chemistry, Candace Pert, says '. . . your mind is in every cell of your body'.[3] Candace Pert, who was formerly Chief of the Brain Biochemistry Section at the American National Institute of Mental Health and is now a Professor at the Center for Molecular and Behavioral Neuroscience at Rutgers University, discovered the opiate receptor and many other peptide receptors in the brain and body. For nearly two decades she has been leading the field in brain chemistry and inspiring a whole generation of scientists, who now recognize that the chemicals in the brain form a continuous circuit not only with receptors in the brain, but with receptors in the immune system, the nervous system and the hormone system. In other words, it is impossible physiologically to separate the mind from the body.

What we are talking about here is peptides – strings of amino acids and the building blocks of proteins. The brain's own morphine, enkephalin, is a mere five amino acids long, while the peptide insulin is a couple of hundred amino acids long. There are about twenty-three different amino acids which, when put together in different arrangements, make different peptides. These peptides connect with receptors on cells, telling them whether or not they should divide, whether or not they should make a particular protein, and whether they should turn on one gene or another – and the thing about all this is that *emotions* and *thoughts* run this system.

When Candace Pert discovered that neuropeptide receptors were found on cells of the immune system, in the 1980s, the scientific community went into shock and denial mode. Only after about fifteen years of further research, and after many other experimenters had replicated her work and carried out more of their own, did it slowly become accepted as fact. Pert describes neuropeptides as 'biochemical units of emotion'.

It no longer seems unbelievable that Jeanne Achterberg, head of research and rehabilitation at the University of Texas Health Science Centre, has found that with visualization techniques people can be trained to increase the level of *particular* types of immune system cells running around in their blood. Depending on what they were asked to do, participants in the trial could increase their T-cell count or their neutrophils (a type of white blood cell).[4]

Stress is now recognized as an important co-factor in the development of cancer while, conversely, some claim to have cured cancer by reducing the degree of stress in their lives. People with cancer are told they can live longer if they keep up a fighting spirit and often take up meditation, or laughter therapy, and re-organize their lives so they can actually do what they really want. Be honest, they are told, admit your problems, air your views, say what you want, get it off your chest, decide your priorities, and act on them – good advice for anyone.

The time has long gone since the mind and body were seen as two different things. According to Michael Talbot in *The Holographic Universe*, 'deeply hypnotized persons can control allergic reactions, blood flow patterns, and nearsightedness. In addition, they can control heart rate, pain, body temperature, and even will away some kinds of birthmarks'.[5] He even reports the case of a sixteen-year-old boy suffering from an advanced case of Brocq's disease, a genetic condition that makes the skin thick and horny – like a reptile, who was cured by hypnosis. This means that the genetic code can be interfered with mentally![6]

Psychosomatic illnesses are defined as 'physical disorders that seem to have been caused, or worsened, by psychological factors'.[7] Eczema, asthma, irritable bowel syndrome and peptic ulcers are among many conditions which are often psychosomatic in origin. The reproductive system can also be sensitive to psychological factors – think of the number of women one hears about who were infertile until they adopted a child, then suddenly become pregnant. And just as the mind can influence life, it can influence death – stress can lead to heart disease, and the grave. Never underestimate the importance of mental health in our lives. By attending to it, we attend to our whole being – mind, body and soul.

DRUG CULTURE

In the modern world, drugs are a way of life. Cigarettes are sold in sweet shops, alcohol is sold in the pub, cocaine is made available at 'sophisticated' parties, crack is sold on the streets, cannabis is smoked in schools, amphetamines and ecstasy are part of the rave scene, while those too young to be allowed out all night may console themselves with glue and other solvents inhaled out of sight of the parents (who are comfort-eating at home). It seems like practically everyone is looking for some addition to their lives, something to make them feel more relaxed, or 'out of it', or in some sense different from their normal selves. To some extent, all this is an extension of our consumer society – we can no more help putting 'extra' things into our mouths or noses than we can help buying things we don't need at the shops. The incentive comes in the form of advertising, peer-pressure or stress. However, much of this is bad for us, and in some cases, it will kill us.

There might have been a time when 'recreational drugs' were relatively harmless, but no longer. The police have found that in some instances, so-called 'amphetamines' sold on the street contain as little as 2 per cent of the drug. These days, cannabis is often cultivated using pesticides which can have a very adverse effect on health. For example, in Mexico they use paraquat which, even in small quantities, can cause irreversible lung damage, while in Jamaica, Colombia and Belize they tend to use glyphosate. Many pot smokers have developed strange illnesses which seem to have no identifiable cause, ranging from temporary loss of sight to loss of strength or swelling in the legs and partial paralysis. Meanwhile hashish is so 'cut' with shoe polish and other non-narcotic substances it can no longer be considered a 'natural' drug. 'Cocaine' is more likely to be rat poison than a derivative of the coca plant, while 'crack' is just junk making the junkie.

So-called 'recreational drugs' have other dangers. Cocaine strips people of their character so they no longer know the difference between right and wrong. Coke-heads become like soulless cadavers, a danger to themselves and everyone around them. Obviously heroin is pure evil and anyone taking it at any time needs his or her head examined.

Alcohol is by far the most widespread drug, legal and taxed, but is said to kill more people than all the other drugs combined. In America, half the accidents on the roads are caused by people under the influence, and because of them, 22,000 people die each year. In 1990 a total of 65,000 Americans died as a result of alcohol – which causes cirrhosis of the liver, heart damage, throat, mouth and tongue cancers, gastritis, pancreatitis, brain damage and many other things. Depression and anxiety are other effects of the drug. Although Europeans tend to think of America as the home of the lush, in fact America consumes a third of the alcohol it did in the 1830s and today, Korea leads the world in per capita alcohol consumption, while the Japanese have doubled their intake since the 1950s. Each country tends to have its own drinking patterns – with the Italians centring the activity around daily meals (20,000 deaths from cirrhosis of the liver each year) while the Finns tend to binge and fall under an oncoming bus.

From all I have said, you might think I'm an old fuddy-duddy who disapproves of people enjoying themselves. Far from it, but drugs in any form are dangerous if not taken in moderation and with caution. There is a worldwide history of people wanting to escape the normal parameters of daily life, but we must somehow strive to lessen the dangers inherent in this activity and find substances which can enhance our normal humdrum lives without killing us or making us ill.

ADDICTION

Although the word 'addict' usually conjures up the image of a pale, skinny, hollow-eyed youth, slumped in an alley with a needle stuck in his arm, the more common addict is a nice old granny with a cup of tea in her hand! At least, it's now becoming clear that millions of people in Britain may be taking in such a quantity of caffeine – in tea, coffee, cola and certain medicines – that they could be classed as addicts. If they don't get their fix, and even when they do, they could become ill. Estimates as to the number of cups of tea or coffee required to classify a person as a caffeine addict vary from five to twelve cups a day – twelve cups of coffee a day represents an intake of about a gram of caffeine. Someone consuming this much caffeine is liable to suffer symptoms that are indistinguishable from those produced by anxiety neurosis – including headaches, poor concentration, irritability, restlessness, insomnia, lethargy, nausea and tremors.

You may not realize that the craving for a nice cup of tea after a hard day's shopping is an aspect of withdrawal symptoms, or that the pick-me-up you feel after that first sip is your 'fix', but caffeine is a drug and if you stop taking it suddenly you will undoubtedly feel rather unwell. However, if you suffer from any of the symptoms above, and want to give it a try, remember to cut down the caffeine *gradually* – and do persevere.

Because caffeine addiction is not often recognized as the root of so many troubles, a sufferer who goes to the doctor is often prescribed tranquillizers – thus exacerbating their problems. Clearly, if you suffer from the symptoms mentioned, before you convince yourself you're heading for a nervous breakdown it might be a good idea to cut down your intake of caffeine by switching to decaffeinated tea or coffee or fruit and herbal teas, and see what happens then – but, please, do it gradually.

Tranquillizer addiction is now, thankfully, a well-recognized problem although vast quantities of drugs are still handed out by doctors who don't know what alternatives there are. In Britain alone, during the year 1992–3, 540 million days' supply of benzodiazepines were dispensed.[8] Drugs classed as hypnotics and anxiolytics, prescribed for insomnia and anxiety respectively, cost the National Health Service about £30 million a year.

Tranquillizer dependence is said to develop after about six weeks. Aside from the horrible effects of withdrawal, which can be as difficult as those arising from alcohol dependency, sufferers report that, on looking back on their tranquillizer-life, they realize they had been 'asleep' – so blocked-in and blocking-out, it was as if that period of time didn't exist. Whole chunks of lives are essentially lost. While on the drugs, people are more detached from life than they were when they had their neurosis and so on. They don't feel numb so much as in a dream-state – watching everything as if it were a film with which they can't consciously relate or interact. They feel invisible.

Clearly, this is an unsatisfactory situation and if anyone reading this is caught in the trap, I suggest you get a copy of the first-ever directory of services for people who want to come off tranquillizers, which is available through the charity MIND.[9] Although I sometimes read that it takes about four weeks to come off tranquillizers, I'd say it takes very much longer than that – months, not weeks. Because the organs seem to have an addictive-type nature, the whole body becomes dependent. Suddenly to stop the drug can cause the organs – like the heart or liver – to go into crisis. Whatever you do, don't get too ambitious and throw the drugs in the bin and say 'that's it'. Give yourself four months, say, and reduce the amount of tranquillizer bit by bit over that time. Eventually you'll reach the point where you are shaving a few crumbs off one pill daily. *Then* take the final step.

In *The Fragrant Mind* we shall be looking at essential oil alternatives to tranquillizers, but there are other options on offer. Health food shops and high street chemists sell a wide range of homeopathic and herbal relaxants such as valerian and passiflora tablets. In general, valerian is calming and will stop the mind racing and is also used to treat hysteria. However, homeopathy is a very individualistic system of medicine and each patient coming to a homeopathic practitioner will be treated very differently. Aromatherapy, likewise, is individualistic, and therapists prescribe different combinations of essential oils for different people.

Tranquillizer addiction is itself so much of a trouble, one cannot sort out the root problems while on them because all they do is put another layer of problem on top of the underlying ones. Step-by-step though, one can reach the ideal situation – living a normal life and having natural helpmates around the house to deal with intermittent stressful situations. (See Chapter 8.)

Alcohol has been brewed by innumerable societies throughout time, with even the Bible referring to a miracle in which water was turned to wine! Poets, painters and writers have created masterpieces with a drink in their hand, and wine buffs have invented a new language to discuss the subtleties of their chosen tipple. Alcohol is an important aspect of the social gathering – it relaxes, makes people more open and forthcoming and can't be all bad. However, there comes a point when a threshold is crossed and instead of being 'a social drinker', an innocent partaker of one of life's little pleasures, one becomes a slave to the drug – in America it's estimated that 10 million people are addicted to alcohol, while in Italy 9 per cent of the population are thought to be alcoholics. However, it's very difficult to convince alcoholics that they have a problem and need to change their habits.

We all know of people whose lives have been ruined by drink, of families that have been broken up by it and the promising futures which have gone down the drain. Some people become alcoholics simply because they are sociable people and the only context available in their community in which they can be sociable is the pub, and at some point their bodies become addicted. Others are driven to the bottle because they have problems which seem insurmountable and the bottle provides the only available solace. If you think you fall into the first group, then beware – you could become an alcoholic just like the millions of socialites who went that way before. The second group are, in a sense, easier to help because there are alternatives when you need help with life's seemingly endless problems, natural alternatives which don't turn you into a slave of the bottle.

Nicotine is a disgusting drug, as most addicts will admit. It makes your hair, clothes and breath smell, makes the children ill, and kills you. While fewer men now smoke than before, women continue to stick to the cigarettes and in many cases I think this is because in their busy lives of remorseless chores – encapsulated in the expression 'a woman's work is never done' – the cigarette break represents a carving out of space for the woman, a little bit of space that says, 'I'm having a break now, I'm going to sit here for five minutes and have a cup of tea and a cigarette.' It isn't the cigarette that's wanted so much as the five-minute break!

Cigarettes are very ritualistic in that some people have to light up just before they sit down to make a phone call, or at other particular times – especially when drinking, for example. Some people convince themselves they can't *think* unless there's a cigarette in their hand, while others carry a cigarette in their hand without it being lit – like having a comfort blanket! And, of course, a cigarette often fills the big boredom void. These days there's plenty of help to get off the evil weed including nicotine patches, hypnotism and acupuncture – all of which work for some people. If you really want to give up, try them!

CONSCIOUSNESS AND CONTROL

Some people seem to float like bits of flotsam adrift on the sea of life, directed by the tide, while others seem to be fully conscious and in control of their lives, aware of what they are doing and why they are doing it. In terms of mental health, being in control is an extremely important factor. Again and again, studies show that those who have little or no control suffer – and that is as true for rats as for people! Research has shown, for example, that patients who are allowed to control the amount of morphine given for pain relief not only achieve better pain control, they use less of the drug. Dr Dean Ornish is rather famous in medical history because he has shown that coronary heart disease can be *reversed* by using a combination of meditation, group therapy, walking, stress-reduction exercises and a vegetarian diet. He says 'If you believe you have some control over your life, and that you have the ability to make choices instead of being the passive recipient of medical care, or the victim of bad luck or bad genes, then you are more likely to make changes that are going to do you good in terms both of your behaviour and of the direct effects of your mind on your body.'[10]

But one cannot take control unless one is conscious – which the Oxford dictionary defines as 'to be aware of what one is doing or intending to do'. In a sense, it is quite easy not to be conscious. Schools and colleges have been criticized for not encouraging creative or original thought – the students are instead forced to learn and repeat whatever version of 'wisdom' is prescribed, and not encouraged to ask the question *why*? As an adult, it is relatively easy to listen to the news but blank it out, to go to work and passively take orders, and come home and let the partner or the children take control. Indeed, the world is full of people who go through life letting the forces of circumstance mould their existence. There's many a passive soul who has woken up at age sixty and asked themselves 'what was it all about?', or bemoaned the fact that they spent so much time pleasing everyone else they never got to please themselves.

However, if one goes through life not fully conscious, a mish-mash of other people's opinions and priorities, what *is* our state of consciousness, which is described as 'the totality of the impressions, thoughts, and feelings, which make up a person's conscious being'? And whose consciousness is it – yours or your teacher's, parent's, lover's or your daily newspaper's? Part of mental health involves being in control – not passive, not a piece of flotsam adrift on the sea of life. Sit down for five minutes, write on the top of a piece of paper

'Me', and underneath make a list of your dreams, priorities, dissatisfactions, satisfactions and so on, and try to establish where exactly you are and where you want to go in this life (as opposed to where everyone else wants you to go). Take stock, be aware, and move forward in the direction you want to go (not where the tide takes you).

THE UNTAPPED MIND

The human mind is a strange, powerful thing. Mothers walking around the supermarket are stopped in their tracks by a 'feeling' that something has happened to their child. Lovers a thousand miles away from each other know when the other is in trouble – and call it 'instinct'. Some people can dream events before they happen – precognition. Uri Geller and many other people can, by sheer force of will, bend spoons. Others can make objects move around the room – without touching them. Archaeology uses the talents of people who can hold an ancient object and give the scientists a full history of it, and lead them to the precise site of an ancient building, far beneath the soil. Under hypnosis people can remember past lives, complete with precise details and even in long-dead languages – which are later proved to be accurate (by amazed professors who have spent their lives studying the subjects). Something is going on – but what?

Works of creation produced by people we would call geniuses are often attributed by the artists themselves to some outside force. Johann Sebastian Bach said, 'I play the notes in order, as they are written. It is God who makes the music.' John Milton said the whole of *Paradise Lost* was dictated to him, while Robert Louis Stevenson received *Dr Jekyll and Mr Hyde* in a dream. Poor Samuel Taylor Coleridge was writing *Kubla Khan* in one long stream of consciousness when he was interrupted, and when he tried to go back to his writing the 'inspiration' was lost, and the work was never completed. In a letter to a friend, Wolfgang Amadeus Mozart wrote that the notes of his music came from outside himself: 'Whence and how they come, I know not, nor can I force them . . . nor do I hear in my imagination the parts successively but I hear them, as it were, all at once.'[11] Many scientists also report that their most brilliant thoughts came to them in a flash of inspiration, as if from outside themselves. Something is going on – but what?

SPIRITUALITY

There is such a thing as 'higher consciousness', which people experience and express in different ways. Tuning in to whatever forces exist outside the normal, humdrum world is an activity human beings have strived to do since the beginning of known time. On the Mediterranean island of Crete, three and a half thousand years ago, the opium poppy was employed to assist in communication with the goddess, while in Mexico for thousands of years the peyote cactus put people in touch with the spiritual realm. In India today people meditate for hours on end – to get in touch with the god within, while in churches and mosques across the world, people pray to a god high up in heaven. In a thousand ways, over thousands of years, people have reached out, and looked within, for that dimension of being we all know is there – the spiritual.

Spirituality and mind are one. To be human, to have a mind, is to be spiritual. In most places at most times the definition of the spiritual realm was pretty straightforward – everyone around believed in the same spiritual concept and one just fell into line. Today, however, there are many spiritual options. Walking down an inner-city street you can pass a church, a Society of Friends (Quakers) meeting house, a synagogue, a mosque, a Hindu temple or a Buddhist centre. Which one are you going to walk into, if any? You might feel more drawn to a goddess-worshipping group, or a Tantric group, or any number of other groups who in their own way seek the spiritual path. On the other hand, you may not like groups, and may want to experience your spirituality in a personal, private way.

People who have a spiritual base, even if it is just a personal idea of their own, have a grounding which is emotionally strengthening. They feel in touch with the wider forces, and linked to other people. Obviously, this can be bad when it turns into moral superiority – 'my religion is the only correct religion and the rest of you are wrong', but it is good to feel links with other people; be part of a wider family. This feeling can be experienced even when all alone – when meditating, for example, or gazing at the stars on a clear night. Even alone, quietly, one can feel a connection with nature, with the natural forces, with the earth, the sky, with animals and people. We are all connected, like a golden web, so try to connect and don't feel so alone.

PSYCHOTHERAPY, COUNSELLING AND OTHER THERAPIES

Sixty years ago in Britain some women who had children out of wedlock were incarcerated in mental institutions – the reasoning being that they must have been mad to get pregnant in such circumstances. Many women spent three and more decades behind bars for actions which today would be considered normal. Likewise, masturbation was once a certifiable offence. We have no way of knowing what judgements will be made in the future of the parameters we now apply to 'sanity' and 'madness' but it is quite likely that for some reason it will be considered in some respects to have been 'wrong'. Society tends to make rules and define 'normal' behaviour, or else how could we operate? But in this, many people get left out of the mainstream because they cannot conform to the rules laid down. Unusual behaviour might be considered mildly eccentric, or out-and-out mad, but who makes the rules? And are *they* sane? Conformity is a strait-jacket we are all forced to wear, but let us not tie the ribbons so tight we squeeze all the life out of ourselves.

There's nothing wrong with seeking help with this life. It is not an indication of failure, rather an indication that you are conscious and want to improve your emotional well-being – which is a responsible, adult, sensible thing to do. The question is, where to go for help?

Psychiatrists are doctors who have been further trained in mental illness and the emotional aspects of life and they can either take a more genetic/biochemical approach or a psycho-analytical one – seeing the source of problems as more to do with environmental factors, like family relationships etc. Psychiatrists can prescribe drugs. *Psychoanalysts* started with Freud, and they're the ones who sit in silence as the client lies on the couch recounting their dreams and remembering their past. Key words in psychoanalysis are the *Oedipus* complex, the *id*, *ego* and *superego*, and a course of treatment can go on for years. There are many different kinds of *psychologists*, like child psychologists, industrial psychologists, clinical psychol-ogists and so on. Carl Jung was a psychologist as much as a psychoanalyst, and took the view that inner mental forces are as much to do with intellectual and spiritual factors, as to do with sexual ones (which is where he differed from Freud). Although some psychologists are medical doctors and others have been through long training, there is nothing in British law to stop anyone opening an office and calling themselves a psy-chologist. *Psychotherapists* may only see a person a few times and give counselling – advice and psychological support – or they may see a patient for years and give classic psycho-analysis. It all depends on the particular psychotherapist and the requirements of the client.

Psychotherapy can be on a one-to-one basis, or involve couples or the whole family. I'd recommend family therapy for any family in which one or more members seems to be having trouble with life. It's surprising what comes out, but it does take a lot of commitment from all sides. Couples also benefit enormously from therapy, and it's well worth trying if the relationship isn't going well.

One-to-one therapy, however, can sometimes be problem-atic in that the client can say whatever they want and there's nobody else there to put another perspective. This is especially likely in post-trauma stress. I recently spoke to one woman, for example, who was in therapy and who, because her records had been subpoenaed for a court case (in which she was the innocent party – but let's not talk about insurance companies and the legal system!), was allowed to see what had been written about her. She was surprised to discover that she had been making things up. I asked her why she did it – 'to please the psychoanalyst', she said, and also it was a self-protective mechanism – if she made up these stories, she wouldn't have to spend time on the things which were true but too painful to discuss. The point is, how is the analyst supposed to know the difference between truth and lies? In the records, it was obvious he had taken all she said at face value – and then assessed her personality on the basis of that!

Another problem with therapy is that it is rather difficult to get referred by your doctor until you are in serious trouble – you might get an appointment with a specialist in aggression, for example, but only after you've killed someone! Places are in short supply. At least, they are if you don't want to pay. If you have not yet gone 'over the hill', so to speak, and just want some general help in sorting yourself out, the doctor is unlikely to be able to help – you must find your own solution, and there is plenty of choice.

Aside from one-to-one therapy, and group therapy, there is dance therapy, art therapy, music therapy, singing therapy, anger therapy, behavioural therapy, grief counselling, rape-victim groups, sexual abuse-victim groups, and 'the wounded male' groups amongst others. Look around and try to identify which type of therapy might be right for you. Many people have started their own groups with people who have had similar experiences; for example there are groups for people who have had a child die of cancer, or who have a particular physical illness.

It will take some homework to find the right group and the way to approach this, I think, is to say to yourself, 'I'm going to make one phone call a day', and carry on until you get through the labyrinth of information to a place that seems right for you. There are several standard reference books which list organizations and they can be found in the large libraries. It might be simpler to start your own group – put an advert in the paper and see who comes forward.

Aromatherapy is being increasingly used in the therapy and counselling situation and specific advice on this is given later. (See Chapter 10.)

MEDITATION AND VISUALIZATION

Meditation and visualization are both very helpful techniques and they can be learned quite easily from books, or even without them. With meditation, you're aiming to clear your mind of all thoughts. This is very difficult at first but it becomes easier with practice and even just ten minutes a day will help improve your health. You will need to focus on something. Some people use a sound – like 'Om' – while others think of an image – a lotus flower for example – while others concentrate on their breathing. The idea is to be very quiet, so silent you can almost hear what's going on within your body. Thoughts will come but let them float away – don't hang on to them.

Sit comfortably with your back straight. Before starting, flex your toes and then release them, then do the same with your calves, thighs, buttocks, tummy, arms, shoulders, neck, head and face. Pre-recorded tapes are available which lead you through a meditation, and they can be very helpful. Unplug the phone or put on the answering machine so you are not disturbed. Burning essential oils in a diffuser can certainly help the meditative process – choose one oil that you like or a combination of oils, perhaps choosing from the list of oils that help with anxiety. (See Chapter 8.)

Like meditation, visualization is an extremely ancient practice. The Hindu yogic texts known as the tantras were written between the fourth and sixth centuries AD and include the advice to visualize the desired lover. By making a precise image in your mind, complete with physical, mental and spiritual attributes, and focusing on it every day, the lover could be conjured up – for real. The Tibetan Tantric texts contain sadhanas, visualization exercises, which could be used to create anything one desired. This method made perfect sense to the Tantrists, who believed everything in the world was created by thought, and continues to be modified by the collective thought of all mankind. To perfect their visualization techniques, the more serious adepts would spend years in a closed room or cave. The Sufis are another group who believe that a person's destiny can be shaped by visualization, which they call 'creative prayer'.

In western culture these days, visualization is being fairly widely used to treat illnesses, especially cancer. In medical visualization, the idea is to imagine a 'killer' destroying the diseased cells. What one imagines doing the 'killing', and how you imagine the bad cells you want to get rid of, is entirely personal. The killer might be a shark progressively eating a school of little fish, or it might be a Pac-Man™ munching through the unwanted cells, or a gun blasting away bits of the tumour.

The crucial thing about visualization is to practise. I don't mean practise doing it (although you have to do that too), but practise visualizing real live objects before you start creative visualization. You can practise with anything – a flower, for example. Look at the colour of the petals, and their texture, and register how many petals the flower has and look at the stamen. Whatever you choose to practise with, just have a good look at the object, close your eyes, try to see it in your mind's eye, and when you lose the image, have another look at the real thing. Keep going like this until your ability to see things clearly, and your ability to remember them, becomes better. Practise looking at and visualizing something interesting and pleasant, real or in two-dimensional picture form – a tree, garden, sea shore or whatever. Don't choose a cup or table or something equally boring because your interest will not be maintained.

If you decide you want to try to get rid of cancer cells inside you, by imagining a shark for example, get a picture of an actual shark and have a good look at it – look at the colours of its skin, the shape and form of its body. And if your cancer is in the colon, for example, get a book on anatomy and have a really good look at the anatomy of a colon. Also, if you are basically a pacifist, don't use imagery which is violent. Instead of thinking of guns blasting away at the tumour, think of it as slowly dissolving, or cracking open like an egg and pouring away, or being baked and gradually shrivelling up.

As you practise visualization, burn six to eight drops of essential oil on a burner or diffuser in the room. Use something pleasant, and relaxing – something you enjoy smelling. Eventually, you'll be able to take your visualization skills out

with you so you can sit on a train and, even with your eyes
wide open, do your visualization exercise. If you also have a
couple of drops of your usual visualization essential oils on a
tissue, or on your sleeve, you can inhale them and it will
remind you of your practising and help focus your mind.

Chapter Four

AROMA-PSYCHOLOGY

WHAT'S IN A WORD?

BEFORE DISCUSSING WHAT AROMA-PSYCHOLOGY MEANS TO YOU or me, I just want to say a few words about the linguistics of aroma, the new language which is expanding by the day. The word *aromatherapy* refers to the clinical use of essential oils combined with physical therapy – usually in the form of massage or inhalations. Aromatherapists go through very different degrees of training – from a few weekend courses to many years of intense anatomy, physiology, chemistry, body-work and massage skills. Fully trained aromatherapists perform work which cannot always be done at home, and their services are sometimes indispensable. A very small minority of aromatherapists have a more medical leaning, while the majority tend towards stress-management. There are also beauticians and cosmetologists who are using essential oils and essential oil products and call what they are doing 'aroma-therapy'. This is the 'beauty and relaxation' end of the aromatherapy spectrum. To some degree, anyone can be an 'aromatherapist' in that much of the information required is available, and the methods do not always need outside help – one can do them at home.

Because there is so much more to essential oils than their use in a 'clinical' setting or even for medicinal use within the home, several other expressions have grown up. The aroma-therapist Professor William Arnold-Taylor first coined the term *aroma-tology* in 1981, and he meant by it 'aromatherapy for the whole person' – body, mind and spirit. This is a very wide term encompassing using the essential oils to reform character and personality characteristics, and to enhance spirituality. It's a good term if you want to indicate the depths of influence essential oils can have.

The word *aroma-chology* is a trademark of the Olfactory Research Fund (formerly the Fragrance Foundation), a research institution that supports the flavours and fragrance industries. Whether referring to the use of synthetics or natural essential oils, aroma-chology is to do with influencing the mind. It encompasses the development of aromas to attract buyers into a shop and make them linger there longer, and of aromas to make keyboard operators more efficient, or customers more relaxed. The research doesn't stop here. Indeed, for many years government defence departments have been exploring ways in which aroma can control crowds or influence the behaviour of the enemy.

Aroma-psychology specifically refers to the use of essential oils to positively affect the mind – such as memory enhancement, learning improvement, mood uplifting, and confidence boosting. These mental stimulations have a direct impact on daily performance and practical applications are currently being utilized by a wide range of organizations.

Because the mind and body are an integrated unit, the term aroma-psychology is somewhat unsatisfactory, as is psycho-aromatherapy, which for some people conjures up images from the shower scene in Alfred Hitchcock's movie, *Psycho*. But they are still useful to denote the degree to which the mental or bodily functions are involved at any one time. For example, if you burn your hand and put lavender oil on it, that's a physical application although the lavender will also help with the shock and make you more relaxed. We would call that aromatherapy. On the other hand, if you're having a party and want the room to smell nice and make your guests relaxed, you might put some geranium, cinnamon and melissa in a room diffuser before they arrive. The fact that these will help prevent one guest passing a nasty flu virus to another is an added bonus! This situation is aroma-psychology bordering on aromatherapy.

Man-made chemical odourants do not have this ability to perform antibacterial or antiviral activities, and although there is now a vast industry which attempts to replicate the aromas of essential oils, what they produce can in no way be compared to essential oils. It is difficult to find analogies to illustrate the difference. Perhaps one could compare essential oils to a music concert, and man-made synthetic aromas to a recording of that concert. Technicians might say the recording can improve on the real event, because in the studio they can over-dub, add echo, and 'drop-in' notes or words which were less than perfect at the time of the performance. This is true, but the concert has an atmosphere, an excitement, and is a total experience in a way a recording can never be. The analogy can never really work, however, because the music in the concert will be different – and *better*, vibrationally and energetically – than the recording. The expression 'chalk and cheese' comes to mind but essential oils are neither chalk nor cheese – they are pure, luxurious, delightful, beneficial substances, designed by God. Synthetic fragrances, on the other hand, were designed by people in laboratories and their benefits (other than to satisfy commercial interests) have yet to be proved. Indeed, synthetics are not even *meant* to be beneficial to us. They're just designed to make us choose one particular product over another, and pay more for it.

The olfactory onslaught is already upon us. Personally, I hate getting into the back of a taxi only to discover there is a horrible chemical air-freshener on the shelf behind my head. The window has to be opened and I practically hold my breath until we get to where we're going. And the massive aroma bombardment that comes from most cosmetics sections in department stores is often overwhelming. But now we have a whole new dimension to aroma as the mind-altering effects of essential oils are being exploited in many so-called 'aromatherapy' products, which you can find in all the major

high street shops. What happens is that research shows a
particular essential oil is relaxing, neroli for example, so the
toiletry manufacturers say 'let's make a relaxing neroli
bubble-bath'. The next thing is you see a product on the shelf
purporting to be a 'relaxing, aromatherapy' bubble bath, but
what you don't know is that the product doesn't have a drop of
neroli oil in it. Instead, it's got some combination of chemicals
that *smells* like neroli.

Now, the chemists will tell you that it makes no difference.
According to them, the chemical cocktails they produce in the
lab and the real thing – neroli oil, say – are more or less the
same thing. Some will even tell you that the chemical version
is better! The logic goes like this: there are 100 components in
neroli oil, say, but only 5 or 10 of these actually produce the
smell, so those 5 or 10 can be tested for safety and combined
to make a 'neroli' product. *Real* neroli, they say, cannot be
tested for safety because it's too complex. Therefore the
chemical 'copy' is safer than the real thing. This logic makes
sense until you realize two other things. First, neroli oil, like
all essential oils, is very complex – too complex to copy. No
laboratory can produce a 'neroli' which does what neroli does
– create well-being, for example, because nobody has yet discovered what all the minuscule components of neroli actually
are. We don't have names for them. The chemists say you
don't *need* the 90 or 95 other components of neroli – but this
really depends on whether you're trying to replicate the *smell*
or the *effect*. Second, it is one thing to test individually a group
of chemicals for inclusion in a product and declare them safe,
but what about the product as a *whole* – how are those chemicals interacting with each other – and, more importantly, with
all the natural chemicals, and cells, within our body?

Chemists are very fond of pointing out that within some
essential oils there are tiny components which may be toxins,
and that if they tried to reproduce them in a product, it wouldn't
be allowed. Yes, maybe, but we're not making essential oils in
a lab. The whole point about essential oils is that they are complex and work as a *whole*. There might be something in an
essential oil which is toxic but in the context of the whole oil,
in synergistic or antagonistic combination with all the other

bits and pieces, it becomes non-toxic. It is this beautiful balance which gives them the extraordinary potency which cannot be replicated. James A. Duke, PhD, one of the world's foremost authorities on natural plant products, makes another, important point:

> Through evolution our genes have already experienced many of the natural compounds, including toxic and medicinal compounds, often equipping us with mechanisms to deal with reasonable doses of these toxins. Our genes have no experience with tomorrow's synthetics ... Through maternal and/or cytoplasmic inheritance, our immune systems have also experienced many of the natural compounds, but not tomorrow's synthetics.[1]

Peppermint

Today, millions of people will apply essential oils to their bodies, in the form of perfume, and other millions will put them into their mouths in the form of drinks and food. Every time you chew a piece of spearmint or peppermint gum, essential oils are involved, while the soft drinks industry purchases by far the largest portion of the citrus essential oils. Even ylang ylang, usually thought of as just a perfume ingredient, is used in confectionery and baking goods. Essential oils are a vast worldwide industry. For example, the 1992 peppermint and spearmint oil production in America alone was worth $95 million and $46 million, respectively. Someone consumes all this, and as far as anyone has ever been able to say, they have suffered no toxic side effects from it. Nor, as far as I am aware, has anyone suffered toxic side effects from potatoes which, as chemists are well aware, contain toxins – especially in the peel.

AROMA-PSYCHOLOGY AND MENTAL STATES

Research into the psychological effects of aroma now attracts major funding. There are four major olfaction research institutions: the Olfactory Research Fund in New York, the Monell Chemical Senses Center in Philadelphia, the Smell and Taste Treatment and Research Foundation in Chicago, and Warwick University's Olfaction Research Department. The Olfactory Research Fund awards grants to doctors who wish to study the psychological aspects of olfaction, and is funded by the fragrance industry, while the Monell employs fifty PhD-level scientists and carries out work on the physiology and psychology of aroma on behalf of various funding agencies – both commercial and governmental.

In addition to these, there are innumerable commercial organizations and education facilities which now look into the psychological effects of aroma, such as International Flavours and Fragrances, the Takasago Central Research Laboratory in Tokyo, the Toho University School of Medicine, Tokyo, and Yale University. Psychology professor, Robert A. Baron, at the

Renselaer Polytechnic Institute in Troy, New York, for example, has found that people in pleasantly scented rooms carry out their work with more confidence, more efficiency and with greater willingness to resolve conflict. From my postbag it is patently clear that tremendous interest in the behaviour-changing potential of aroma exists among the new generation of psychology students.

As a subject, olfaction has become a hot item among a whole range of scientific researchers for several reasons. The fact that olfactory cells regenerate every thirty to forty days makes them unique among brain and central nervous system cells, and rather exciting components of neurobiology. The olfactory receptor system also involves P-proteins, G-proteins and GABA receptors, which are interesting for various reasons, and by understanding how they work, many other physiological mysteries may be revealed. However, a vast body of research is also being done on the psychological effects of aroma because these have powerful commercial implications, and projects can easily attract funding.

When I read research papers involving essential oils I am more often than not surprised at the choice of oils, and the volumes at which they are used. For example, one trial exploring the sedative effects of lavender on elderly patients involved putting three drops of lavender on their pillows. Lavender is an adaptogen which means it can have one effect in low dosage and another in a high dosage. Depending on the person on whom it is being used, one drop of lavender oil should be quite sufficient to make anyone sleep, while three could have the opposite – stimulant – effect.

Another problem, of course, is that you cannot patent nature. Sorry, but Mother Nature Inc. has got the patent already. To register a patent you've got to *invent* something, and essential oils were invented a very long time ago. The people who fund research into the psychological effects of odour want to be able to exploit the information they get. To do this, they've got to come up with a new combination of chemicals and register it for a particular purpose. Man-made aromas (like drugs) can also elicit behavioural change, a fact which pleases commercial interests, who find dealing in natural products – which are prone to the vicissitudes of the weather and pests, and liable to degrade quicker – more troublesome than synthetically produced products. Consequently, the research is directed at finding which combination of man-made chemicals elicit certain responses. The end result, of course, is that you and I are increasingly going to be exposed to these chemicals as the research turns into practical applications. The important question for the future is not 'are we going to use aroma to change behaviour?', which is going to happen anyway, but, 'are we going to use man-made chemicals, or essential oils?'

HOSPITALS, HOSPICES AND NURSING HOMES

Hospitals and hospices need all the cheering up they can get, and essential oils are the perfect way to do it. Aside from the fact that they deodorize the clinical and organic smells, and make the place smell fresh and charming, they can (if you use the right ones) cut down cross-infections. Mr Fred Dale of Dale Air Products, who has twelve years' experience in installing essential oil diffusion-systems in hospitals, museums and other public buildings, says that 'synthetic materials, when interacting with certain other smells, won't get rid of those smells and you'll end up with a worse smell than you started with'.

Essential oils, on the other hand, work very well. And they have other benefits. At the Worcester Hospital in Hereford a six-month trial showed that vaporizing lavender through the air caused patients to sleep in a more natural pattern, and made them less aggressive during the day. More than that, over the six months, some patients were weaned off their tranquillizers – simply by substituting lavender in the atmosphere, which has a calming effect on the brain.

Mr Dale has devised a 'Reminiscence Pack' which he supplies to day-care centres for the elderly. Five aromas are used together with a script by care staff to elicit memories from the old folk. As you may know, elderly people tend to have bad short-term memory but a very good long-term one, and if that long-term memory can be evoked, through aroma, their minds can be kept active recollecting their school days, youth, and happier times. It is, apparently, very effective and much appreciated by all concerned. Meanwhile, an American diffuser-system company – AromaSys of Minneapolis – are also working with nursing homes for the elderly to explore ways of reducing 'wandering'. Here too, aromas are being used to create a nostalgic stimulus to kindle more dynamic mental states.

Lavender

AromaSys has installed six hundred aroma-diffusion systems in the United States, including one at the St Croix Valley Memorial Hospital in Wisconsin. In this fully registered general hospital, essential oils are diffused throughout the lobby, at a nurses' station and in the emergency waiting room. Here, family members wait to hear news of their sick relatives and it is obviously an extremely stressful place, made more bearable by the anxiety-relieving essential oils which are diffused in the atmosphere. The hospital also has two 'floaters', mobile systems, which can be taken to any areas where they are particularly required, including the chemical dependency unit where people with drinking or drug problems are seen. Various aromas are used in different areas, at different times, depending on the requirements. The hospital administrator, Steve Urosevich, says his aim is to make the patient's hospital stay 'more humanizing, more personal and demystifying'.[2]

In 1992 Drs William Redd and Sharon Manne at the Memorial Sloan-Kettering Cancer Center in New York conducted tests to see whether aroma could reduce the anxiety of patients undergoing magnetic resonance imaging procedures. They compared stress levels between forty-two patients who breathed normal air with thirty-eight who breathed air containing molecules of heliotropin – a sweet, vanilla-like fragrance naturally occuring in pepper oil. Sixty-three per cent of those exposed to the aroma experienced reduced anxiety levels.

Stress reduction is a major concern of the London Lighthouse – a specialist facility for those with HIV-related problems. For many years now they have been offering complementary therapies in addition to the usual medical treatments. Aromatherapy treatments have an extremely high uptake rate, but because of financial restrictions demand outstrips supply. The main benefits are perceived to be general relaxation and stress and anxiety relief, which in turn positively affect the immune system. Wendy Peters of the medical and complementary health services department says that aromatherapy treatments seem to prevent the onset of the disease, although this can only be an anecdotal observation as each client will be undergoing several different treatments at the same time. I find it very touching that many clients, or their family and friends, ask that essential oils are diffused in the atmosphere during the death process itself.

At the St John's and St Elizabeth's Hospital in London all eleven midwives have become trained aromatherapists. They have no doubt as to the benefits of essential oils. They offer them to women during the antenatal stage, during the birth itself, and in after-care – for both mother and child. They use essential oils for physical ailments such as nausea, swollen legs, muscular pains, mastitis and infections. (See *The Fragrant Pharmacy*.[3]) But anxiety, stress and tension may also accompany pregnancy and birth, particularly for women who have had previous bad experiences, and blood-pressure levels must also be controlled.

There is a growing interest in aromatherapy on the part of nurses, who were inspired by the good work done by members of the International Federation of Aromatherapists, as part of the 'Aromatherapy in Care' project. These practitioners worked with children, cancer and AIDS patients, among others. The Royal College of Nursing, in recognition of the interest, has produced its own literature on the subject, and many small-scale studies are being carried out all over the country. At the Royal Sussex County Hospital in Brighton, for example, a trial involving thirty-six patients in the intensive care and coronary care units were put into three groups which would receive either aromatherapy massage, massage without oils and nothing – i.e. the control group. (Massage was done to the feet.) Over a five-week period various measurements were taken. Systolic blood pressure measurements showed a reduction in the control group of 16 per cent over the five weeks, while the aromatherapy group decreased by 50 per cent (massage alone was 40 per cent); decrease in respiratory rate was 16 per cent in the control and 75 per cent in the aromatherapy group (41 per cent massage alone); while reduction in heart rate was 41 per cent for the control and 91 per cent for the aromatherapy group (58 per cent massage alone).

Hopefully, as ignorance and prejudice breaks down, more trials should be instigated. Experience has shown that no harm comes of aromatherapy, and that patients very much appreciate its benefits. As 'patient care' becomes a buzz-word in the restructured National Health Service, we should see more attention being given to aromatherapy.

OFFICES

The Japanese have a long tradition of using aroma, and they have much respect for it. Perhaps then, it is not so surprising that it should be the Japanese who have most easily accepted the logic of using aroma as a management tool. In 1985 research into the mind-altering effects of essential oils was started in Japan by Dr Shizuo Torii who, by measuring brain waves, showed that some aromas can have a stimulating effect and some can have a relaxing effect. Things have progressed somewhat since then, and to my knowledge there are now fifty aroma diffusion systems in place in both commercial and municipal offices.

Japan's third largest construction company, the Shimizu Corporation, has specialist engineers who incorporate aroma systems into the new 'intelligent' buildings which use aroma to improve efficiency and relieve stress. In one bank, designed by the company, lavender or rosemary are diffused into the customer areas, while lemon or eucalyptus are used to keep workers alert at their VDUs. Commercial diffuser systems are capable of pumping different aromas into the atmosphere at different times of the day, to relax or stimulate as required. The fragrance company Takasago have shown that keyboard punching errors fell by 20 per cent when lavender was diffused in the atmosphere, by 33 per cent with jasmine and 54 per cent with lemon. By changing the aromas around periodically, smell sensitivity (tolerance) – and efficiency – can be maintained.

Another Japanese construction company which has taken aroma to heart is the Kajima Corporation, which now also sells aroma diffusion systems. In their state-of-the-art 'intelligent' head office in Akasaka, Tokyo, sensors monitor atmospheric conditions like temperature and humidity and the building's computers blend appropriate fragrances which are diffused into different areas of the building, taking the time of day and the male–female ratio of any one department into consideration. While a lavender and rose combination creates a calming, stress-relieving and blood-pressure reducing effect for general purposes, the after-lunch drowsiness is combated, they say, with lemon and jasmine, which have a refreshing and reviving effect. Many combinations of aroma are possible, and Kajima are using lemon in the morning, floral and wood aromas during the day to maintain a relaxed atmosphere, with a final flourish of lemon at the end of the day to give workers the boost they need to fight their way home through the traffic. And after a good night's sleep they can be woken by Seiko's Hattori clock, which releases the aroma of pine and eucalyptus just before the alarm goes off – to create the impression of waking in a lovely natural environment, and to invigorate the worker to get going again.

The logic of using aroma to keep workers happy, relaxed and efficient has not been lost on certain American companies either. In Ohio, the 10,000 square feet offices of Frederick's Inc – hair care distributors – have been fitted with an adjustable aroma-diffusion system. Their chairman, Frederick Holzberger, says 'I have seen an absolute major attitude change.'[4]

Lemon

RETAIL OUTLETS

Retail Planning Associates of Seattle, USA, are one of the new breed of companies who specialize in creating fragrances for retail outlets. Their president, J'Amy Owens, says that aroma is '. . . one of the best ways to influence the customer that's legal . . . It's the "come into my parlor" approach, one more piece of netting in the web.'[5] A unique, personalized store aroma, which can be used in the air conditioning system, can cost anything up to $20,000 to create.

Aroma diffusion does not have to be an expensive business, however. Anyone can create their own, unique, personal range of preferred aromas when they have a few bottles of essential oils with which to work. There is a very effective diffuser available, which doesn't use electricity or candle-heat, and because it's portable, can be used in your office as well as your home.[6] Even on a commercial scale, using essential oils, the cost is not excessive. The Radisson Mart Plaza Hotel in Miami, for example, fragrances its 7,000 square-foot lobby for $21 a day.

According to Alan R. Hirsch, Neurologic Director of the Smell and Taste Treatment and Research Foundation in Chicago, USA, 'Odorants are potentially more efficacious than any other modality in increasing saleability of consumer products. This is true regardless of whether the odor is actually related to or synergistic with the product.' In other words, you can put a false aroma of popcorn into the environment, a cinema foyer for example, and increase your sales of actual popcorn, or you can use a floral aroma to make the customer buy something that has nothing to do with flowers – a pair of trainer shoes, for example.

In 1990 Dr Hirsch recruited thirty-one people at a shopping centre and asked them to look at trainer shoes in two rooms. The Nike trainers used in the trial were identical, but one of the rooms was perfumed with a light, mixed floral aroma. Twenty-six or 84 per cent of the people indicated that they were more likely to buy the shoes in the scented room, and on average, they said they'd pay $10.33 more for them. Although the test attempted to make the aroma detectable to the participants, many couldn't smell it although they too preferred the product in the perfumed room. This means the 'buy-me' reflex is operating at a subliminal level too. All this is very tantalizing to sales managers, especially as the technology now exists to release a variety of odorants into a closed atmosphere in standardized but adjustable concentrations.

In another trial, in a gambling casino in Las Vegas, Hirsch discovered that if a particular aroma was put into the atmosphere around a group of slot-machines, the amount of money put into them by gamblers increased by an average of 45.11 per cent. As part of the trial, Hirsch had also used a second aroma around another group of machines and taken a non-perfumed area as his control. Neither of these areas saw any increase in their takings, so obviously there was something in 'aroma #1' causing the increased sales effect. Finding exactly what makes people spend their money so freely is what the new aroma research is all about, and what more and more businesses will find themselves having to pay for, as aroma-competition hots up.

Although Japan does not at present use aroma to an extensive degree in retailing, Toyota does use floral aromas to attract women into its showrooms. Meanwhile, an unnamed American car manufacturer is supporting research to find a scent which makes its salesmen appear 'more honest and trustworthy to customers'.[7]

Of course, making a sale is only half the problem – then you've got to collect the money. Aroma can help here too. Imagine if there was an aroma you could spray on your invoices to induce the customer to pay up. There is. It's called *Aeolus 7* and smells like sweat. Apparently, it is a much faster way to get payment than sending a lawyer's letter and, of course, *very* much cheaper.

SCHOOLS AND COLLEGES

The first hard proof that aroma can be used to improve memory (and thus learning and passing exams) came from psychologist Frank Schaub at Yale University. He gave seventy-two undergraduates a list of forty adjectives and asked them to write down their opposites. They were not told that the next day they would be required to remember them. At various stages of the experiment, some students were given the aroma of chocolate and some were not. On average, those not given the aroma remembered 17 per cent of the answers and those given it, 21 per cent. These results were replicated later using the aroma of mothballs. The crucial factor, apparently, is that the same scent is used in each session – remembering and recalling. Aromatherapists believe essential oils can improve on 21 per cent, but then we don't use mothballs!

More recently, Dr Hirsch and his team in Chicago found that students in the senior calculus class at Lincoln High School, Portland, Oregon, could be made to increase their speed of learning by using a chemical mixed floral aroma in the room. The students had to do a test three times, wearing a mask, either with or without the odorant. When the same test had been done on adults, they improved their score from 14 to 31 per cent, while the high-school students improved their scores from 14 to 54 per cent. Dr Hirsch has proposed several mechanisms which may explain why aroma should have a positive impact on learning, as the exact reason is not yet clear. Indeed, what is most clear is that there is still much work to be done. However, if these findings can be replicated, the implications for education are staggering.

It is not too hard to imagine a future in which our children are exposed to aroma in the classroom – but what aromas are they to be – natural or chemical? Already, our children (and we ourselves) are exposed to pollutants in the water, to pesticide, herbicide, and fungicide residues in vegetables, and metals and hormones in meat, as well as to air pollution, chemical air-fresheners, cleaners and toiletries. There has to come a point at which we say 'too much'. And the classroom has to be it. On the other hand, it is true that aroma can enhance memory, and there is a way to do it – using essential oils. Although one is adding something to the room, it is something which can be found in nature – which is, after all, where children throughout the aeons have sat and learned their lessons. With essential oils, we're putting back some of the benefits of the natural environment, things you would experience in the country –

trees like pine, eucalyptus or cypress, fruits like bergamot or grapefruit, herbs like basil or rosemary, flowers like geranium or rose.

THE FUTURE

In the case of aroma-psychology, we are standing on the threshold of a new era and there is no reason not to take the natural route.

From a worldwide supply and demand point of view, one might say that if all the products, which now use fragrances, were to switch to naturals, there wouldn't be enough space on the planet to grow them. The answer to this may be in bio-technology, which the perfumery and cosmetics house, Estée Lauder, are looking into as a way of producing rose and jasmine oil – which are notoriously expensive. The method their research and development department is exploring involves isolating the oil-producing cells in the flower petals and culturing them in a soup of nutrients. If this method works, it may be a good thing in that it will provide a source of 'rose' and 'jasmine' which can be used in perfumery. However, these would not be substances which I or my collegues would use for traditional aromatherapy. Whatever science may tell us, we believe that real essential oils can only be produced by chlorophyll-bearing plants which absorb the sun's rays and synthesize organic compounds. We prefer bio-dynamics over bio-technology. However, for fragrancing alone, the new biotechnology may provide a solution to supply problems.

From the future of the planet point of view, plants are already being explored as a means of helping the ozone layer. Much international interest is being taken in *Vernonia gala-mensis*, from the Compositae family (which includes chamomile and helichrysum) because its oil can be used in paint manufacture and reduce the pollutants in the atmosphere. Because of its low viscosity, *Vernonia* can be used as a solvent which, uniquely, actually becomes part of the dry paint surface and does not evaporate to pollute the air. In America and Germany, according to a report in *Herbalgram*, 'research is

Jasmine

under way in university and industry laboratories on its use for
lubricants and lubricant additives, adhesives, and epoxy resins
and in the synthesis of dilbasic acids currently obtained from
petroleum and used in the manufacture of industrial nylons.'[8]
As a cash crop for the Third World *Vernonia* has the distinct
advantage of being able to grow in as little as eight inches of
annual rainfall and is distasteful to animals. As a benefit for
the whole world, consider the fact that in the Los Angeles
basin alone 22 tons of volatile organic compound emissions
from paints and varnishes rise to deplete the ozone layer each
day.[9] Any reduction in that has to be a blessing.

Citrus essential oils, meanwhile, are a good alternative for
petrochemicals used in paints, household cleaners and solvents
used to clean computer chips. This is good news for the 20 per
cent of people who suffer headaches caused by the common
solvent, trichloroethylene.[10]

The human mind was not designed to inhale the plethora of man-made chemicals and we are only just beginning to understand what effects they are having on us. In the year 2020, children may not know what it feels like to walk, exhilarated, through a pine forest, and they may associate the aroma of pine with synthetic cleaning fluids. Already olfactory researchers are having difficulty finding people who make natural associations with aroma. For example, because of its widespread use in confectionery, synthetic strawberry flavour is more often identified as 'real' than the real (i.e. natural) thing. Natural aromatic connections are in danger of being lost!

Part Two

EMOTIONAL HEALING AND AROMATHERAPY

'Miracles occur naturally as expessions of love.
The real miracle is the love that inspires them.
In this sense everything that comes from love is a miracle.'

A Course in Miracles

Chapter Five

HOW TO USE ESSENTIAL OILS FOR THE FRAGRANT MIND

THERE'S ALWAYS BEEN SOMETHING FOR PEOPLE TO GET depressed about. When there weren't any supermarkets filled with foreign goods, the crops were all-important. If they failed, or the pests came, life became hell. People starved. And you might hear rumours about a strange army moving towards your area, on horses, carrying weapons, intent to pillage and rape. You might spend half your life anxious about what might happen to your children – now and in the future. People have been under stress for as long as we can imagine and, in among the balms, unguents, ointments and salves of ancient times, you can be sure there were plant essences being used specifically to ease the burdens of the mind. Even the frankincense given to Jesus was (and is) a mind alterant – in fact, it uplifts the spirit and helps dispel earthly problems. By the time Dioscorides came along in AD 60, he could name 1,500 medicinal plants, many of which were in aromatic oil form. This was the *materia medica* with which our ancestors grew up, and which we have developed to the point where we can see the rich diversity of help nature can provide, including that for the mind.

Over the years many different systems of medicine have developed. These are not necessarily in conflict, as a wise person somewhere once said – you can take many routes to get to the same place. In India, the traditional method of medicine is Ayurvedic, and in that the personality and character of the patient is taken as part of the diagnostic procedure. The type of person would (and still does) determine the particular plant prescribed. This diagnosis by character is today routine in homeopathy and herbalism, while personality, in all its forms, is a routine subject of discussion for perfumers. Personality and character, in relation to essential oils, is the subject of Part Three of this book.

Part Two deals with all those things for which aromatherapy is best known – stress, tension and so on. They are included within the A-Z of emotional problems – which goes from abuse, addiction, aggression through to trauma, withdrawal and worthlessness. In between the downs, there are ups – confidence, contentment and joy. It is these potentials which have contributed so much to the growth of aromatherapy in recent years. Essential oils are positive additions to one's life, including one's mental life. And the great thing is, one doesn't have to be sick or even troubled to use them. They are there to enhance, to strengthen and to delight.

COMPLEXITY AND FLEXIBILITY

Essential oils are like people – complex. One person called Rosemary might be a fabulous ballet dancer, and a computer buff, a mother, a cook, a driver, a chess player, a tennis player and a poet. Likewise, the essential oil, rosemary, can do many different things. Just because you might have read somewhere that rosemary oil is used for rheumatism, for example, don't assume that is its only use. It's also good for depression and fatigue. Essential oils are flexible and adaptable – like people.

In a clinical setting, an aromatherapist will individualize the formula of essential oils she or he uses on a client. No two people are alike, and even if they were, circumstances or situations can be different. In a book it is obviously impossible to individualize, but the format of this book allows us to get around this problem to a certain degree. Alongside the standard clinical formulations I give for each situation, you will find a list of essential oils from which you can choose to design your own formula, tailor-made for you. Look at the individual oils listed for a particular problem, emotional violence say, and cross-reference them with what else is said about them throughout the book. Smell the actual oil next time you go into a shop. If you like it, buy it. You can personalize a formula for yourself, which might change with time and circumstances. There are many possibilities because essential oils are so flexible; there are lots of options to try.

One of the great things about aromatherapy is how you get a synergistic effect when you blend two or more oils together. Bergamot is a great confidence booster, but blend it with geranium which is an emotional balancer, and you have a winner. Single essential oils can be vibrant and dynamic on their own but put in a blend, they become more than the sum of their component parts – with a unique character of their own, and with an extra energizing and harmonizing potential. With approximately 300 essential oils available, you can see how many permutations there are to try! Two of this and one of that, two of that and one of this, or two of each – all these are different blends. It would take a mathematical genius to work out all the possible permutations, even given certain restrictions.

SYNERGY AND CREATIVE BLENDING

When you put two essential oils together you create an entirely new compound. The number of permutations – using blends of two, three or more – are incalculable. Throughout this book you will find blends which contain several essential oils but, because these blends are meant to be taken as a *whole*, and because particular essential oils cannot be taken out of context of the entire blend, do not assume that if a particular oil is included in a blend for stress, say, then that oil can be used on its own for the same purpose. Sometimes this is indeed true, but not always. Please therefore use *either* the blend given in particular sections, *or* a single oil listed for that purpose

(which may also be in a blend), *or* a combination of oils from
that list, made up to suit your choice.

ADAPTOGENS

Many herbs, roots and essential oils are adaptogens – natural
balancers. Lemon works on the nervous system, active as a
sedative or tonic, as required. Lavender is another adaptogen –
small quantities are usually relaxing, while high concentrations can be stimulating. With essential oils, balance is all,
and when balanced, the body and mind can perform to their
best. Bear all this in mind when you see a particular oil
appearing on two lists of opposing conditions – the *quantities*
of these oils can be all-important, as is the *quality* or nature of
an individual person at any given time.

CHEMOTYPES

The same species of plant, grown in different growing conditions, produces a different essential oil with unique properties.
Altitude, water quality, soil fertility, the magnetic pull of the
earth, methods of growing and weather are all factors which
have an effect on the way the plant develops, and thereby influence the properties a particular batch from a particular country
produces. Think of it like wine. People transport vines with
them as they emigrate, and produce a wine that is related to,
but not exactly the same, as that produced in the valley from
which the vine came. The word *chemotypes* describes these
branches of the same family, which can do somewhat different
jobs, and gives another indication of the broadness of the
possibilities inherent in essential oils use.

PURITY AND QUALITY

It used to be the case that you could be pretty sure where a
particular species of plant was grown and from where the

essential oil came – lavender used to come from either England or France, for example. Lavender still comes from England and France but now it also comes from China, from where it is sometimes shipped to France – and re-exported as 'French'. It used to be the case that French lavender was grown under clear skies, fresh and clean. Now you can see lavender growing in fields adjacent to motorways, under skies thick with the smoke rising from nuclear plants. It now makes a great deal of difference from where, *exactly*, in France the lavender comes – the high Alps are preferred partly because the air is cleaner there. For an aromatherapist it is also important to know whether a helichrysum, for example, is grown in Corsica or the former Yugoslavia, because the two essential oils have different therapeutic qualities.

It used to be the case that some essential oils were sold at auction. Nowadays, wholesalers tend to have a more direct access to the source – the field in which the crop is grown, and the farmer – often through a middleman. This gives purchasers more control, which is necessary, because there are more factors to consider. Aside from the question of which country, and *exactly* from where in that country the oils come, aromatherapists who use essential oils for clinical use want to know which, if any, chemical pesticide, fungicide or herbicide is used on the crop. Bear in mind here that we are talking about tiny quantities of biocide residues. These things also exist – in very much larger quantities – in the foods we eat every day. Plagued as they are by insects, insect eggs, snails, rodents, weeds and fungi, farmers are tempted to use chemicals (known as 'biocides'), and it is the job of the middleman or direct buyer to make sure they don't. Just how much biocide residue is left in any particular essential oil depends on the integrity of the line of supply. For serious aromatherapists, this is the thing they look for when choosing essential oils. The various aromatherapy oil trade organizations recognize the public's desire for purity and as the acceptance of biocides grows less, growers are responding by trying to cut down on them, or omit them altogether.

Essential oils are tested by gas chromatography, mass spectroscopy, thin layer chromatography and high performance liquid chromatography, which are methods for separating essential oils (and other things) into their component parts and analysing them. The gas chromatograph (GC) is basically a hollow column which is lined inside with a chemical resin. A tiny amount of essential oil is diluted with a solvent and injected into one end of the column and then a gas – hydrogen or helium – is forced through the column, under constant pressure, forcing the components of the essential oil to stick to the sides. The most sophisticated machines have columns which are just 0.25mm in diameter and 100 metres long. A detector at the other end identifies each component as it releases from the resin and comes to the other end of the column, the most volatile being evaporated first. Then the column is heated, releasing more components, which are likewise registered, one after the other. As they arrive at the detector, the components are burned, which causes electrical activity, which is recorded as a series of peaks on a piece of paper. The unique pattern of the peaks, showing the relative positions of the components, creates a 'fingerprint' of the oil.

There are several problems with this, and other, methods of analysis. As we have already noted elsewhere, each machine responds somewhat differently, and records differently, so fingerprints cannot be accurately compared from one machine to another. That means that a library of characteristic fingerprint patterns has to be built up, for each machine, so that there are accurate fingerprints against which the tested material can be compared. However, what tends to happen is that the fingerprint is compared with one of the set of 'standard' fingerprints used as a reference by the industry, so the idiosyncrasies of each machine are not always taken into account. Also, interpreting the fingerprint is done by humans, who can take different opinions on the matter. Nevertheless, the GC can help to a certain extent to identify adulteration of essential oils. For example, a common adulterant is linalol, an alcohol found in many essential oils. Linalol, produced artificially, contains traces of other compounds, dihydrolinalol for example, while natural linalol does not, so if any dihydrolinalol shows up on the fingerprint, it shows the oil has been adulterated. However, it is also possible to add a naturally produced linalol, extracted from another plant, and this form of adulteration cannot be detected by this method. Once the essential oil components have been separated by the GC, there are other machines which can further help identify them, including mass spectrometers and infrared spectrometers. However, essential oils contain hundreds of components and not all of them have been identified by science yet. Because of this, certain peaks on the printouts that come from the various machines cannot be named.

If one were to apply all the known technology to an essential oil to be analysed, although one couldn't get a *complete* picture, a fair enough picture would emerge – of its age and chemical composition, albeit limited. However, this process would be very expensive. What often happens instead is that a substance is tested for the main constituents that are supposed to be in it. 'Eucalyptus essential oil' will be tested to see whether it has the correct proportions of eucalyptol and 1,8-cineol for example. However, this doesn't tell us much about the tested material, which might even be an entirely man-made composition.

The term 'essential oil' can, in law, be applied to a liquid that has nothing whatsoever to do with nature. Also, bottles can be labelled 'essential oil', but bear no relation to what description is given on the bottle – 'tuberose absolute' could, in fact, be a mixture of other absolutes and essential oils cleverly blended to smell like tuberose. It is also possible to buy bottles labelled 'aromatherapy essential oils' which have a few drops of essential oils blended in with carrier vegetable oils. In some cases these mislead people into thinking they are buying undiluted essential oils.

Most essential oils are distilled from the plant material which is placed in a still and exposed to steam, forced through from below, which makes the volatile aromatic molecules detach from the plant. These rise with the steam and after condensation, turn into liquid form. At this point, the essential oil is separated from the water – as it is lighter than water it is siphoned off the top. Citrus essential oils are produced by another method known as *expression* which involves highly sensitive machines extracting the essential oil from the rind, without using heat. In this process, whatever biocides were used on the fruits are inevitably included with the essential oils. All these aspects of cultivation and extraction have to be considered by wholesale purchasers of essential oils, who are more and more coming to the conclusion that it is better to lease your own fields, so control over growing methods can be maintained, and the biocides eliminated. Ultimately, they all know the end-user would prefer to use organically grown essential oils, and by collectively pressing this point home we, the consumers, can pressurize suppliers to aim for the highest purity.

Professor George Dodd at the olfaction research department at Warwick University has developed an electronic nose capable of picking up and identifying small components of aroma. Perhaps in the future this will be a tool in essential oil analysis but until then, despite all the latest technological developments in essential oil analysis, the human nose is still the most sensitive aroma-detector going, and it is sometimes still used, instead of a machine, at the receiving end of the GC column. The best way to assess an essential oil is to smell it but, like the GC machines, each of us has to build up our own library of aromas. Obviously this takes time, but the powers of discrimination should soon build up providing you have access to pure fresh essential oils. At the end of this book you will find the addresses of suppliers that I recommend.

THE ART OF SMELLING

The professional 'noses' employed by perfumers and essential oil houses go through many years of training before they are able to identify which components are in a particular product, but apparently any healthy human nose can be trained to distinguish between 10,000 different aromas. It does take experience and practice to develop a nose capable of distinguishing between essential oils, and determining the country of origin and quality of them but, also, one needs to know something about the art of smelling.

Take an open bottle of essential oil, or a perfumer's smelling strip (simply a thin strip of blotting-like paper on which a smear of essential oil has been put), in your hand and swing it around in a circle about six inches under your nose. This creates a vortex in which the aroma molecules become 'excited' and more easily detectable. Then move the bottle or strip under your right nostril and sniff, then under your left and sniff, and then under both and sniff. When you sniff, inhale the aroma so you can feel it at the very top of your nose, then take it (visually) to the crown of your head, and through the whole body. To do this, you must have a fully conscious intent about what you're doing. Really concentrate to experience the aroma. If you do it correctly, you can feel the aroma in the back of the mouth, and feel its effect on the brain. After trying four oils, take a rest from concentrated sniffing – olfactory overload will reduce the ability to perceive accurately. The smelling strips can be used afterwards as book markers or put in drawers to fragrance clothes.

HOW MUCH?

Less is sometimes best. It is not the case that by doubling a quantity of essential oils being used, double the effect is achieved. Also, if you are looking at a choice of blends in a particular section and you see that the first blend has 30 drops, say, and the second has 28 and the third 26, do not assume that the one with 30 drops is the stronger. Each oil has its own potency, so fewer drops of certain oils may be required in particular blends. Also, when essential oils are mixed with each other, an energetic potency is achieved, through the synergistic effect. If you stick to the proportions used in any one blend, you'll be fine whatever quantity you make up.

Unless you are a qualified practitioner, do not use essential oils neat (undiluted) massaged on the skin. There are a few medicinal circumstances when essential oils are used neat – lavender on a burn, for example – but this is a particular situation. There is *no need* to use essential oils neat on the skin for emotional problems, no matter how desperate you may be feeling. Don't worry – the problem can be sorted out – just be patient and stop panicking!

HOW LONG?

There are no hard and fast rules about how long a particular blend or essential oil should be used for a particular purpose. It all depends on the person, the problem and the root cause of that problem. For the purposes outlined in this book, try a blend or oil for a couple of days and if it doesn't work, simply switch to another.

WHICH METHOD?

There are many methods of using essential oils, as you can see from the following chart. When you visit an aromatherapy clinic you are most likely to be massaged – using a system *particular* to aromatherapy. A more general massage can also be done at home and this is a very effective method because, as we have seen in an earlier section, the essential oils are absorbed through the skin and dispersed through the body, and the aroma molecules can also be inhaled at the same time. It is thought that essential oils get into the body when they're used in baths, although in lesser quantity, through the process known as osmosis. Water molecules are too large to penetrate the skin but the molecules of essential oils are tiny, and easily pass through. One also gets the benefits of the aroma molecules as they rise with the steam, and are inhaled. But simply sniffing the oil – direct from the bottle, from a tissue or handkerchief – is also very effective. The subtle way to use essential oils is in the room methods – diffusers, candles, room sprays, water bowls, humidifiers and heat-sources. Which method you use depends upon your degree of requirement and also the particular circumstances you happen to be in. If you're at the office, for example, it is impractical to have a bath – obviously – so you can use a diffuser or simply inhale from a tissue or bottle. The diversity of methods-of-use match perfectly the diversity of situations we find ourselves in over the course of the day. Experiment!

SPOONS, BOTTLES AND DROPPERS

Throughout this book I advise you to make blends or use individual oils diluted in base oils which can be measured by spoonfuls. Spoons do vary in size so buy a set of accurate measuring spoons from a chemist, cooking shop or hardware store. Generally, however, modern cutlery measures are as follows: 1 teaspoon=5 ml; 1 dessertspoon=10 ml; and 1 tablespoon=15 ml.

You will need clean, brown, glass bottles in which to mix your massage oils. You can wash thoroughly and then sterilize bottles you happen to have in the house, or obtain them from any pharmacy. The volume of the bottle is usually imprinted on the base – the figures '20', '30' or '50' refer to millilitres. In this book I usually refer to blends mixed in 30 millilitres of base oil, and for these you only need a bottle with 30 ml capacity because the essential oil addition will not increase the volume substantially and this size of bottle is perfectly sufficient. Bottles are made so that the intended capacity, written on the base, will reach to the shoulder of the bottle, not to the neck.

If you are purchasing them, try to get round bottles because these are much easier to roll between the hands – an important component in the blending process. The bottles must be stored in a cool, dark, dry place. Keep any bottle with essential oil in it, or any essential oils, well away from homeopathic preparations because the essential oils may alter the homeopathic preparations if kept too close to them. This is the case whether or not the essential oils are well sealed. (Also, do not buy homeopathic preparations that have been kept near essential oils, or near strong smelling perfumes, soaps or other toiletries. Classical homeopathic preparations are very subtle, and are said to be adversely affected by any strong aroma.)

Most essential oil bottles have a dropper in the lid. In the rim of the dropper-top there is a little hole. This should always be uppermost because it allows air in, and the essential oil to come out in nice, equal drops. If you don't do this, the essential oil may not come out of the bottle or the drops will fall out in a long stream – and ruin your calculations – and you'll have to start again! Some essential oils are sold without a dropper-top and this is against the guidelines of the Aromatherapy Trade Council because if children find the bottle they may drink from it. Also, of course, it makes it difficult to measure drops. However, pharmacies do sell droppers on their own, and these can be used in this case. But you'll have to have many droppers – one for each essential oil. Do not use one dropper for all your essential oils because small residues may still be left in the dropper and these will get mixed in the next time you use it.

BASE OR CARRIER OILS FOR MASSAGE

Aromatherapists use a wide range of base oils including sweet almond, apricot kernel, grape seed, macadamia and hazelnut oils. We also use wheatgerm, avocado, carrot extract oil, borage and evening primrose oil for certain medical conditions, and rose-hip oil for regenerative purposes. There are many other carrier oils available, from the mundane – like corn oil, to the exotic – like Karapa oil from the Amazon. And there are many other oils which have been around for some time, like cherry seed oil, kukui nut oil, kiwi seed oil, coprah oil, camellia oil, passion flower oil and orchid oil, whose benefits are being rediscovered by aromatherapy.

Because the various benefits of these carrier oils do not directly relate to the workings of the brain (although almond oil is used in India to heighten intellectual ability), I do not intend to go into any detail on them here. A few pages of *The Fragrant Pharmacy*[2] have been devoted to this subject, and the interested reader may want to refer to them.

When choosing a base oil, almond is the easiest to obtain, although you could also try sunflower, safflower or grape seed oil. Buy the one which looks the most pure – that is to say, any one labelled 'organic' – that is grown without biocides (without pesticides), and/or 'cold pressed' or 'virgin'. If you can find an oil that is labelled with all three, that would be perfect.

METHODS OF USE AND DOSAGES

One of the great things about essential oils is that there are so many ways to use them. If you don't have a diffuser for dispersing the aroma around the room, simply put a few drops on a cotton wool ball and tuck it behind a hot radiator, which will heat up the aroma molecules and release them into the atmosphere. If you don't have a radiator, you can put a few drops into a bowl of hot water, which again heats the aroma molecules and releases them into the room. If you don't have a bath, they can be used in the shower, and if you don't have time to see an aromatherapist, you can massage yourself.

The quantities recommended for use in the room methods may seem rather small, and if you prepare them and wait to experience the effect, they may seem hardly perceptible. In fact, the aroma is there but the olfactory tricks we play on ourselves makes it seem that it isn't. Think of how the smell of cigarette smoke can seem completely overpowering when you walk into a smoky bar or party, and yet after a few minutes it is not so noticeable. Likewise with essential oils, we get used to them quickly. When you come to prepare a room method, therefore, do what has to be done and then leave the room, closing the door behind you. When you return a few minutes later you will get a much clearer idea of their true impact on the atmosphere, and you'll be better able to judge whether you have used too little or too much.

Chart 5.1 outlines the various methods, and gives the dosages you should use. Following this there is another chart (Chart 5.2) which gives the quantities of essential oil that should be used in various amounts of carrier oil for massage.

ESSENTIAL OIL FORMULAS USED IN CHAPTERS 7 AND 8

All the blends used in this book are in the amounts one would expect to use for initial aromatherapy bodywork. However, there are those who may wish to use lower amounts of essential oil. This can be done simply and effectively by halving the number of drops in the blends while keeping to the correct proportions, and using the same amount of base oil specified. By using lower amounts of essential oils it is often the case that one must use the blend more often and for a longer period of time.

CHART 5.1: METHODS OF USE AND DOSAGE

METHOD	DOSAGE	
Bath	As directed or a maximum of 8 drops	Run the bath and then add the essential oil. Close the door so the vapour doesn't escape. Soak for at least ten minutes, relaxing and inhaling deeply through the nose. The essential oil can be diluted in a small amount of vegetable oil before being added to the bath. Unless otherwise indicated, certain essential oils should *not* be used in baths. They are: basil, cinnamon, clove, peppermint, thyme, ginger and eucalyptus piperita.
Shower	As directed or a maximum of 2 drops	Wash as usual. Then put the essential oil onto a wet wash-cloth or sponge and rub it over yourself briskly, still standing under the hot water, inhaling deeply through the nose.
Jacuzzi	3 drops per person	Same as for bath.

Sauna	2 drops per 600 ml water (approx 1 pint)	Only use eucalyptus, tea tree or pine as these three enter the body with inhalation. They are excellent cleansers and detoxifiers. Mix the oil with the water beforehand and put on heat source as usual.
Massage oil	As directed or a maximum of 1 drop to each ml base (vegetable) oil.

See chart at end of section for complete guide of amounts to use. | Add the essential oil to the base oil: use sweet almond, hazelnut, peach kernel, grape seed, soya, peanut, sunflower or safflower, etc. Mix in a clean, brown glass bottle – available from any chemist (the volume it contains should be imprinted on the base). If using more than one essential oil, blend those in the bottle before adding base oil. Blend essential oils into base oil by turning the bottle upside down a few times and rolling briskly between the hands. To ascertain how much to use for a body-massage, pour oil into cupped hand. The amount held there without pouring over the sides of the hand or into the finger creases is adequate. As hand size is relative to body size the amount used will vary. Generally, one dessertspoon should be sufficient. *If you have allergies* to soaps, perfumes or cosmetics, do a skin test twenty-four hours before using massage oil. |
| **Tissue or handkerchief** | 1 drop | Just inhale when required. |

Inhaled as vapour	2–3 drops	Pour hot water into a bowl and add the essential oil. Place your head over the bowl, about 10 inches away, and cover with a towel so the sides are completely closed. Eyes must be shut. Breathe deeply through nose for about one minute. Mainly used for medicinal purposes.
Water bowl	1–9 drops	Room method. Pour hot water into a small bowl, add essential oil. Make sure windows and doors are closed. Allow 5–10 minutes for aroma to permeate atmosphere; replenish if required, but the aroma should not be overpowering.
Diffusers	1–6 drops	Diffusers are especially designed for use with essential oils. They have a bowl section which is heated by candle flame or electricity. This bowl should be made of non-porous material so it can be wiped clean after use, ready to take a different aroma if required. Usually diffusers are made of pottery. Always put water in the bowl before adding the essential oil. Diffusers heat and release aroma molecules into the atmosphere. There is now a model which does not use a heat-source – of particular interest to those with children or pets. See suppliers for details.
Radiators	1–9 drops	Put the essential oil onto a cotton wool ball and lodge it either on the radiator or by the pipe.

Humidifiers	1–9 drops	Add the essential oil to the water.
Room sprays	4 or more drops per half-pint (280 ml) water	Use a new plant-sprayer. Put in warm (not boiling) water, add the essential oil and shake. Spray high in the air. Do not spray over polished wooden furniture or velvet – as you would avoid putting water on these or other vulnerable items.
Light bulbs	4–6 drops	You can buy specially designed rings – usually made of metal or pottery – which can sit on top of a lightbulb in a table-standing lamp. They have a hollow section which can take the essential oil. Always put the ring on the light bulb when it is turned off and cool. Take care not to spill the essential oil onto the attachment because essential oils are flammable (as well as wet).
Log fires	1 drop per log	Use pine, cypress, sandalwood or cedarwood essential oils. Put 1 drop on each log half an hour before using although the essential oil will still be effective if the log is used many weeks later. Three drops of essential oil per log fire is sufficient.
Silk and paper flowers	1 drop per flower	Simply put the essential oil onto the flowers and place in a vase. Some essential oils are colourless and have the texture of water, others have a slight colour and are more viscous so depending on which oil you use, and the

colour(s) of the flowers, place
the essential oil on a petal,
stamen or stem.

Pillows	1–3 drops per pillow or pillows	Some essential oils will leave a mark on pillows (and other cloth material) so, depending on the essential oil you use, place it directly onto the corner of a pillowcase or onto a cotton wool ball which can be placed in the corner between the pillow and pillowcase. Alternatively, the cotton wool ball can be tucked under the pillow.
Clothing	1–2 drops	Some essential oils are colourless and have the texture of water, others have a slight colour and are more viscous. Bear this in mind when choosing the oil to use by this method as it may damage material. The essential oil needs to be placed where its aroma can be appreciated. If it is put on the cuff, it can be smelled easily when required. If it is put on a collar, the aroma will rise to the nose over the course of the day (or evening).
Perfume		Essential oils can be used as a perfume. For the purposes outlined in this book, they can be diluted either in jojoba oil or vodka (alcohol). Use one third volume essential oil to two thirds *either* jojoba or vodka. If it's in vodka, it can be further diluted in 50 per cent water. The bottle can also simply be opened and sniffed from when required.

Jewellery		With the rise in interest in aromatherapy more manufacturers are producing neck pendants and even earrings in the shape of a little bottle – designed to hold perfume or essential oils. The bottle can be opened at any time and sniffed.
Lotions and creams	10–15 drops per 50 mls or grams	Essential oils can be added to pre-packaged lotions and creams or you can make up your own (see *The Fragrant Pharmacy*). If adding to a pre-packaged product, it must be perfume-free. Buy the simplest, purest product you can find. Pots: add the essential oil and stir. Bottles: empty the contents into a bowl, add the essential oil, mix and replace in the bottle.

Pregnant or Lactating Women
Such women should always use the minimum quantity of essential oil stated here, and reduce the number of essential oils used in formulae or blends by half. Please also see page 554 for the list of oils you should not use at all during pregnancy or while lactating.

CHART 5.2: BLENDING ESSENTIAL OILS WITH BASE OR CARRIER OILS – QUANTITIES TO USE

Number of drops of essential oils to use			Blend the number of essential oils on the left into the volume of base oil on the right.			
Essential Oils				**Vegetable Oil**		
MIN	to	MAX drops	Per ml.	teaspoon	dessertspoon	tablespoon
½	–	1	1	1	–	–
1	–	5	5	1	1	1
2	–	10	10	2	1	1
3	–	15	15	3	1	1
4	–	20	20	4	2	1
5	–	25	25	5	2	1
6	–	30	30	6	3	2

These are the minimum–maximum quantities that should be used, unless otherwise stated in blends mentioned elsewhere.

People on medication	For all methods use up to half the maximum recommended dosages. If you are using them as medicines inform your doctor. If using homeopathic medicines, inform your homeopath. It is thought that essential oil use may negate the effect of homeopathy.
Tranquillizer addiction	During addiction all essential oil dosages should be half the maximum general dosage.
Substance addiction	During addiction all essential oil dosages should be half the maximum general dosage.
Alcoholism	When using alcohol to excess all essential oil dosages should be half the maximum general dosage.
Chronic or long-term conditions	Use formulations at half the minimum to maximum strengths.

When buying essential oils it is useful to know how many drops there are in a bottle. These can only be approximations because droppers do vary slightly. Here is a guide:

1 ml essential oil =   20 drops
2 ml essential oil =   40 drops
5 ml essential oil = 100 drops
10 ml essential oil = 200 drops

Many of the expensive essential oils and absolutes are sold in 2.5 to 5 ml bottles.
Most essential oils are sold in 10 ml bottles.

Blending and Mixing

The very fact that you can smell the aroma of essential oils being used as a massage oil proves the point that they evaporate. Indeed, *most* of the essential oils being used will evaporate before they have a chance to penetrate the skin. For this reason it is wasteful to mix essential oils in an open bowl. The essential oils start to oxidize on contact with air so it is also wasteful to leave the bottle of essential oil open while treating yourself or others. These factors have been taken into consideration in the blends and volumes suggested in this book for home use and if you follow the guidelines above sufficient quantities will be absorbed.

How to make a diluted oil using more than one essential oil.

Collect the things you will be using: essential oils; empty bottle; and base (vegetable carrier) oil.

Drop the various essential oils into the empty bottle. Put the top back on and roll the bottle between your hands to thoroughly blend the essential oil molecules together.

Then add the base oil to just above the level of the bottle's 'shoulder'.

Put the top on the bottle and roll between the hands vigorously to thoroughly mix the essential oil and base oil together.

How to make a synergistic blend concentrate of essential oils.

Collect the things you will be using: essential oils; and small empty brown bottle.

Put the required number of essential oil drops into the empty bottle, starting with the more viscous essential oils first.

Put top on the bottle and roll well between your hands, to thoroughly blend the essential oil molecules together.

Turn bottle upside down.

Turn bottle right way up.

Using one essential oil in a massage oil.

Pour the base oil into your empty brown bottle so it reaches to the 'shoulder'.

Add the essential oil.

Put the top on the bottle and roll between the hands vigorously to thoroughly mix the essential oil and base oil together.

Chapter Six

HOW TO GET THROUGH LIFE IN ONE PIECE

SOMEONE SOMEWHERE ONCE SAID 'LIFE'S A BITCH AND THEN YOU die'! I'm not sure it's quite that bad, but it does have its moments. I think we can all agree that if you can get through it in one piece with your sanity intact, you're doing OK. In this chapter I shall discuss a few areas of particular stress in which essential oils can help: education, offices, industry, farming, plane and car travel, the police and prison services.

SCHOOLS AND COLLEGES

Essential oils can play several roles in helping us get through the education process – happily, confidently, efficiently and healthily. To a large extent, of course, just how well we perform within the education system depends on factors we can't control. If we come from a family of ten children and live in a small overcrowded flat, it's going to be more difficult to find the peace and quiet needed to study, and our parents will have less time to apportion to each of us when it comes to helping with homework. Essential oils can't do much about that. What they can do in a general sense is help us maintain good health so we don't have to take time off. If we catch 'flu and miss school for three weeks, that can be a setback from which it's difficult to recover. However, physical health is not the subject of this book and I have covered in another publication, *The Fragrant Pharmacy,* quite a bit that could be said on that subject. But the other factors too – happiness, confidence and efficiency – are certainly things with which essential oils can help.

Again, in a general sense, the mood we feel in when we arrive at school or college goes a long way to determining how we approach the material being supplied to us, and how we absorb it. In the next chapter there are many formulas and suggested essential oils which will help you to overcome the negativity that prevents us performing to our maximum potential. Included among these, for example, is enhanced confidence, which can help if you're on the receiving end of bullying, as it can help when you're sitting in a classroom of thirty people listening to every word you say, and every mistake you make.

Of course the main objective of education is to fill your head with as many facts as possible, in a way that you'll be able to remember them later – in an exam, or in the work situation. This is very much a matter of memory, an area in which essential oils are well known to be very helpful. It also depends on the teachers being in a frame of mind best suited for the communication of ideas. Essential oils used in the staff room can help here too. Then there is the larger environment, the buildings themselves, in which everyone has to operate for a large portion of the week. As we shall see, essential oils can have a beneficial effect on this in various ways, not least in the control of infections. If one person comes into the building with 'flu a week before exam time, with the domino effect, by the time the big day arrives half the school or college – both students and staff – could be out of action. Even during other times in the term, lost time still has to be made up – only putting more pressure on everyone concerned.

Memory Enhancement, Mental Clarity and Efficiency

As we saw in Chapter 2 in *The Sense of Smell*, when an aroma molecule hits the olfaction receptors on the cilia of the olfactory bulbs, they are actually connecting with a part of the brain. The olfactory bulbs are embedded in the 'limbic system', a part of the brain that deals with, among other things, memory. Usually we experience this connection *passively*, when an aroma reminds us of something that happened in the past. In aromatherapy we use this connection in an *active* way, by stimulating the memory to recall information we previously studied.

Basically, what happens is this: while you study, and your mind is absorbing information, you use a particular essential oil nearby – in a diffuser or on a tissue or hanky from which you can occasionally sniff. The information thus becomes associated with this particular aroma. When the exam comes along, you use that same aroma nearby – this time not in a diffuser, but again, on a tissue or handkerchief. You can discreetly sniff the aroma, an action which transports you back to the time when you were studying, and this helps your memory recall the information. There are several rules to follow in this process:

1) Try to use a fragrance you have never used before because an aroma used previously may have associations that probably have nothing to do with the subject being absorbed. Make a unique formula especially for each subject.

2) If possible use one fragrance (or formula) per subject, and then not too much.

3) Only inhale the aroma when you need to remember the studied information – in a test or exam for example, and not at other times. If you use it all the time, your memory will get confused. Be very precise about this.

4) Be discreet. There are no rules, as far as I know, forbidding the use of essential oils during exams, but it could be construed as an unfair advantage!

5) Do not rely solely on this method. The aroma-memory

connection is meant to be an additional aid, not a replacement for hard work. Don't just scan your textbooks expecting everything magically to go in. Sorry, it's not that easy. You'll have to put in the time and read your material thoroughly, and check with your tutors that you have understood it.

The memory has a horrible habit of slipping away. You can listen to a general knowledge quiz on TV, merrily shouting out the answers but, if you were actually in the studio, in front of TV cameras and glaring lights, aware that millions of people were watching, that same information you *know*, slips away. You go blank! Essential oils won't make you remember things you simply don't know, but they'll help you bridge the gap between knowledge and recall. This advantage can be the difference between pass and fail. As I have said, you can use any essential oil to do this but good choices, for example, would be basil, bergamot, lemon or rosemary – or a blend of two or more of these. Basil gives the mind tremendous clarity while bergamot is terrific for giving confidence. Rosemary is renowned for memory and lemon is great for concentration.

Years ago I heard a young man being interviewed on radio. He'd just passed fifteen 'O' levels in that school year – the highest number passed in Britain by one student. The interviewer asked him how he'd done it. Apparently, he'd put a tall pile of books and papers relating to all his homework on his right, on the desk, and took the first book off the pile, opened it, and worked at it until he got to the point where he couldn't continue. Without wasting time worrying about his inability to finish, he moved that book to the left of him. He then took the next book/papers and carried on with them until he got stuck, immediately putting them to the left, and so on. So he worked through the pile on the right, actually finishing a couple of homework projects, leaving him with the pile on the left. He moved the whole lot to the right, and continued the process again. By the time he'd gone through this process a few times, he was left with a couple of subjects he was truly stuck on and the next day he referred to the teachers for help. The point was, when he came to look at the sticky subjects, either on the second look, the third or fourth or fifth, his mind could approach them slightly differently – the 'lateral thinking' effect I suppose it would be called – and on these subsequent looks he could grasp the point, solve the problem, or whatever. When you're completely overburdened (as I have been myself on occasion) his advice comes in really handy. Try it.

The Staff Room

Trying to keep thirty and more children under control and actively engaged in useful activity is a really hard task, and I take my hat off to all those who do it. Using essential oils in the staff room should be directed at reducing the 'frazzled' element in the day by creating a little peaceful haven where teachers can relax and recharge their batteries. With the agreement of all those concerned, I suggest using the relaxing and calming essential oils in a diffuser. The relevant oils are listed in the main chart at the back of this book.

Also, because the staff room is an enclosed space, it is the perfect environment for the transmission of germs, especially those that cause coughs, colds and 'flu. Essential oils used in a diffuser can prevent infection spreading, if they are of the antibacterial and/or antiviral type. I would suggest using eucalyptus, rosemary, thyme, clove, cinnamon or, especially in times of major 'flu epidemic, a special mixture called 'Dermatect' (see *Suppliers* on page 558).

The School Buildings and Halls of Residence

In Japan large offices are using essential oils diffused throughout the building to enhance efficiency and create a relaxing environment. Different aromas are used at different times of the day to create different moods (see Chapter 4, *Aromapsychology*) and there's no reason why this principle shouldn't be applied to education facilities. For a stimulating effect, especially perhaps after lunch when everyone is feeling a bit deflated and needs a bit of a boost, I suggest using one of the citrus essential oils – lemon or grapefruit, lemon eucalyptus (*E citriodora*), or a light floral. These would not be irritating, and most children like them. The aroma should not be over-powering, but barely perceptible.

Leaving home for the first time to go to university or college can be stressful, if liberating. Everything is new – the place, the people, the home and the work. The temptations to go out every night and socialize are powerful, and while there is no harm in it, that's only so long as it doesn't blind you from the object of the exercise – study. Central to study is the ability to concentrate – to focus your mind – and essential oils are useful in this. What you can do is use one oil or a special blend of oils in your room at the halls of residence or in your digs, as an environmental cue to 'this is my study time'. Set the scene: arrange your desk and make your coffee and try to forget what happened at the pub last night, what dramas and gossip are still cluttering up your brain, and then light your diffuser, or arrange whatever room method you're going to use, add the essential oils and say to yourself 'now I'm going to concentrate on this' – and do it! Having an aroma around can focus your mind on the task in hand – pull you in, as it were.

OFFICES

Offices are more stressed out than they ever were, with the threat of redundancy hanging over everyone and the new technology buzzing away all day. As we all know, work-related stress is a major problem for this country, as for others, and the number of days lost through it costs every large company a small for-tune. Some of the more forward-thinking companies employ in-house aromatherapists who give treatments to stressed-out executives and other favoured personnel. When an executive is earning a small fortune a year, you can see the financial logic in doing what you can to make sure he or she is actually sitting behind their desk every day, and not lying in bed suffering from stress-related disorders. However, there is no joy in anyone being ill, and no advantage in it as companies more and more keep a tight check on the number of days taken off for illness. Being ill these days can easily lose you your job. It makes sense then, all round, to employ the benefits of essential oils in the work place.

The crucial thing to bear in mind about essential oils is that people have different reactions to aromas. Because of the memory connection, someone might have a negative association with one particular aroma, for a multitude of reasons, and you have no way of knowing which aromas may cause a bad reaction, and to whom. For this reason, if you share an office, you must get the agreement of all concerned before putting a diffuser on your desk which will, of course, let the aroma into an area extending beyond the confines of your desk. Bring several aromas into the office for everyone to sniff before actually using them in the shared space. As there are so many essential oils to choose from, it should be easy to find something that suits everyone and still does something positive for you. If you have your own office, obviously you can use whichever oil you like.

Which particular oils you use rather depends on the situation. If there's a bad 'flu doing the rounds then use something which is antiviral and protective. If you are under constant pressure, use something relaxing, and if you've got a rush job on, use something stimulating. As we have already seen in the chapter entitled *Aroma-psychology*, essential oils have been shown to reduce keyboard errors significantly. You will find information as to which oils to use in chapters 7 and 8 and also in Charts 11.1 and 11.2, but you may consider grapefruit or eucalyptus lemon (*E citriodora*) to combat lethargy, and basil, cardamon or bergamot to help concentration. Stale air is another problem in offices, and I'd suggest any of the following to combat this: lemon, lavender, rosemary, grapefruit, eucalyptus lemon or cypress.

If you work in sales, you should really be aware of the recent work into the effect of aroma on clients, as discussed in *Retail Outlets* in Chapter 4, *Aroma-psychology*. As researcher Dr Hirsch says, 'odorants are potentially more efficacious than any other modality in increasing sales ability of consumer products'. The thing about aroma is that it's subtle – it can work on the subconscious – and people can be favourably impressed without even knowing why. This dynamic can be used in all sorts of ways. Essential oils can be diffused through the atmosphere when you show clients your latest products

Basil

and they can be used to infuse brochures and other paperwork with an aromatic impact. Light florals have been shown to be particularly effective.

INDUSTRY

All the problems and solutions discussed above are relevant for industry in general, and as time goes on, with everyone looking for things to give them the market edge, aroma is being used more and more. The process known as 'micro-encapsulation', best known for the 'scratch and sniff' perfume samples we find in our magazines, is shortly going to arrive on supermarket shelves. Your bleach container will be micro-encapsulated with the aroma of the bleach inside, and released when you pick up the product from the shelf and squeeze that area with your hand. In five years time we'll probably be able to walk into huge supermarkets and find the toiletries department or the coffee shelf simply by following our noses – there's going to be a major aromatic experience in-store!

Aromatherapy works in a different way. It's not about informing you of the aroma inside a bottle before you open the top, it's about convincing the customer, subliminally, that your product is best, and your product doesn't have to have any aroma whatsoever – although, as Dr Hirsch showed in Chicago, if it does, it's more likely to sell, and at a higher price!

Companies spend a fortune sending out catalogues and promotional literature – and much of it ends up in the bin, so anything you can do to make sales literature more appealing has got to be a help. It's been shown in various trials that people will linger longer when there is a pleasant aroma in the atmosphere so if there's a pleasant aroma on your paperwork it stands a better chance of lingering on your potential customer's desk! Essential oils can do better than this, however. Certain essential oils instil confidence. Now think of the possibilities. The client gets your brochure and for some reason unbeknown to them, feels compelled to keep it out on the desk; and for some reason (unbeknown to them) they feel confident when they pick it up. 'Let's use this company,' they say, 'I have a good feeling about it' . . . and you're halfway there!

To make brochures and other paperwork aromatic, simply drop some essential oil on the cardboard box in which they're packed, then wrap the box in a black plastic bin liner for at least twenty-four hours. Keep it closed, of course. The aroma will permeate the box and, eventually, the papers inside. Although the aroma may seem hardly perceptible, especially when it has been through the postal system, remember that aroma works subliminally – it doesn't *have* to be perceptible. As an experiment, aromatize one box of catalogues and keep another un-aromatized box for a control. It's no good using a floral essential oil if your firm doesn't want to project a feminine image so choose something that reflects confidence and prosperity. In this case I'd suggest using cardamon, petitgrain, coriander, lemon or bergamot. When you send both boxes of brochures out keep a record of which potential customers each type of brochure was sent to, and see which brochure – aromatic or not – produces the most enquiries. What have you got to lose? I'll tell you – sales!

In the future I'm sure we're going to see aroma used in many more subtle ways. Already in America, fragrance houses produce 'corporate aromas' for clients who use it in their customer waiting rooms and on their paperwork. If, let's say, there is an element of lemon in that corporate aroma, each time a customer smells lemon (in other contexts) they will be reminded of the company. Now that's clever. If you can get your potential customers to think about you when they're cooking dinner, out at a restaurant, walking through a market or washing their hands with a lemon-scented bar of soap, you are really in their mind – where you want to be!

Smart corporations have already grasped the fact that aroma can be diffused into their offices to make their workers relax when they come in at nine in the morning after struggling through the rush-hour, or perk up after lunch. Errors on keyboards are reduced with aroma, customers are relaxed, sales staff made more confident, and illness is reduced by pumping anti-microbial essential oils into the air conditioning system. All this is happening now throughout the world. Factory floors may seem difficult to aromatize in this way because the floor areas are usually so large, and the ceilings so high. However, there are commercial diffuser systems which can get around these problems and workers on factory floors can also reap the benefits of essential oils. Some factory jobs are very tedious and if you drift off to sleep after lunch while on an assembly line, you could lose your hand, as well as your job. Accidents at work are often caused by a moment's loss of concentration and anything that can be done to reduce them has got to be a good thing.

FARMING

The growing interest in aromatherapy is creating a greater demand for essential oils but meanwhile farmers in Europe are being paid subsidies by the European Community (EC) to let their fields lie idle. It doesn't make sense. British growing conditions are ideal for certain species of plants from which essential oils are distilled including chamomile roman, lavender, clary-sage, sage, rosemary, peppermint, spearmint, rose, melissa, marjoram and thyme. We also need base oils, which are extracted from borage and evening primrose, just for example. Some of these plants grow so fast one would hardly have to do much to propagate them – such as melissa and borage – while others are easily propagated from cuttings, such as lavender and rosemary. The seeds of some species, such as chamomile roman, are harvested simply by putting bags over the flower heads at the right time of year.

The growing demand now is for oils distilled from organically grown plants, and if farmers turned their attention to this method of farming, I'm sure they could easily find a market. Indeed, it would help all of us if farmers approached essential oil distributors directly and asked if they'd like to lease their fields for this use, with the farmers doing the work required. It would cut out the middlemen and reduce prices, give the essential oil company a guaranteed source of supply and the farmers a guaranteed buyer. As I have previously discussed in *The Fragrant Pharmacy* the system of inter-cropping known as companion gardening can easily be applied to essential oil production and it does away with the need for biocides – pesticides, herbicides and fungicides – which just destroy the environment. It can't be very pleasant being a farmer when you're obliged to use these products because the food-seed companies (which are nowadays owned by chemical companies) engineer food plants so they *require* certain chemicals (which are supplied, of course, by the chemical companies!).

Essential oil production is a very environmentally friendly occupation. Not only is there no need to use biocides, the unrequired and dried part of the plant can be used to fuel the fire in the still. The ashes can go back onto the land, as fertilizer. Stills in Egypt are cleaned using dried basil, followed by lots of water, and that basil is also grown on the land – again, no need to buy expensive, environmentally unfriendly, chemical cleaning solutions. In many parts of the world farmers club together and buy

a still as a co-operative. They share it, so the initial financial out-
lay is not too great. All in all, essential oil production is a very
viable alternative to the production of foodstuffs at times when
the market doesn't require them. Plus, the farmers would be producing something which does everyone so much good.

PLANES AND CAR TRAVEL

If you travel in Virgin Airways 'Upper Class' you can stop off
at the 'Club House' at Heathrow Airport and get an aromatherapy treatment. On selected flights they also provide 'Upper
Class' passengers with in-flight beauty therapists who can give
an aromatherapy neck and scalp massage, as well as a mani-
cure. They're also looking into the possibility of providing
essential-oil impregnated pillows which, on request, can be
given to those who'd like to have a sleep, helped along by the
relaxing properties of the chosen essential oils. Next time you
detect a delicious aroma coming from the Upper Class section,
you'll know how the other half lives! Passengers in 'First
Class' or 'Club Class' on British Airways flights, meanwhile,
are given, along with other goodies, miniature aromatherapy
products – rehydration face and hand gel and rose-water face
spray. Aromatherapy has clearly taken off!

Flying is a very stressful experience for some people – so
much so that they simply won't do it. This is a major nuisance
if you dream of going to visit relatives in Australia. Airlines
fully appreciate this and would, if it were practicable, diffuse
relaxing essential oils into the atmosphere – they are certainly
aware of their potential – but the problem is that each person
has a unique reaction to aromas and there is no way of anticipating which aroma might bring back unpleasant memories for
one or more passengers. On an individual basis, however, the
stress and anxiety related to air travel can be alleviated by having a relaxing essential oil bath or shower before leaving for
the airport, and taking with you a tissue or handkerchief which
can be taken from your pocket and inhaled when required. I
would suggest you use one of the following oils singly or in a
combination of your choice: marjoram, lavender, clary-sage,

bergamot, ormenis flower (chamomile maroc), chamomile roman, nutmeg or the more expensive linden blossom. Although by all means use any essential oil or combination that you have found relaxing previously. I find the combination of clary-sage, marjoram and lavender particularly effective. Bear in mind though that you are in an enclosed space with other people so don't wave your hanky around the place. Just keep it in your pocket and take it out and hold it to your nose as and when required.

When travelling by car, as a driver or passenger, you definitely don't want to use essential oils that are going to make you feel relaxed – and make the driver fall asleep at the wheel. Avoid lavender essential oil and other relaxing oils which could slow down reactions. Yet driving is a stressful experience, especially in traffic jams, and there are essential oils that can help deal with this while, at the same time, keeping you alert. The only essential oils that should be used in cars are peppermint, lemon, lime, grapefruit, cypress, bergamot, juniper, rosemary, petitgrain, eucalyptus lemon (*E citriodora*) and eucalyptus peppermint (*E piperata*).

THE POLICE AND PRISONS

Nobody goes into police stations or prisons for fun. Police stations are places you go to when you've been robbed, raped or mugged, and if you go to a prison it's because you or somebody you know has (allegedly) been naughty. To say they are stressful environments would be an understatement, perhaps especially for the people who have to work in them day after day. In Essex the police are regular clients of aromatherapists, who try to relieve the stress associated with being on alert all day and having to deal with some very nasty characters. Indeed, the police forces need to have special counsellors to help police officers come to terms with some of the unpleasant experiences they go through in their job which, in point of fact, puts them in life-threatening situations on a regular basis. When you're a police officer, the unexpected is to be expected and if you don't keep your wits about you, you could easily end up dead. On top of that, you have an enormous amount of paperwork to deal with! Stressful? Yes!

I know of at least one police counsellor who has trained as an aromatherapist, who gives officers massages as they recount the dramas of their day. I hope in the future there will be more trained aromatherapists within the police service. Macho police officers certainly don't have to worry about aromatherapy being a cissie namby-pamby treatment – I can assure them that there are some very macho, successful businessmen who have regular aromatherapy treatments to alleviate their different kind of stress – like doing deals which could make them a million or lose them a million. Keeping your nerve can take several forms!

Precisely because police stations are stressful environments, they would be ideal candidates for the benefits of essential oils. Lavender would be inappropriate in police personnel areas because officers need to be alert, but lemon or grapefruit would take the edge off things when a whole pile of paperwork is looming after a hard night on the beat. The waiting room, on the other hand, where distressed victims of crime wait to be seen would be far more pleasant environments if anxiety-relieving essential oils were gently diffused in the atmosphere. You could try lavender, bergamot, geranium or clary sage. These same oils could be used in interview rooms where victims must recount their unpleasant experiences, sometimes for hours on end. This gruesome procedure, on top of the crime itself, is a tortuous nightmare, often carried out when the victim is extremely tired, both physically and emotionally, and I know if it were me, I'd find the essential oils a tremendous help.

There was, unfortunately, a time not so long ago when rape victims were made to feel as though they were the guilty party – by the police as well as by the courts and society at large. These days police authorities make an effort to make the victim feel more relaxed, even to the extent of creating less institutional environments in which the victim will be seen by the doctor, be interviewed and counselled. Because the day a woman is raped will probably be the most traumatic and terrifying day of her life, it is extremely important to take a sensitive approach to the use of essential oils. The woman *must* be given a choice in the matter. For one thing, by using a particular essential oil, no matter how relaxing she may find it at the time, it may in the future be associated with this horrific event. Some women may prefer to go through the interview and counselling procedure without essential oils being diffused in the atmosphere for the simple reason that they don't want the aroma to become negatively associated. Yet essential oils can help alleviate stress, give courage and, moreover, give a gentle air of femininity and humanity to what is an otherwise crudely masculinist and inhuman experience. Therefore, if essential oils are to be used in a rape counselling environment, they must be placed openly where the woman can see them, she must be given a choice of oils and, above all, the choice of whether she wants them used at all. When I acted as a victim supporter on one occasion we used essential oils that helped the victim be open and expressive about the experience. She found this invaluable, especially in the long term.

As for the criminals, there are no essential oils which will make them spill the beans, although research is currently being carried out into aromas that can break down resistance. The police cells, however, are another matter. The enclosed space is enough to drive anyone to distraction and, even though belts and shoelaces are taken away, people do hang themselves or somehow kill themselves in there. Others just scream and shout all night or throw themselves against the wall – all of which helps no-one. An essential oil like lavender, gently diffused in this environment, would help to keep everyone calm and quiet.

Essential oils used in prisons to keep prisoners calm and less violent seems a better option than giving them drugs. What essential oils do is give a positive attitude. They don't just numb, they bring out the best in people. Anyone who is in prison needs all the positivity they can get, to get through the experience and consider their future role in life. British prisons are today overcrowded not only with lawbreakers but with people who have been released from mental institutions and, basically, have nowhere to go. Any prison doctor will tell you they are their most serious problem. Those who are in charge of our prisons should seriously consider (aside from relocating those who really shouldn't be there) using essential oils to diffuse this situation. They could start with prisons for women because the prisoners, being female, will have less resistance to essential oils – which may be perceived by some men as 'feminine'.

Chapter Seven

EMOTIONAL HEALING

'A journey of a thousand miles
must begin with a single step.'

LAO TSE
Chinese Proverb

INTRODUCTION

THE BRAIN DRIVES EVERYTHING: EVERY WORD IS PROJECTED
from it, every mood emanates from it, and every feeling
passes through the brain at some point. But the brain and body
are one, they work together all the time, part of the same
system. The brain says 'get up' and the legs swing out of bed.
But, also, as discussed in Chapter 3, *The Modern Mind*, there
are receptors throughout the body which are directly connected with chemicals we also find in the brain. It is no longer
possible to discuss neurology, immunology and endocrinology
as three different fields because they are all related, like bits of
a telephone system. You can't have one without the other.
Psychoneuroimmunologists are now telling us that, scientifically,

body and brain are one and the same.

What happens in the brain decides whether you're going to be happy or sad; it decides whether or not life is worth living. But we are very passive about the brain, we don't pay much attention to our emotions until something goes wrong. We don't take our brain to the emotional gym for a work-out, like we exercise our body to feel fit and stay well. But, with a strong mind, we can do anything, even cure disease in our own body, and with a weak mind, we can't do a thing. Some people do, of course, control their brain, or at least attend to its well-being: meditation, yoga and tai chi are just three practices which are carried out by millions of people each day around the world. And no doubt it has a beneficial effect on the emotions of them all. Other people go to counselling or therapy of some sort, and clearly this is extremely helpful to many people. Essential oils have a different approach (that is clearly complementary to the others), which is to help a person obtain emotional equilibrium – which allows the happiness and joy, our birthright, to come out. Essential oils are facilitators, balancers and, at the risk of sounding poetic, drops of pure positivity. They can put the sparkle back into life.

Essential oils are a chest of goodies you can dip into at any time. Got a tough interview ahead? – just put a drop of bergamot on a tissue and take a deep sniff before you go in. Feeling really vulnerable but got to get through the day as usual? – sniff some rose otto – it will help. Just want to feel bright and on top of it today? – have a grapefruit shower. The variety of essential oils are there to dip into, for a variety of different emotions and feelings, a rich treasury courtesy of mother nature.

This chapter explains how essential oils can help us keep in tip-top emotional condition, under the headings *Alertness, Assertiveness, Concentration, Confidence, Contentment, Creativity, Focus, Happiness, Joy, Memory Enhancement*, etc. Then comes a much larger chapter, concerned with the negative emotions which exist in this world, *The A–Z of Emotional Problems*. Under 'A', for example, you'll find *Abuse, Addictions, Aggression, Amnesia, Anger, Anxiety* and *Apathy*. There are so many entries under this negative emotion section because there are so many problems out there in the world, and at home. And, as we need all the help we can get, in Chapter 9 I briefly discuss *Auto-Genic Training, Breathing, Massage, Meditation,* and *Relaxation and Visualization.*

In an ideal world, happiness would be the norm. We'd all go around smiling. As it is, we sit on an underground train each morning with our heads hung low, like everyone else! There is so much to worry about. Rapists stalk the streets; jobs can go; people get ill; and war is ubiquitous. And here comes the post-man with another bill in his hand. How is one supposed to find happiness in all this? Ironically, it is those who have been through a near-death experience who usually have the answer to this question, and we read their stories in magazines and newspapers every day. For example, there's the man who had a heart attack and realized he was wasting time taking an antagonistic approach to people close to him. He realized he loved them, and that they were more important than his job. From that moment he lived life to the full; before he was walk-ing around saying 'How is one supposed to find the happiness in all this?' Now he knew, you look to your loved ones, and treat them right. That is happiness.

Love is the most important formula we have for solving problems – it dissolves them away like mist in the sun. Love is an energy that radiates from every person, young and old, and lifts the darkness. It is instinctive, the blossoming flower with-in, the opener of hearts, the bringer of joy. The vibration of love is the greatest gift we can bring to this life, if we contribute a good share of that, our life has purpose. Ideally, none of us would be emotionally damaged in our youth, and our hearts would be open to love – love of our neighbour as well as our family and friends. But it is not an ideal world and many of us arrive in it damaged in some way. Essential oils can help a person recog-nize and repair this damage, allowing the love to recover, and strengthen the soul.

The problem with love, of course, is that it opens us up to emotional pain. To love is to hurt. Children are hurt by the parents they love; and children hurt parents in return. Lovers hurt each other, with a careless word or more. We are all vulnerable to emotional pain and sometimes we hurt. That is unfortunate, but our pain is not unique, it is a part of the human heritage, something we know and, to a certain extent, something essential oils can help deal with. They can assist us as we repair the damage, and get us back on our feet. Their job is not to numb, but to put us back into our feeling selves. Being alive *is* to feel – to feel sad watching a sad movie, or feel a rush of adrenalin with fear. These are the feelings of life, they are to be expected now and again. But to be overcome with a negative feeling a lot of the time, this is not good.

We seem to have got in a mind-set which says 'being miserable is normal, life is so hard, if only I had this-or-that I'd be happy'. Happiness is like the butterfly we never quite catch. But being happy is normal – it's normal to babies and children, and normal to many poor people, and rich people, around the world. What is it exactly that stops us, too, being happy? I don't think it is the number and severity of life's knocks that makes the difference, from my experience of people, rather the attitude they take towards life. Those who realize that life is short and precious, see the good things in life – of which there are many. Each day people set off to do voluntary work for people less well off than themselves, in terms of money, physical health, or whatever. Each day people pull out their cheque books and send money to charity. We all do each other 'favours' all the time. If we can see this as the norm – people being kind, people showing love, life going on, then the bad episodes can be put in perspective – small windows in the long wall of happy normality.

It does sometimes seem indulgent to think about oneself and do something for oneself, and it might seem altogether easier to use essential oils, for example, to help make a friend feel better. Ourselves, we forget. But we deserve attention too. The fact is, we are born alone and will die alone, and must take care of ourselves in between. Only we can find the purpose of our lives; only we can make sense of it. We have the right to deal with problems in our own way. If that involves sitting on a sofa for three weeks, hugging a cushion and crying, so be it. If that involves three weeks of cleaning the house from top to bottom, so be it. Just be yourself, and you will be beautiful. Indulge yourself, be good to yourself . . . it is not a crime! You could say it's your *responsibility* to make yourself happy, because when you're happy, those around you are too.

It helps to have a philosophy of life, and some people have religion. But anyone can have a reverence for the beauty of nature – the design of a flower, the call of the birds, the wind in the trees, or the moving shadows of clouds on a hill. How magnificent it all is, there, a constant reminder of the beauty in life. And nature is full of surprises, and lessons too. I remember one day driving in Europe – a long and tiring haul towards a destination and meeting I didn't want to reach – fed up, when I saw a huge, perfect rainbow ending right there, in the grass between the road and a wood. I pulled the car over and leapt out, looking up at the huge miracle reaching across the sky above me. It was so close and real I could jump into it, I thought, and did. But the rainbow moved away, again and again, and then I realized that rewards are not the goal – if one seeks the ulti-mate, it will elude you. The reward is life itself, in its richness, in its sadness and joy. Humbled, but happier, I continued my journey and did what I had to do.

All experience is good because that is the truth, the reality of our life. We must embrace it and make it work for us, trans-mutate the bad experiences into lessons for the future, wisdom for our soul, compassion for others, and understanding for the world. Good experiences are the icing on the cake, the bit that makes life sweet. But it is all real, and there is purpose in it all, even if we cannot see it now.

If we could expect nothing more than to be happy, we would be happy. But we expect too much. Some of the happiest people I know have nothing, or have lived and worked among people who have nothing. Every small thing then becomes a gift, not an expectation. Let us stop and thank our lucky stars for what we do have, for the people we love (and tell them), for our humble home, our memories. We can't expect to go through the hurdle race of life without getting a few knocks – that's what it's about. All we can do is appreciate the people around us, be kind to them and ourselves, and hang on tight during the rough patches. Essential oils appreciate the drama of life – they have been there, so to speak, they are part of it. We're all in this together, and essential oils are there to help.

It is our birthright to be spontaneous, joyful, confident, loving, trusting and free – free in mind and spirit, free to soar and create and laugh. And it is our human responsibility to be compassionate, sympathetic and aware. Deep inside us, there is a spiritual connection which we can find if we just stand still long enough, quietly absorbed. That spiritual connection is the reference point we should take as 'normality', that quiet, re-assuring wholeness, more soothing than mother's breast. If this could be our normality, rather than 'depressed', 'anxious' or 'stressed', how much happier our lives would be. It is not a question of how many knocks one has because those who have had more than anyone, are often the first to say that the knocks are not what's important – the good is what we should focus on.

The mind comes with certain gifts – like intuition. Our in-tuition says of someone 'not aura friendly' – so we keep away, to protect ourselves. Our mind gives us individuality, to approach things our own unique way. That is good. By con-trast, co-dependency, relying on others for gratification, a form of vicarious living, is a bit of a cop-out, like hitching a lift through life on the back of somebody else's lorry. Patience is a gift we often ignore and even feel contempt for, calling it passivity. But impatience causes frustration and anger. Patience is the better quality, along with positivity, hope, enthusiasm and the capacity for enjoyment. These are the gifts within us that essential oils seek to bring out, philosoph-ically, deeply, naturally. And, by seeking a solution to our problems, we show our awareness – that we are alive and kicking, confident and optimistic.

POSITIVE MIND, MOOD AND EMOTION

Alertness

Twenty thousand years ago, being alert was the difference between life and death. You couldn't wander around the country-side ignoring the sound of a twig cracking behind the bush (an animal about to charge) or the sight of a plant crushed on the ground ahead (potential dinner nearby). Well you could, but you might not have lasted very long or had much to eat. Being alert is a survival mechanism, now as ever. Women walk down the street late at night acutely aware of the footsteps behind them, and alert to shadows in the alley up ahead. Drivers are alert to the vehicles in front and behind and mothers are alert to their children's movements in the playground. We are all alert, to greater or lesser degree, because our life or someone else's life might depend on it. Also, our future and job might depend on it and managers make sure they're alert in meetings while students must be alert to what the tutor says if they want to stay on the course. Certain jobs require more alertness than others. If a pilot, air-traffic controller or train-driver is not alert, just for a minute, a major disaster can result.

Being alert is more than vigilance and attention, like soldiers on guard. It's about mental responsiveness, being alive in the head. Alertness extends beyond our physical surroundings, it's about being alive to the people around us too. Can we hear the twig breaking and can we sense what people are feel-

ESSENTIAL OILS THAT HELP TO BRING ABOUT ALERTNESS

Basil, Black Pepper, Cardamon, Coriander, Cinnamon, Juniper, Petitgrain, Thyme Linalol, Eucalyptus, Peppermint, Rosemary, Pine, Grapefruit, Bergamot, Lime

ing? Alertness is not just about staying alive, it's about *being* alive – on the ball, in the game, sensitive.

See methods of use Chart 5.1 for oils which should not be used in baths. The following two blends can each be diluted into 30 ml base oil and made into stimulating massage oils, or made up into a synergistic blend using these proportions and use 1 to 3 drops in inhalations, or 8 drops in one of the room methods. Blend 1 can be used in baths – 5 drops.

ALERTNESS 1 BLEND 1		ALERTNESS 2 BLEND 2	
Juniper	14 drops	Grapefruit	10 drops
Pine	8 drops	Lime	10 drops
Rosemary	8 drops	Black Pepper	5 drops
		Peppermint	5 drops

The following blend is for use in diffusers only. Again, it is stimulating, and helps make one alert:

DIFFUSER BLEND – ALERTNESS	
Eucalyptus citriodora	15 drops
Peppermint	5 drops
Basil	5 drops

Assertiveness

I once overheard someone in hospital say, 'The trouble with being ill is I'm not my usual assertive self. I can't seem to get the staff to tell me anything and I'm fobbed off all the time.' This happens to sick people a lot, in and out of hospital, because they're so busy fighting the illness there's nothing left over to fight for their rights. Assertiveness is all about not being afraid to ask for what you want, or feel is rightfully yours. It's about doing what you feel instinctively should be done, whatever anyone else says; and it's about defending your right to be who you are, not what someone else wants you to be. Assertiveness is about defending your integrity and, at times, maintaining your sense of who you actually are.

Assertive people get what they want. They stand their ground when they've been given shoddy service, and get recompensed by the manager they insist on seeing; and they're not frightened to ask the man or woman of their dreams out for a date, and may find true love. In women assertiveness is often mistaken for aggression, but these are two entirely different things.

Essential oils are wonderful in the way they work to bring out assertiveness, and I really don't know how they do it – but they do! Over the years I've seen countless people coming to their first aromatherapy treatment all meek and mild, but blossoming into frank and open, assertive people after several sessions. One particularly unforgettable case was an elderly lady who'd been under the thumb of her family for years, who wouldn't say 'boo' to a goose but who, after a few months of aromatherapy found herself walking into a friend's house, straight over to the fruit bowl, from which she picked up a peach and promptly bit into it. At this point she 'woke up' and realized what a cheeky thing she'd done, unimaginable a few months ago – and the elderly lady and her friend had a good laugh over it.

All the following oils have been used successfully to bring out the assertiveness in people. Choose individual oils from the list, or combinations from the list to suit your choice, or try one of the blends below. They can be used in a bath, massage oil, diffusers or other room methods, in the steam inhalation method or inhaled from a tissue. The change will not happen overnight, and will take about two weeks of regular use. You may not recognize the change yourself until someone says to you 'Oh, I liked the way you handled that, what's come over *you*?'

ESSENTIAL OILS FOR ASSERTION

Sweet Fennel, Basil, Jasmine, Cedarwood, Cypress, Frankincense, Ginger, Patchouli, Ylang Ylang, Black Pepper, Ormenis Flower, Bergamot, Coriander, Carnation, Tuberose, Pimento Berry, Lime, Cardamon, Cistus, Litsea Cubeba

Basil and ginger should not be used in baths. For the blend overleaf, use these quantities each diluted with 30 ml base oil for a massage oil, or make a synergistic blend using these proportions. See Chart 5.1 for quantities to use and methods.

ASSERTIVE BLEND 1		ASSERTIVE BLEND 2	
Cistus	2 drops	Patchouli	10 drops
Litsea Cubeba	10 drops	Frankincense	10 drops
Jasmine	6 drops	Bergamot	10 drops

ASSERTIVE BLEND 3	
Cedarwood	15 drops
Cypress	5 drops
Lime	10 drops

Concentration

There's a lot to be said for concentration. It certainly helps to get jobs done more efficiently, and it's more fun doing them too. There's nothing worse than a stream of interruptions when writing, for example, and I'm sure a mechanic banging away under a car bonnet needs to be able to concentrate just as much. Lives may depend on it. But people have different requirements for concentration – some can do it with a radio in the background, and teenagers seem *only* to be able to do it with the volume turned up high! It is difficult to concentrate when children are running around demanding things, but I've seen women concentrating on complicated lace work at the same time as giving instructions to half a dozen kids.

Others have immense difficulty finding the quiet to concentrate. One writer friend was plagued by roadworks outside her window and then a guinea fowl settled in a large tree in the garden and started squawking from five o'clock in the morning. Concentration was difficult to achieve. The phone rings; the doorbell goes; so many distractions – programmes we *must* watch on TV and phone calls we must make. Finding the time to concentrate is difficult and jobs are often rushed. What we've learned to do is concentrate on several things at once. I knew a woman, for example, a mother of four, who wrote TV screenplays, who could hold a conversation, accurately scan the credits on the TV screen after a show, read the paper – and tell you stories from it, *and* paint her nails . . . all at the same time.

Lemongrass

Whatever it is you do, it helps to be able to concentrate – to cut outside interference and direct your mental energy to the subject in question. The job is done better, and gives a greater sense of satisfaction. It's also much easier to organize life when you can concentrate on a job long enough to get it done. Concentration helps towards clarity of thought, which is a marvellous thing.

Essential oils have been well documented for their ability to enhance powers of concentration. They can be inhaled from a tissue, gently diffused throughout the room, perhaps during work or meditation. They can also be used in the bath, which is a good time to concentrate on oneself. To help overall concentration, use the essential oils in a massage oil. There are many approaches to take. Also, aside from the oils listed below, people find certain other essential oils help their concentration, for example jasmine and rose are great for getting the mind to concentrate on romance. (See *Fragrant Sensuality*.[1]) For concentrating on efficiency, better choices would be lemon, basil, litsea cubeba or frankincense.

ESSENTIAL OILS FOR CONCENTRATION

Lemon, Basil, Lemongrass, Litsea Cubeba, Cardamon, Bergamot, Orange, Cedarwood, Rosemary, Eucalyptus Radiata, Peppermint

The following can be used in all the usual ways except basil and peppermint should not be used in baths. See Chart 5.1 for quantities to use and methods.

CONCENTRATION BLEND 1		CONCENTRATION BLEND 2	
Lemon	*20 drops*	*Litsea Cubeba*	*10 drops*
Basil	*6 drops*	*Cardamon*	*10 drops*
Rosemary	*2 drops*	*Lemon*	*10 drops*
Peppermint	*2 drops*		

ESSENTIAL OILS FOR SPIRITUAL CONCENTRATION

Frankincense, Neroli, Chamomile Roman, Rose Otto, Narcissus, Hyacinth

Confidence

Self-confidence makes us sure of ourselves, unafraid to walk tall, go anywhere or do anything, feeling free. Confidence means you don't let opportunities pass you by, and generally make the best of what life has to offer. Confidence is attractive, and we all know it when we see a confident person walk into the room. They have an air about them that says 'take me or leave me as I am'. Being confident gets us the job, and makes us bold enough to buy that fabulous dress the less confident woman wouldn't dare splash out on. In some sense, to have confidence is to allow us to enjoy life to the full.

Essential oils can't do it all for you, but they can certainly boost confidence, a fact established by countless people who have had aromatherapy treatments over the years. From the list choose an essential oil that you feel akin to when you breathe it in deeply through the nose. You will feel something emotionally, and if that feeling is negative, don't use that particular oil because it won't work. The oil you choose should make you feel good, and you should like it. Essential oils work on confidence by relieving the fear, stress and nervous tension that often prevents us from doing things.

ESSENTIAL OILS FOR CONFIDENCE

Cedarwood, Cypress, Linden Blossom, Cardamon, Sweet Fennel, Ginger, Bergamot, Grapefruit, Jasmine, Pine, Rosemary, Orange, Coriander

In the blends below, add the quantities in each to 30 ml base oil, to make a massage oil, or use these proportions to make a synergistic blend of oils, which can be used in baths, inhaled direct from a tissue, or diffused in the room. See Chart 5.1 for quantities to use.

CONFIDENCE BLEND 1		CONFIDENCE BLEND 2	
Orange	*10 drops*	*Grapefruit*	*10 drops*
Cedarwood	*5 drops*	*Orange*	*10 drops*
Ginger	*5 drops*	*Bergamot*	*5 drops*
Jasmine	*6 drops*		

CONFIDENCE BLEND 3		CONFIDENCE BLEND 4	
Cedarwood	*10 drops*	*Rosemary*	*20 drops*
Cypress	*12 drops*	*Sweet Fennel*	*10 drops*
Pine	*8 drops*		

CONFIDENCE BLEND 5		CONFIDENCE BLEND 6	
Cardamon	*5 drops*	*In 30 ml base oil use 15 drops*	
Ginger	*15 drops*	*of either Jasmine or*	
Coriander	*10 drops*	*Linden Blossom*	

Contentment

When people are asked what they want out of life one of the things high up on the list is 'contentment'. For some reason, contentment conjures up images of animals – the cat that got the cream lounging in front of the open fire, a big dog sitting at your feet. We might feel content after a good meal, especially if we prepared it. Contentment isn't being complacent, it's about being satisfied with your life, or with a job well done – whether finishing the ironing, tidying up the tool shed or mowing the lawn.

Few people go through an entire day feeling content, and some might say that would be boring anyway because a whole range of other feelings would be missed out. But there has to be some kind of balance. Consider the extreme – the discontented soul, dissatisfied with everything and everybody, who dismisses contentment as an impossibility. Some people don't want to believe they can be content, and may have unreal ideals or expectations. To them I say look at your life and name one small area with which you could say you feel content, love of music say, and build on that, extend your contentments one by one.

Don't expect essential oils to do your inner work for you, but they can help by reducing the tenseness that discontented people feel, and any other stress or unhappiness. The person may then be able to see clearly enough to find at least a small piece of contentment. Use the oils in all the usual ways.

ESSENTIAL OILS FOR CONTENTMENT

Rose Otto, Cypress, Lavender, Neroli, Bergamot, Orange, Sandalwood, Patchouli, Yland Ylang, Chamomile Roman, Clove, Benzoin

The quantities in the blends below could each be diluted with 30 ml of vegetable oil to make a massage oil, or make a synergistic blend using these proportions. See Chart 5.1 for quantities to use and methods.

CONTENTMENT BLEND 1		CONTENTMENT BLEND 2	
Bergamot	*10 drops*	*Chamomile Roman*	*5 drops*
Clove	*5 drops*	*Orange*	*10 drops*
Sandalwood	*10 drops*	*Lavender*	*10 drops*
Ylang Ylang	*5 drops*	*Cypress*	*5 drops*

Creativity

Apart from nature, the delights of this world are due to the creative spark in the human spirit. The things that make life a joy are music, paintings, books and for some, designer dresses and a good dinner! Imagine a world with no creative people – no TV or movies, no computers, no cars, no planes, no news-papers, no radio. Hang on, it's starting to sound good! But no beautiful buildings and gardens? It all sounds a bit bland.

Creativity is like shaking hands with tomorrow. It's the interface between the known and the unknown, and about the art of the possible. To be creative, the imagination has to soar. It can be painfully satisfying but takes confidence and belief in oneself, especially when treading into an area nobody has ever gone before. Creativity is a joy and delight, both to the creative person, and to the one who enjoys the fruits of that creativity. Art saves lives. It is the thing people turn to when under most pressure – a piece of music, a book, a picture; these things hold us tight in a sometimes difficult world.

We are all creative, to some degree or other. Look about you, isn't there something you've created – a piece of sewing, a model, a picture, a photograph, a garden? But some people seem better able to access those parts of the brain which facilitate the flow of ideas. They have gone beyond focus and concentration, and tapped into that gem, intuition. Baudelaire, the French writer, loved his essential oils, and it's reported that Leonardo da Vinci liked to have 'perfumes' around, particularly neroli. William Shakespeare's father was a glover, and that was a profession that used liberal amounts of perfumes which, at that time of course, were essential oils. Perhaps they were a contributing factor in Shakespeare's prodigious and brilliant output – they certainly didn't hurt! These days, rock musicians write songs while using essential oils and I even know a vicar who writes his sermons with the help of their fragrance. They are just as uplifting as ever they were.

When it comes to choosing a single oil or oils to blend, pick aromas that appeal to you, that feel right. Choosing essential oils here is almost as individual as creativity is, however, the oils listed below have been found useful by both people I know as well as by other colleagues. The following can be used in all the usual ways except clove should not be used in baths – see Chart 5.1 for quantities to use and methods.

ESSENTIAL OILS FOR CREATIVITY

Bergamot, Lemon, Frankincense, Geranium, Neroli, Rose Otto, Rose Maroc, Jasmine, Bay, Clove, Carnation, Mimosa, Litsea Cubeba, Sandalwood, Cypress, Juniper

Focus

Being able to focus on the task ahead is often the difference between doing well and just scraping through, and gives a great sense of satisfaction. To focus is being able to direct all your attention and energy to one place, focused on the job in hand. Meditation teaches people to focus – both when doing meditation and, as a 'side' benefit, throughout their daily lives. Focus is a great attribute, and we owe many of our inventions and creations to people's ability to do it.

In this noisy world it is difficult to find a quiet place to focus the mind: neighbours play loud music, children slam doors, kittens climb up large house plants. And, given all that, there is only one word to think about – 'selfish'. *You* need to be self-ish so take the phone off the hook, ignore the doorbell, send everyone away and meditate, or at least sit still for five min-utes and focus the mind on what you are doing, and why. Identify the side-tracks and determine to ignore them.

The following essential oils are renowned for helping people to focus. Use them in all the usual methods, following the dosages recommended in Chart 5.1 in Chapter 5. It's not going to help to use aromas which already have a memory-connection because those memories will flood in, and not allow focus on the job or thought in hand. So it might be bet-ter to choose essential oils which have no previous connota-tions.

ESSENTIAL OILS FOR FOCUS

Thyme Linalol, Lemon, Fennel, Bergamot, Basil, Cedarwood, Cypress, Juniper, Lemongrass, Litsea Cubeba, Ginger, Cinnamon, Clove, Ylang Ylang, Linden Blossom, Nutmeg, Rosemary

Use the quantities in the blends below, each with 30 ml base oil for a massage oil, or make a synergistic blend using these proportions. See Chart 5.1 for quantities to use and the list of oils which should not be used in baths.

FOCUS BLEND 1		FOCUS BLEND 2	
Thyme Linalol	10 drops	Fennel	5 drops
Lemon	6 drops	Cypress	5 drops
Rosemary	10 drops	Juniper	10 drops
Basil	4 drops	Litsea Cubeba	10 drops

Happiness

Happiness is that magic state we all aspire to, and if we achieve it, we've clinched life, got it right. The happy person exudes a radiance and seems to have found a philosophical position which banishes misery from the soul. Their aura is a delight – but happy people can sometimes attract unhappy people, energy vampires of whom one should beware.

Happiness is a very personal thing – what makes one person happy would not necessarily make another one happy. However it comes though, happiness is glorious. In a sense, it is nothing more than the ability to accept who we are and how we are living, instead of striving to be someone we could never be. Accepting our limitations is one door to happiness; having self-worth is another.

Essential oils will not put a person in a happy state if they have been miserable all their lives, but they will certainly help in a subtle way to bring out happiness. Traditionally, of course, aromas have been used for celebrations and other happy occasions. When it comes to choosing a single oil or oils to blend, pick aromas that appeal to you, that feel right. You might want to refer to other sections in the book.

On the list below, clove and cinnamon should not be used in baths, although if you use 4 drops of one of the blends below, their inclusion is actually tiny – much less than half a drop, and OK to use when included in such blends. See Chart 5.1 for quantities to use and methods.

SOME ESSENTIAL OILS FOR HAPPINESS

Orange, Rose Otto, Rose Maroc, Jasmine, Coriander, Ginger, Clove, Cinnamon, Benzoin, Carnation, Pimento Berry, Geranium

HAPPINESS BLEND 1		HAPPINESS BLEND 2	
Orange	19 drops	Pimento Berry	5 drops
Rose Maroc	5 drops	Geranium	10 drops
Jasmine	5 drops	Cinnamon	5 drops
Clove	1 drop	Ginger	10 drops

Joy

Joy is pure, unadulterated delight. It is the feeling a small child has when they see the parcels Father Christmas left under the tree. It is the feeling the young person gets when a parent hands over the keys to the car. Joy can be felt in a football stadium when the home team makes a goal. Joy is when you open the envelope containing the exam results, and find that you have passed; and it's the feeling someone gets when they finally get a date with the love of their lives. Joy is boarding a plane to a dream destination; and for those travelling the spiritual path, the ecstatic joy of becoming one with the universe. And with joy, comes peace. Joy is healing too – it makes every cell in the body feel good – a tremendous pleasure, a gift!

Use the essential oils in all the usual ways, and create your own formula for joy!

ESSENTIAL OILS FOR JOY

Sandalwood, Lemon, Bergamot, Orange, Rose Otto, Neroli, Ylang Ylang, Frankincense, Chamomile Roman, Petitgrain, Linden Blossom, Mimosa

Memory Enhancement

This section is not intended for people who have memory loss or forgetfulness, amnesia and so on, but for people who wish to improve upon what they already have – perhaps at certain times, like before starting a new job or college, or just in general. No magical memory tricks will appear, to do them you'll have to read a book on mnemonics and other aids to memory, and do some practice, but essential oils will have cumulative benefits, perhaps not noticed at first, when things will become easier to recall, and the details of situations and events will be remembered in more detail. Creative people in particular appreciate being able to recall the details of a landscape or the design of a flower.

Essential oils can be diffused, inhaled, used in a bath or massage oil. A world-famous artist told me that he uses essential oils to prepare himself before looking, and also during the creative process, and a business man told me he diffused them on his desk when writing a report, so he would remember all the little details he wanted to put in. Using essential oils regularly seems to give access to areas of our memory that might otherwise be overloaded with the plethora of daily events, or ignored by a conscious mind that has its own ideas about what is important. Aromas are the direct route of access into the brain, stimulating brain cells to respond. Aroma probably works well to retrieve memorized information because it stimulates the hippocampus, which seems to be responsible for storing information, both about experiences (*episodic memories*) and facts (*semantic memories*), in the brain. Aroma evokes memories – it presses a button and flash!, the memory is there. How it does this, we do not know. The following essential oils have been found by essential oil users and therapists to be particularly useful in enhancing memory:

ESSENTIAL OILS FOR MEMORY ENHANCEMENT

Ginger, Basil, Lemon, Grapefruit, Rosemary, Thyme Linalol, Cardamon, Black Pepper, Coriander, Pimento Berry

The essential oils can be diffused, inhaled, used in the bath (except basil and thyme unless only a small part of one drop, taken from a blend) or in a massage oil. Use the oils singly or in blends. The quantities in the blends below should each be blended with 30 ml base oil if making a massage oil, or mixed in these proportions if making a synergistic blend. For quantities to use, see Chart 5.1.

MEMORY ENHANCEMENT BLEND 1		MEMORY ENHANCEMENT BLEND 2	
Ginger	*7 drops*	*Rosemary*	*10 drops*
Lemon	*8 drops*	*Basil*	*5 drops*
Cardamon	*10 drops*	*Thyme Linalol*	*7 drops*
Pimento Berry	*5 drops*	*Grapefruit*	*8 drops*

Peace

Ah, peace, how magnificent it is! Peace is a state of grace, a spiritual restfulness that reaches to every cell in a body. It can come anytime, even standing in a crowded commuter train. Peace may be the view from the top of the mountain, the reward for a job well done. It might be the peace of knowing we have tried our best to mend a rift or put right a wrong. But how many of us have 'tied up the loose ends' of our life, or as regression expert Dr Roger Woolger says, 'finished our unfinished business'? Until we do this, will there ever be peace in our hearts?

Having inner peace doesn't mean you don't get angry at injustices, or never shout, and it doesn't mean being passive either. But it is about having an all-embracing stillness inside – in the muscles and nerves, in our minds, and spirits – the still vibration of the universe. It may be fleeting, but peace will be unforgettable. It may come when fully absorbed reading a book, or during meditation. Peace is there within us, like a quiet pool beneath the rocks, there for us to draw on when we take the time to find it. And we can find it if we listen with every cell in our body, not just the ears, and feel with every atom of our being, not just our hands.

The following essential oils create a peaceful environment, which encourages peace within. Use them in a massage oil or diffuser, inhaled, or in the bath method. Aroma is so individual and subtle, what might be a peaceful oil for one person will not be so for another, so these can only be guidelines. Smell the aroma of them and see what they do for you, or perhaps use another unlisted oil.

ESSENTIAL OILS FOR PEACE

Chamomile Roman, Neroli, Juniper, Frankincense, Rose Otto, Melissa, Angelica Seed, Spikenard, Yarrow, Jasmine, Carnation

Performance

Cars 'perform' well, we say, by which we mean they achieve towards the upper limit of their mechanical ability. Humans 'perform' too, but we don't know what our upper limits of performance are, and there are few 'mechanical' limitations to us. Who knows what we could do if we were trained, and if we tried. Perhaps we could become astronauts flying to the moon!

Professional performers give immense pleasure to others, whether they act or dance on stage, or play in an orchestra or rock band, and they try to excel themselves each time. It is onwards and upwards for them. But we all strive to perform better, whether we're performing for others, or performing for ourselves. Being able to perform well gives us confidence and self-esteem, and enables us to focus and channel our creative nature into an ever better performance of skill and control.

Essential oils will not make a person perform to an ability they do not possess, but by giving confidence, they allow a person to perform to their maximum potential, if they apply themselves. Professional performers use essential oils to overcome stage fright, to give confidence and assurance, and make them feel good.

ESSENTIAL OILS FOR BETTER PERFORMANCE

Lemon, Bergamot, Lavender, Grapefruit, Helichrysum, Rose Otto, Rose Maroc, Jasmine, Geranium, Eucalyptus, Citriodora, Bay, Ormensis Flower, Frankincense, Cypress

Use the quantities in the following blends each diluted in 30 ml base oil for a massage oil or make a synergistic blend using these proportions. For quantities to use, and methods, see Chart 5.1.

PERFORMANCE BLEND 1		PERFORMANCE BLEND 2	
Helichrysum	*8 drops*	*Frankincense*	*4 drops*
Geranium	*12 drops*	*Orange*	*8 drops*
Bergamot	*10 drops*	*Lemon*	*10 drops*
		Ormenis Flower	*8 drops*

Positivity

Thought is perhaps the most powerful tool we have. Some say you can think up your future – determine whether it will be full of happiness and cash, or miserable and lonely, and workshops are held on this subject every day of the year. We are the architects of our own future, we are told, so think positive. Anticipate a positive outcome to get one, and take control. The classic test of a positive or negative personality is to show the person a half-full bottle of wine and ask how much is in it. If they say 'it's half empty', they're negative, and if they say 'half-full', they're positive. This simple test does make an important point – our view of reality is altered by our attitude, whether positive or negative. We know this from our own experience, and from watching other people. The trick is *to get* a positive attitude, so how is it to be done?

Dr Seymour Epstein, of the Psychology Department of the University of Massachusetts, is one of the new breed of positivity gurus, and one of his pieces of advice is to 'dispute' a destructive thought every time it occurs. To help you do this he suggests you wear a rubber band on your wrist, then each time a negative thought comes up you shout 'stop' and snap the elastic at the same time. This kind of thinking-programming could be thought pointless because we're human and going to react in an emotional way to whatever happens. This is the 'you can't stop negativity, it's human' theory. I might once have agreed with that but over the years I have seen people deliberately adopt a positive attitude and, sure enough, change for the better. I can think of a couple, for example, who determined ten years ago never to argue, and they haven't, despite all the usual ups and downs that could give a couple an excuse. But not only do they not argue, they don't gripe, complain, criticize or make bitchy comments towards each other and, they tell me, their relationship gets easier and more respectful all the time . . . and is more blissful by the day!

Another piece of advice from Dr Epstein is to accept your failures without judging yourself too harshly which 'only feeds your mind's habit of thinking destructively'.[2] As another guru said many years ago, 'today is the first day of the rest of your life', so don't labour over past misfortunes, take the lessons from them and move on. All is not lost.

Interestingly, eccentricity could put ten years on your life. At least, research carried out by psychologist Dr David Weeks of the Royal Edinburgh Hospital has shown that unconventional people live longer than their staid counterparts – by between five and ten years longer. 'Unconventional' is defined as having a strong sense of purpose, robust sense of humour, and curiosity (which doesn't say much for 'conventional'!). Staying involved and stimulated is important for a long life, we are told.

One of the qualities that distinguishes 'winners' from 'losers', apparently, is that winners know when to extricate themselves from situations which are leading them nowhere while losers, on the other hand, tenaciously hang on to a project even when it is worthless. But persistence is not always a virtue, and like gamblers we have to know when to quit, and let things go. This can be difficult if there are few other options, which reminds me of a piece of advice given by a very positive American lawyer lady – 'put all your pots on the stove'. What she means by this is explore all the avenues and let the projects roll, put them on the stove, and see which ones come to fruition and which fizzle out. Because that's the point – not all projects will work out well, so don't rely on one pot!

Positive people construct strategies to improve their chances of success – they are pro-active. Rather than leaving things to chance, they put the odds in their favour by careful planning and learning to deal with different situations. Positive people don't day-dream that one day it's all going to get better, they set themselves realistic goals and go for them, step by small step, and they don't blame themselves for every little mishap. Mishaps are to be expected, they are part of the drama, so expect them but just don't expect them to rule your life.

Life is about good and bad and the trick is to find a balance in which there is more good than bad. That is all one can do. According to the Oxford Dictionary, 'optimism' is a word 'applied to any view which supposes that good must ultimately prevail over evil in the universe'. Pessimists tend to see the worst aspects of everything, which we can all do – the bottle is half empty syndrome. But how can we think good must prevail over evil when the world is such a rotten place? We can read, hear and see *that* on the news. But forget the news for five minutes and phone those long lost dear friends, and make good contacts again. There is positivity out there, but one has to reach out for it.

Because I work with essential oils every day, and see them dispel negativity, I find it easy to say good will prevail over bad. Positivity is part of my day. But the essential oils are there for anyone to use and they're like little packages of positivity, a helping aid in the move towards optimism. They gently nudge a person with positivity, and you find yourself saying 'Oh, maybe things aren't so bad' or 'Oh, maybe I can get out of this'. You'll have to help yourself too. Because it's easier to deal with small problems, cut a large problem into several smaller ones. Think of your successes, not your failures. Know what you want and why you want it then write it down, and draw up a plan of how you're going to get it. Don't wait till tomorrow – if you do just one small thing towards your goal every day you will get there.

I don't know of an essential oil that *doesn't* add positivity, but the following have been chosen for their traditional use in this area. Like other things in life, essential oils work better with positivity. Use them with positive thought, intent and purpose. In the diffuser method they create a positive atmosphere, at work or at home, and they can also be used in massage oils and inhaled from a tissue.

ESSENTIAL OILS FOR POSITIVITY

Basil, Lemon, Grapefruit, Cedarwood, Pine, Vetiver, Patchouli, Juniper, Cypress, Cardamon, Petitgrain, Geranium, Frankincense, Rosemary, Pimento Berry, Bay

Basil should not be used in baths. The quantities in the following blends can each be diluted with 30 ml base oil for a massage oil, or make a synergistic blend using these proportions. For quantities to use see Chart 5.1.

POSITIVE BLEND 1		POSITIVE BLEND 2	
Geranium	10 drops	Cedarwood	10 drops
Pimento Berry	8 drops	Pine	5 drops
Bay	8 drops	Cypress	5 drops
Frankincense	4 drops	Petitgrain	10 drops

Restfulness

We all need to rest, not only to sleep but to balance, and ease our minds. Restfulness is a joy, as we allow our minds to drift and the equilibrium to return. But some minds never rest – they are constantly filling with new ideas, projects, things to do, ever searching, learning, probing, ever on the move. There's nothing wrong with having an active mind, providing it's smart enough to know the benefits of rest. As a wise person once said, to be a perfect human being one needs the stillness of a sage and the action of a king. Balance is all, and restfulness is part of the equation. Any of the following oils will work equally well on their own or in mixes:

ESSENTIAL OILS FOR RESTFULNESS

Lavender, Geranium, Rose Maroc, Clary Sage, Linden Blossom, Neroli, Marjoram, Petitgrain, Rosewood, Sandalwood, Mimosa

The quantities in the following blends can each be diluted with 30 ml of base oil to make a massage oil, or make a synergistic blend of oils using these proportions and use in all room methods, inhalation methods, and in the bath. See Chart 5.1 for quantities to use.

RESTFUL BLEND 1		RESTFUL BLEND 2	
Neroli	10 drops	Geranium	20 drops
Petitgrain	20 drops	Lavender	5 drops
		Clary Sage	5 drops

Self-Awareness

Being able to connect with who we really are is a useful tool in the striving for fulfilment. Not only does self-awareness bring us closer to our spiritual selves, it helps identify our hopes, fears and joys. If we have an awareness of how we feel and react, a strong sense of who we really are, it contributes to emotional well-being. There are many routes to self-awareness, including Gestalt therapy, which is based on the idea that a person reflects his or her true personality through the things they do or need to do, and tries to make the person aware of their thoughts, feelings and actions. The aim is to view the life clearly, uncluttered by outside thoughts, and try to understand what it is that is wanted from it. People are encouraged to feel free to be who they are, and to feel content with themselves. The message is, *appreciate yourself.*

We don't all need to go into therapy and a great deal of self-awareness can be had from simply observing ourselves, and asking other people how they see us. By understanding the effect we have on other people, we can gain an insight into our motives and hidden agendas. What the essential oils can do is help bring out parts of ourselves we may not have recognized, or been aware of, before.

ESSENTIAL OILS FOR SELF-AWARENESS

Clary Sage, Ylang Ylang, Cypress, Geranium, Pine, Sandalwood, Bay, Ormenis Flower, Jasmine, Clove, Pimento Berry, Mandarin, Coriander, Angelica Seed, Sage, Cistus, Myrtle

Self-Esteem

There's nothing wrong with having a favourable appreciation or opinion of oneself. If you can't appreciate yourself, who else can? But I am constantly amazed at the number of people who put themselves down with comments like 'I could never do that' or 'I'm not smart enough for that'. In fact, they are perfectly capable of meeting the challenge, or at least having a jolly good go, but have low self-esteem, so do nothing.

Simply, self-esteem is recognizing your potential and worth, taking pride in what you do, and trusting your judgement in most things. When you have self-esteem you are secure in yourself, despite the weak points, because you recognize your strong points and appreciate them. OK, you're not perfect, but who is? – and you're as good as the next person. So Mr Jones next door grows bigger cabbages – so what? Your potatoes are bigger than his! We cannot go around making value judgements about other people in comparison to ourselves, it is a totally useless exercise. Everyone is different, that is the beauty of it, and we all have our good points, which should give us self-esteem.

Essential oils won't miraculously turn you overnight from someone with low self-esteem into someone brimming over with high expectations of themselves, but they will subtly and gently help you deal with any corner of your life with which you feel unhappy, and so build up your self-esteem and your estimate of what you can do in this world. Use an oil or oils with no previous memory connection which could have negative associations.

ESSENTIAL OILS FOR SELF-ESTEEM

Hyacinth, Sandalwood, Vetiver, Ylang Ylang, Rose Maroc, Jasmine, Carnation, Bergamot, Geranium, Ormenis Flower, Cedarwood

The quantities in the following blends can each be diluted with 30 ml of base oil to make a massage oil, or make a synergistic blend of oils using these proportions and use the synergistic blend in baths, room methods and inhalation methods. For quantities to use see Chart 5.1.

SELF-ESTEEM BLEND 1		SELF-ESTEEM BLEND 2	
Ylang Ylang	*10 drops*	*Hyacinth*	*8 drops*
Bergamot	*4 drops*	*Bergamot*	*4 drops*
Vetiver	*2 drops*	*Rose Maroc*	*8 drops*
Sandalwood	*12 drops*		

(The second blend here uses a particularly powerful combination of oils and only 20 drops are needed in 30ml.)

Self-Image

If we can see ourselves as a positive, happy, vibrant, radiant person, other people will be more likely to see us in the same way. Of course, having a good self-image isn't very easy if you've been battered down by life's events, but it is possible to raise oneself out of this hole by thinking positively. In the early 1970s practically everyone wore a yellow badge with a smiling face on it, and the word 'smile' underneath. This icon of an era worked – people wore it and smiled! Smiling makes you happy, just as being happy makes you smile. If we can visualize ourselves as positive, smiling people, and project that image into the outside world, perhaps that is exactly what we shall become!

Essential oils can help in raising self-image by seeking out the hidden reserves we have within us, and bringing them forward. They find our best qualities and fortify them, which improves our self-image. This is an intensely personal area and so only use those oils to which you feel drawn. Certain aromas could already have a memory connection which is negative – associated, for example, with someone who put you down – so obviously don't use them. The following oils can be used either singly, or in blends:

ESSENTIAL OILS FOR SELF-IMAGE

Orange, Lavender, Melissa, Neroli, Chamomile Roman, Ylang Ylang, Rose Maroc, Jasmine, Sandalwood, Cypress, Juniper, Cedarwood, Pine, Black Pepper, Frankincense, Mandarin, Nutmeg, Myrtle, Bay

The quantities in the following blends can each be diluted with 30 ml of base oil to make a massage oil, or make a synergistic blend of oils using these proportions, and use diffused in the atmosphere and in the inhalation methods. For quantities to use see Chart 5.1. Blend 1 can be used in baths.

SELF-IMAGE BLEND 1		SELF-IMAGE BLEND 2	
Rose Maroc	10 drops	Sandalwood	5 drops
Orange	5 drops	Black Pepper	5 drops
Mandarin	10 drops	Frankincense	5 drops
Ylang Ylang	5 drops	Jasmine	5 drops

Chapter Eight

THE A–Z OF EMOTIONAL PROBLEMS

ABUSE
(Emotional and Physical)

THE WORD 'ABUSE' IS EXPECTED TO EXPLAIN A WHOLE RANGE OF experiences suffered by an individual – from regular violent beatings from a so-called 'partner', or daily sexual violation as a child, to verbal attacks or put downs which are within the boundary of so-called 'normal' behaviour. For example, countless parents all over this country say of their child 'they're a monster' or say 'come here you little monster' – half-jokingly, half meaning it. If, as an adult, someone called you a monster, you'd be pretty upset, but children are expected to take this abuse – as some kind of punishment for crying as babies, demanding food at inconvenient times, producing dirty nappies or taking the parent's freedom away. But if a child is called 'a monster' just four times a day, by the time they reach five years of age, they've been called a monster 7,300 times and the danger is, the child may come to believe that they are, in fact, a monster. When one includes this kind of verbal abuse in with the discussion of 'abuse', and add in the nastiness siblings can inflict upon each other, one could come to the conclusion that there are few people in our society who have

Rose

not been through some kind of abuse or other!

Of course, some forms of abuse are more damaging than others but it is most often inflicted upon us by someone we love; babies get called a 'monster' by the mummy they love, little girls are abused by the fathers they love, and lovers are abused by each other – both physically and verbally. It is this, the mixing of hate and love, that is so damaging in the long term because later, in other relationships, it can become difficult to extricate the hate from the love and future love becomes a love-hate relationship, somehow never entirely satisfactory.

As the word 'abuse' covers so many experiences, which could affect us all to some degree or other, it is impossible to say what emotional damage results from it. However, these may include the inability to accept love, or feel love, the inability to share, lack of self-confidence, low self-esteem, insecurity, shame, inferiority complex, depression, fear and guilt. It may express itself as a general feeling of anxiety – inexplicable perhaps, and general, a sort of permanent discomfort with life. If any of these feelings are left unexpressed, they can eat away at the very fabric of a soul or personality, like woodworm silently eating away a timber-framed house, which one day may fall.

Thankfully, abuse is now a widely discussed subject, partly thanks to the frankness of certain famous people, and it's no longer thought to be the victim's fault. However, although it might be easy to understand *intellectually* that abuse was not our fault, coming to understand that *emotionally* is another thing altogether – and much more difficult. Help is often required, and although there are now counselling services available for people who have experienced sexual abuse as a child, and domestic violence, it is very difficult to find a context in which to discuss the less dramatic types of abuse, the type that is part of 'normal' behaviour. Doctors aren't as a rule very sympathetic when a person goes to them and says, 'Doctor, I feel permanently anxious because my big sister used to verbally abuse me remorselessly, until I left home at eighteen, and now I just feel permanently anxious and lack confidence.' He or she is unlikely to consider the case important enough to refer to a free counselling service, and may just tell the person to 'buck up'. What they need to do, however, is discuss the problem, get to the root of it, look at it, examine it and, having done that, throw it away like so much garbage.

Sexual abuse is altogether more difficult because it is *so* appalling, often 'blanked out' altogether – until something triggers off the memory, perhaps decades after the events. One dreadful aspect of sexual abuse is that the abuser often makes the abusee think they are responsible or somehow compliant in the acts. It is not only physical invasion but mental manipulation too. Figures show that it is very widespread – horrifyingly so. In *Women: A World Report*, the authors looked at statistics from Britain, America, Australia, Israel, Egypt and India and extended them worldwide, coming to the conclusion that they could imply that 'as many as 100 million young girls may be being raped by adult men – usually their father – often day after day, week after week, year in, year out'.[1] These men aren't obvious demons, they're men we see walking down the street, men we work with, men we see driving cars or on the bus. They *look* and, disconcertingly for the children concerned, behave normally for most of the time. One woman I know, whom I shall call Linda, was regularly abused by her father on the evening her mother went to an evening class. Like most abusers he made her feel as if it were her fault, that she had somehow invited it or deserved it. She couldn't tell her mother, then or even to the present day, because she knew and knows it would destroy her, and still feels she should somehow get through the experience without putting her mother through the anguish, and that is her choice. I recently went to Linda's wedding and marvelled at the way she got through the whole event without once looking at her father, embracing him or in any way recognizing him. If he was standing on her right, she talked to someone on her left. If he stood on her left, she talked to someone on her right. It was a masterstroke of polite avoidance! But, I wonder, hasn't her mother noticed that Linda never actually looks at her father or speaks to him? It is not only the abusee that 'blanks' it out! Like many abusers, Linda's father is a respectable, professional man, and one would never guess from looking at him that he was capable of such ghastly deeds. Another abusee I know, whom I shall call Jill, grew up on a farm with three brothers, a mother, and violent father. He would beat Jill's brothers on the slightest excuse – so badly they would often have to miss school for a whole week to allow their physical marks to heal. Like many mothers and wives, Jill's mother was so passive (and terrified), she just let the whole business pass. As Jill entered adolescence she discovered that she could prevent her father beating the brothers by interrupting him and becoming like a young Lolita, stroking his face, kissing him, saying, 'Please daddy, stop'. This calmed him down long enough to stop the beating. However, being a nasty, manipulative man, he also saw that Jill's 'solution' could be exploited and as time went on he wanted more than a kiss on the cheek and a hug. By the time she turned fourteen, only full intercourse would 'calm' the man down and, predictably, Jill's father would find more and more excuses to thrash the boys, knowing that Jill would 'placate' him.

It's easy enough to say children or young girls or boys should 'tell', but very difficult for them actually to do it. I know of a recent case involving two eleven-year-old boys who were regularly 'touched up' by a classmate's father who came along to 'help' when that class went swimming. The boys kept it all a secret for about six months, and then one told his mother. All hell was let loose, the man was taken to court but, because it was their word against his (and he was a highly respectable member of the community) he got off the charge. In his summing up, the judge noted that the boys hadn't mentioned the first (alleged) incident and apparently thought the boys were having pre-adolescent fantasies, and advised the jury accordingly. The whole experience has left the boys devastated, distrustful of both men and authority.

I know of so many cases of sexual abuse it is quite easy for me to believe the horrifying statistics, and difficult to find the space here to recall them all. But one thing that recurs through all these experiences is the fact that the abusee, for many reasons, doesn't tell, or makes the one person they tell *promise* not to tell. *Not telling* and abuse seem to go hand in hand. It is then, precisely *telling* that's required before the events can be 'processed' by the mind, allowing the abusee to continue with their life without this experience gnawing away at them. This is where essential oils can help. We know that aroma molecules do reach and activate the limbic system, which is the home of memories and emotions, thereby facilitating the release of pent-up experiences, while at the same time certain essential oils are calming, seemingly, as research shows, because they expedite the production of beta-waves in the brain.

Someone who has been abused needs to discuss it and work it through. It is irrelevant how long ago it all was. Not everyone needs to go to counselling or to a special therapist. Linda, mentioned above, kept her experience a secret until she was thirty years old, then went through a crisis period during which she discussed it with a few close friends, and came out of it all a much more confident and assertive person. She no longer apologized for everything she did, and felt she deserved the little space she took up in the world (which was a profound change for her). After much thought, she decided group counselling was not for her. But the point is, she had to discuss it with *someone* to get it off her chest, and it didn't much matter who that someone was, or who those somebodies were, so long as they were genuinely supportive.

Of course, it is upsetting to recall the abuse, and it often involves coming to the realization that the abuser is a horrible person, even if he is your father. However, it has to be done. The alternative may be to live with a whole range of feelings which slowly destroy the abusee – and nobody deserves that to happen. Abuse generates feelings of betrayal, suspicion, mistrust, self-doubt, dread, terror, panic, resentment, violation, guilt and many other things which could perhaps be dissipated with sympathetic help.

Some essential oils are better suited to use in cases of abuse and have been empirically shown to help the wounded child or adult. Also, refer to other sections in this book – those dealing with emotional hurt, anxiety, depression, lack of self-confidence and so on – and see which essential oils seem most relevant to each particular experience.

ESSENTIAL OILS TO HELP OVERCOME EMOTIONAL ABUSE

Ormenis Flower, Chamomile Roman, Melissa, Rose Otto, Neroli, Mandarin, Benzoin

ESSENTIAL OILS TO HELP THE HURT INNER CHILD

Geranium, Lavender, Neroli, Melissa, Mandarin, Rose Otto, Chamomile Roman

Abuse – Using a Blend

As each case of abuse is so individual, create a formulation using essential oils particular to your needs. For example, if you experience a lot of panic, see that section and include an oil or oils from that list. Make up a synergistic blend of essential oils in a bottle and from that you can use the oils in various methods, in the quantities given below. For example, you might put into your synergistic blend bottle some mandarin or chamomile roman for gentleness, some rose or neroli to deal with the sadness, and some geranium to deal with the insecurity. Here are a couple of suggested blends you might like to try, remembering that these quantities indicate proportions to be used when making a synergistic blend, and not the maximum number of drops:

SYNERGISTIC BLEND 1		SYNERGISTIC BLEND 2	
Chamomile Roman	2 drops	Rose Otto	4 drops
Mandarin	4 drops	Geranium	2 drops
Neroli	6 drops	Mandarin	4 drops

Once you have made your synergistic blend of oils you can use it in several ways. Use 5 drops to a teaspoon of base oil for a massage. This doesn't sound like much, but it will go further than you think, and it can be effective if massaged into the solar plexus area (middle, where the ribcage separates), upper chest and across the shoulders. Alternatively, use 3 drops of synergistic blend in a bath. Also use the synergistic blend in any of the room methods. Using the essential oils in this way will help you express yourself during counselling, or help you generally as you try to deal with the problem by facing it and expressing your feelings about it. Use the essential oils daily and change the blend as you progress.

ADDICTIONS

When the body cannot react normally without a particular substance, it's said to be 'dependent' upon it, and the body will go through 'withdrawal symptoms' if that substance is not provided. This is addiction, and it can be caused by many substances – heroin, cocaine, diazepam and other tranquillizers, amphetamines, alcohol, the nicotine in cigarettes and the caffeine in tea and coffee. Addiction involves physical processes and is not simply a psychological demand – like a baby crying because their comfort blanket is not in their hands. It is even possible to become addicted to chocolate – don't blame yourself, it's the chemicals in the chocolate!

Whether the addictive substance comes in the form of little pills from the doctor or in the form of tea-bags from the supermarket, it is a drug. By taking it into the body on a regular basis, the cells in a body adjust themselves to it, so they then *expect* it. When the head decides to 'give up', the body may not be ready so, whatever the drug, unless the person is prepared to go through rather unpleasant 'withdrawal symptoms', they'll have to reduce their intake of the drug slowly, allowing the cells gradually to adjust back to their old selves. With some drugs, the cells adjust and keep adjusting so that as time goes on they require more and more of the drug to achieve the same effect. Heroin is a classic example of this, but so is alcohol. One becomes inexorably drawn into addiction, deeper and deeper, day by day.

This section is arranged as *Drug Addiction, Alcohol Addiction* and *Nicotine Addiction*, and please refer to the section which applies to you, but most addictive substances are poisons and they need to be cleared out of the system. Fruit juices, water, fresh foods and vitamins are all useful aids in the process of withdrawal. Change to a wholefood diet, avoiding junk foods, refined food products and soda drinks (which can themselves be addictive if they contain caffeine). Eat plenty of fresh green vegetables, salads and fruits, and drink sparkling water combined with fruit juices, as this lifts low blood sugar levels. It's important to eat three meals a day, especially breakfast: have cereal or an egg on toast with fruit juice, something light but nutritious. Also consider going to an acupuncturist, who might be able to help.

Use the following oils in diffusers, in massage oils, inhaled in the water-bowl method or, indeed, in any way that is found helpful, following the dosage guidelines in Chart 5.1 in Chapter 5.

ESSENTIAL OILS TO USE IN THE FIGHT AGAINST ADDICTION

Vetiver, Narcissus, Helichrysum, Basil, Rose Otto, Frankincense, Spikenard, Benzoin

HYPNOTICS THAT CAN BE USEFUL IN THE FIGHT AGAINST ADDICTION

Narcissus, Jonquil, Rose Maroc, Hyacinth, Carnation, Jasmine, Hops, Valerian, Tonka Bean, Vanilla, Tuberose, Spikenard

OTHER ESSENTIAL OILS THAT MAY BE OF USE TO COMBAT ADDICTION

Marjoram, Bergamot, Chamomile Roman, Juniper, Patchouli, Bay, Clary Sage, Nutmeg, Cistus

Drug Addiction

When tranquillizers first came on the market, nobody knew they were addictive, not even the companies that made them – who are currently embroiled in expensive legal battles with people who were prescribed the drugs by their GPs. Now we all know what trouble they can be. As the dangers of tran-quillizers were becoming known, people were reassured that anti-depressants were not addictive, but now of course we know that they are. Patients are told that the panic, anxiety and depression they may feel when they stop taking anti-depressants is a symptom of *withdrawal*, and not a sign of relapse, and to reduce the dose gradually over a four-week period, at least. It's got to be worth a try. In an article in the magazine *She*, one woman gave a very moving account of anti-depressant dependency. Her memory was like porridge, she said, she couldn't remember what happened yesterday. And decisions took days. She experienced mental confusion – 'like being hopelessly drunk', her thinking 'fogged and slow', her limbs 'leaden', and her joints 'aching'. Plus her life was full of dread – as in dreadful.

When you're addicted to drugs, your whole life revolves around them. Are they in your handbag when you go out? Where is the next fix coming from? Likewise, withdrawal takes over the life. How am I going to get through the next five minutes? The addict needs support. There are several useful addresses, at the end of this book, of organizations that advise on support groups people can join.

There are two ways to get addicted to drugs. Tranquillizers are often prescribed for far too long. Instead of seeing the person through a rough patch of anxiety or depression, the pills are continued because the problem itself isn't being sorted out, and even when time has passed and dissolved it anyway, the tranquillizer addiction remains – probably causing more problems than the original problem! Of course tranquillizers, sleeping pills and anti-depressants have their place in the pharmacopoeia, but to take them over long periods when they are no longer required is to use them incorrectly. Another way to get into drugs is to be drawn to them, like an animal to water, because of some very hurtful dynamic in the early family life, or a traumatic experience. Drugs provide comfort. If this is the case there is only one answer – counselling, in some form or other.

People often become addicted to drugs because they were mistreated as children. Not in dramatic ways necessarily, but in ways that hurt. Simone, for example, was brought up by her grandmother because her mother was sixteen and single when she had Simone, and couldn't cope. The father was nowhere to be seen, and the grandmother resented Simone for having 'ruined' her daughter's life. Not surprisingly, Simone grew up feeling unloved and later turned to drugs – including heroin. David's parents were similarly unloving, but in a different way. His father was a sparkling, successful professional man – charming, liked, amusing and rich, and was much adored by the mother. David and his siblings were always second in line – 'stop that now, your father's talking', or working or whatever it was. Not that David had much time to interrupt his perfect father, because like many other middle-class boys of his generation, he was packed off to boarding school at the age of seven. Because father was the centre of the domestic universe, mother dismissed David like a little inconsequential boy, even when he was thirty years old. He too turned to drugs. Many problems like this are still unresolved in the minds of junkie-type personalities, and it's not really their fault. I know David's family and to look at them you'd say, 'Oh what a perfect family', so it's difficult for David openly to blame them for his indulgent behaviour, or at least it may seem so to him. But his situation is real, and unresolved, something trained counsellors would recognize, and have sympathy with. That's what they're there for.

As for the physical effects of withdrawal, these must be overseen by a medical practitioner because it can be dangerous to do it on your own. Plan to cut down over a long period, cutting down the number of pills taken each day, cutting them in half, then into quarters, then scraping small bits off, gradually – and very slowly – reducing the amount of drug that is taken in each day. Withdrawal from drugs such as the opiates morphine and heroin, or amphetamines, synthetic slimming tablets, and the barbiturates, tranquillizers and sleeping pills, causes the body to go into crisis. It's tough for all those little junkie cells. They're not used to it and they have to readjust. People think of drugs as 'head' things. They're not. Benzodiazepam receptors (and benzodiazepines are the most commonly prescribed drugs for anxiety and stress) are found all over the body, not just in the head, and more drug receptors are being found every day – in the least expected places. The whole body is into drugs, not just the head, and consequently the whole body is going to react with a whole range of symptoms that might include sweating, or palpitations, shaking, nausea, breathing difficulties, tremors, rashes, aches and pains, diarrhoea or constipation. The brain, meanwhile, could be suffering with headaches, distorted vision, anxiety, confusion, panic attacks, insomnia, paranoia and hallucinations. No wonder addicts trying to come off drugs wonder if it's worth the trouble! But it is . . . well worth it.

During the withdrawal process essential oils can help in two ways – by contributing to a sense of well-being, and by treating the physical problems that go along with it. The essential oils listed below can be used to supplement and support any other treatment. Use the oils in warm baths, inhaled as a vapour and diffused in the room. If possible, arrange to see an aromatherapist, at least once a week to begin with, and then monthly. This may not be possible for financial reasons, but you can massage the oils in yourself. (See *Massage*, p. 282.)

ESSENTIAL OILS FOR USE DURING WITHDRAWAL FROM DRUGS

Vetiver, Helichrysum, Spikenard, Valerian, Ormenis Flower, Nutmeg, Juniper, Bergamot, Basil, Clary Sage, Geranium, Hyacinth, Narcissus, Tuberose

There are many essential oils to choose from. As well as those listed above, refer to particular sections throughout this book, or try one of the blends below. They are synergistic blends, use these quantities each diluted with 30 ml of vegetable oil to make a massage oil, or make up a synergistic blend using these proportions and use in the inhalation or diffuser methods. See Chart 5.1 for quantities to use. Blend 2 can be used in baths.

DURING DRUG WITHDRAWAL

SYNERGISTIC BLEND 1		SYNERGISTIC BLEND 2	
Vetiver	*10 drops*	*Nutmeg*	*10 drops*
Basil	*5 drops*	*Ormenis Flower*	*5 drops*
Bergamot	*5 drops*	*Spikenard*	*4 drops*
Clary Sage	*10 drops*	*Bergamot*	*5 drops*
		Juniper	*6 drops*

These blends can be altered as time goes on, when a lighter emotional blend may be needed. The essential oil of helichrysum has been used on its own very successfully in some cases of withdrawal, as have the floral absolutes – which are very expensive but as a very small amount is required, they need not be as expensive as they first appear.

When withdrawing from drugs, as well as using the essential oils suggested in the lists and blends in this section, take 100 grams of vitamin B complex twice a day, and 500 grams of vitamin C complex twice a day, or a multi-vitamin and mineral supplement. Homeopathic remedies may help as well, such as capsicum, ignatia or nux vomica (x6). Also, consider going along to the meetings of Narcotics Anonymous, or contacting the organizations Tranx or MIND, who can give advice about coming off drugs and put people in touch with local support groups.

Alcohol Addiction

There seems to be something in human nature that drives people to brew up alcoholic drinks, which we make from just about every grain, berry and fruit going. Even grannies brew up elderflower champagne and plum wine in their back kitchens! Drinking is a part of life and we flock to the pubs for a tipple, are encouraged to buy wine with our meal in restaurants, and cannot avoid it at parties. It's not all bad, of course, and alcohol can help us to relax and communicate, it keeps us warm in winter and, according to some doctors, drinking two glasses of red wine a day is actually good for the heart and digestive system, something the French and Italians have been saying for years.

So much is drinking a part of life, that 'to go out' is synonymous with 'let's have a drink'! But for some people, a social drink becomes a problem drink, from which there is no going back. Once an alcoholic, they say, always an alcoholic – it's as if the body can let you give up for ten years and then, a couple of drinks' lapse, and you're in its grip again. That's why they say drink is evil.

People get driven to drink by the manifold pressures that

face the average human soul – financial problems, marital breakup, depression, unemployment, boredom, frustration, lack of confidence, insecurity and so on and so on. The drink is in the cupboard, it's there in that friendly pub, and so it draws us to it, solace in a bottle. Some people, we are told, have a genetic pre-disposition to alcoholism – it's wired in the genes. As many people who are married to alcoholics know, from trying over and over again to get their loved ones to stop, alcohol is a deep dark abyss from which it is difficult to escape.

In Los Angeles today, the Alcoholics Anonymous meetings are full of movie stars, and all over the world other less famous people stand up in AA meetings and bravely admit they too are hooked. AA is a wonderful organization but families need sup-port too, and Al Anon are there to do that. Doctors can prescribe a drug such as Antabuse, which makes the person feel sick if they have a drink, but it usually takes more than this to get to the root of the problems.

As with drug addiction, essential oils have been shown to be very helpful, especially during the first stages of withdrawal. You might like to try the following oils, used singly or in blends:

ESSENTIAL OILS FOR USE IN WITHDRAWAL FROM ALCOHOL

Helichrysum, Juniper, Lemon, Bergamot, Marjoram, Clary Sage, Eucalyptus Citriodora

Or try either of the following blends, which are both syner-gistic blends. Either add one of the blends to 30 ml of base oil for a massage oil, or mix the essential oils in these proportions for a synergistic blend to be diffused in the atmosphere, or add 8 drops to the bath. See Chart 5.1.

DURING ALCOHOL WITHDRAWAL

BLEND 1		BLEND 2	
Helichrysum	10 drops	Marjoram	10 drops
Lemon	10 drops	Bergamot	10 drops
Juniper	10 drops	Clary Sage	10 drops

After a while, different oils should be substituted to deal with the withdrawal symptoms – try chamomile roman for a calming effect and geranium to ease anxiety. But look at the other sections through this book and find what is specific for each person, during the various stages. (Refer to *The Fragrant Pharmacy* for various physical reactions that may occur.) This is one of the great advantages with essential oils – aside from detoxifying, and making one feel positive, they can run with you – providing specific help every step of the way.

Nicotine Addiction

Cigarettes are so dangerous, manufacturers are obliged to print 'Cigarettes can kill you', and other such warnings on the packet and advertisements. This doesn't stop people buying them! Indeed, people buy nicotine sticks by the zillion, despite the fact that there isn't a good word to be said about them, even by the people who smoke them. Cigarettes cause all kinds of cancer, heart disease, strokes and respiratory tract disorders including bronchitis and emphysema – sufferers of which often have to carry their own life-saving supply of oxygen around with them. Cigarettes make the skin grey or yellow and the breath, hair and clothes stink. Plus, aside from killing yourself you may be killing somebody else, who passively inhales your smoke – and increasingly, court cases are being fought and won on this point. It's a myth that smoking reduces stress – and that's official. Clinical psychologists have shown that smoking at the same time as experiencing stress just compounds the bad effects on the heart. You can't even console yourself with the thought that at least tobacco is a crop which provides a living for someone somewhere, because tobacco is an invidious crop, which sucks all nutrients from the earth and leaves it useless, and farmers say it requires much more tedious manual work than almost any other crop and the work must go on right throughout the year. Other crops would be more useful, in more ways than one.

Nicotine is highly addictive, and rumour has it that manufacturers are putting more and more chemicals into the tobacco and rolling paper each passing year. Old grandad smoking his pure roll-ups for eighty years might have survived, but I don't know that smokers will live that long in the future. However, giving up isn't easy, and help is required. Essential oils can provide relief for some of the specific symptoms of withdrawal such as grumpy moods, depression, anger, nervousness and sheer panic – and please look to those sections to see what is required with each passing day, if not hour. Also try vitamin therapy to build up your strength, and replenish some of the supplies smoking inevitably drains. Vitamins B1, B6, B12, and vitamin C are especially important now, or get a daily multi-vitamin with B-complex and mineral supplement, and take it with a minimum of 200 grams of Vitamin C each day.

AGGRESSION

Aggression is part of our survival system and shouldn't be entirely wiped out because aggressive tendencies can actually help protect us from what the world throws at us today, as ever. Nevertheless, it's perfectly clear that some people are too aggressive. You can see it in certain children, in men who get in a fight, and people who seem to thrash it out with the wall when they hang wallpaper. Supposedly, aggression is due to the hormone testosterone, of which men have more than women. We expect men to be more aggressive than women, to the point where if a man and woman were behaving in exactly the same way, he would be called assertive, and she would be called aggressive! Aggression is hostile action or behaviour – rough, hard and unpleasant. It may only become a problem when it is already well and truly established as part of the personality. Little Billy is 'a bit of a rebel', then he grows up into a thug.

In some cases, we know which components in essential oils bring down the level of aggression, in some we don't. But they are proven to do so, in animals as well as in people. Thankfully, essential oils quite easily reduce aggression in most cases. Relaxation exercises are also most helpful, particularly the tension-release ones, which make one very aware of the mind-body connection. It is very effective under these circumstances to use essential oils in a diffuser at the same time as doing breathing exercises. Also, take a regular warm bath using one of the essential oils listed below (or a blend of oils) and then take that same oil (or blend) out with you on a tissue or handkerchief and whenever you feel the aggression coming on, just pull it out and inhale. Think of the nice, relaxing bath you had last night.

ESSENTIAL OILS TO HELP REDUCE GENERAL AGGRESSION

Geranium, Frankincense, Sandalwood, Grapefruit, Cedarwood, Vetiver

---

OTHER ESSENTIAL OILS THAT HAVE A SOOTHING EFFECT

Neroli, Lavender, Clary Sage, Chamomile Roman, Benzoin, Marjoram, Coriander, Litsea Cubeba, Valerian, Spikenard

plus the more expensive absolutes of Rose Maroc, Tuberose, Mimosa and Carnation

---

Aggression can also turn inwards, and there may be feelings of aggression towards oneself. Try the soothing essential oils for this – lavender and litsea cubeba are also useful for this situation. Alternatively, try one of the following blends – adding these quantities to 30 ml base oil for a massage oil, or making up a synergistic blend using these proportions and using 8 drops in a bath, or in a room diffuser method, or 3 drops inhaled direct from a tissue.

AGGRESSION TOWARDS SELF

BLEND 1		BLEND 2	
Clary Sage	*10 drops*	*Frankincense*	*15 drops*
Vetiver	*8 drops*	*Geranium*	*5 drops*
Grapefruit	*12 drops*	*Sandalwood*	*5 drops*

In the case of aggression towards other people, use suggestions made elsewhere in this section, or one of the blends below. Use these quantities added in 30 ml base oil for a massage oil, or make a synergistic blend using these proportions and then add 8 drops to a bath, or in a diffuser, or 3 drops on a tissue or hanky to be inhaled when required.

AGGRESSION TOWARDS OTHER PEOPLE			
BLEND 1		BLEND 2	
Cedarwood	5 drops	Chamomile Roman	10 drops
Grapefruit	15 drops	Litsea Cubeba	6 drops
Frankincense	5 drops	Clary Sage	2 drops
Geranium	10 drops	Sandalwood	12 drops

Children can be aggressive too, and it's a bad habit for them to acquire. Those under five years of age should only be exposed to chamomile roman and lavender, while those over fifteen years of age can follow the adult lists and blends. Children in between – over five and under fifteen – can use the one below:

CHILDHOOD AGGRESSION AGES 5–15	
Chamomile Roman	5 drops
Lavender	5 drops
Frankincense	2 drops
Geranium	3 drops

Blend these quantities with 30 ml base oil to make a massage oil or make a synergistic blend using these proportions and use 4 drops in a bath.

AMNESIA

It's bad enough to wake up after a wild night out and not remember where you went, or who with, but try to imagine what it's like to wake up in a hospital after a car crash and not remember a thing about last night, the night before that, and all the days and nights of your life. Even your mother is a stranger. It is truly terrifying.

Forty per cent of people involved in road accidents suffer brain damage and some degree of amnesia. Most of these victims are under twenty-five. Amnesia can also come about as a result of various illnesses, such as meningitis or encephalitis; alcoholics can have it as a result of their thiamine deficiency; drug addiction can cause it; as can epilepsy, stroke and brain tumours. Amnesia can also come about for no apparent, physical cause, but because of emotional trauma. Perhaps something so painful happened in the past, that a period of one's life is simply wiped out as a self-protection mechanism. Shock or hysteria can also cause amnesia.

There's retrograde amnesia – forgetting things that happened before the incident that caused the amnesia, and anterograde amnesia – forgetting things that happen after the incident. People who have retrograde amnesia also often cannot remember things that happen after the incident very well. Amnesiacs have dreadful problems with which to deal, frustrating, exasperating and debilitating. Essential oils obviously cannot help all these problems but where they may be able to help some people is in alleviating some of the confusion that results from the condition. Also, if the amnesia was caused by shock or fear, essential oils can work on them, and thus may perhaps beneficially affect the amnesia. It's certainly worth a try.

ESSENTIAL OILS THAT HELP THE CONFUSION OF AMNESIA

Cardamon, Tuberose, Ginger, Black Pepper, Bergamot, Geranium, Petitgrain, Helichrysum, Grapefruit, Basil

The two following blends can be added to 30 ml base oil and made into massage oils, or they can be made into a synergistic blend and used in diffusers or other methods. See Chart 5.1 for quantities to use.

AMNESIAC CONFUSION			
BLEND 1		BLEND 2	
Cardamon	10 drops	Helichrysum	10 drops
Bergamot	10 drops	Petitgrain	5 drops
Ginger	5 drops	Geranium	2 drops
Petitgrain	5 drops	Grapefruit	10 drops

ESSENTIAL OILS TO HELP SHOCK-INDUCED AMNESIA

Mandarin, Ylang Ylang, Rose Maroc, Rose Otto, Neroli, Melissa, Peppermint, Lavender

Also see the essential oils listed under the *Trauma* section.

Both the following blends can be made into a massage oil by adding each to 30 ml base oil. They can also both be made into a synergistic blend and used in a diffuser or sniffed from a tissue or the bottle. The Emotional-Shock blend can also be used in a bath – use 8 drops. However, the Trauma-Shock blend should *not* be used in a bath.

TRAUMA-SHOCK		EMOTIONAL-SHOCK	
Peppermint	10 drops	Rose Otto	5 drops
Lavender	20 drops	Neroli	5 drops
		Mandarin	15 drops

ESSENTIAL OILS TO HELP FEAR-INDUCED AMNESIA

Sandalwood, Chamomile Roman, Cypress, Vetiver, Lemon, Bergamot, Orange, Cedarwood, Neroli, Geranium

Also see the essential oils listed under the *Fear* section.

The following two blends can be each added to 30 ml base oil for a massage oil; they can both also be made into a synergistic blend and used in the usual methods including diffusers and baths – 8 drops per bath.

FEAR-INDUCED AMNESIA 1		FEAR-INDUCED AMNESIA 2	
Chamomile Roman	15 drops	Sandalwood	15 drops
Cypress	10 drops	Lemon	5 drops
Vetiver	5 drops	Orange	10 drops

ANGER

Many people working in the medical and therapy fields have commented that unexpressed anger can result in many chronic symptoms including chronic tiredness, apathy, the inability to concentrate, back ache, intestinal problems, rashes, skin disorders and many other more serious physical problems, including heart disease. At the same time, too much anger can cause a rise in blood pressure and the possibility of a stroke. Just as it can kill you, anger can make you lose control and kill someone else. The French recognize that anger is a safety-valve, built into our programme for psychological well-being and have tolerance for crimes of passion, but not every country is so broad-minded and anger can send you straight to the electric chair if you don't watch out!

Clearly, the trick with anger is to keep it in balance – have enough to express what is really felt, but not enough to get someone into trouble. We know we shouldn't bottle it up, but when a job is at stake it might seem more sensible to bite our tongue and pretend nothing happened. Inevitably, perhaps, in our nice civilized world, much anger remains unexpressed, festering away in our body and soul.

The colours of anger are red, black and white – as in 'to see red' and have a red face, have a black scowl of fury, or white clenched knuckles and a face white with rage. People can go very still and quiet – seething with anger, while others shake, tremble or feel weak. Some people express their anger at a moment's provocation, others bottle it up and explode like a volcano hours, days or weeks later while others still tuck it away and pretend they don't have it. Everyone reacts in a different way. And there are people who seem to be angry for no reason at all, or no reason they have yet understood. And there are people who are angry with others; and those who are angry with themselves.

The essential oils have been arranged in this section under three categories: essential oils to calm down anger; essential oils to help cope with anger; and essential oils to help express anger. We start with the oils which can help calm an angry person down, long enough for them to look at the heart of the matter and hopefully try to find help:

ESSENTIAL OILS TO CALM DOWN FEELINGS OF ANGER

Chamomile Roman, Chamomile German, Tuberose, Linden Blossom, Vetiver, Lavender, Bergamot, Rose Maroc, Rose Otto, Petitgrain, Patchouli

There are many ways of coping with anger, from relaxation techniques, yoga, holding your breath, doing deep breathing exercises, counting to ten and punching a cushion instead of a head. I know a man who used to jump in his fast car when he had an angry row with his wife and drive like a maniac until he cooled down. He and quite a few other people were lucky they didn't end up dead. Essential oils are a much safer bet! Choose from the following list:

ESSENTIAL OILS TO HELP COPE WITH ANGER

Chamomile Roman, Linden Bossom, Vetiver, Ylang Ylang, Rose Maroc, Valerian, Black Pepper, Spikenard, Myrtle, Benzoin, Bergamot

The following quantities of oils can each be blended with 30 ml of base oil for a massage, or made into a synergistic blend and used in other methods – for quantities to use see Chart 5.1.

COPING WITH ANGER 1		COPING WITH ANGER 2	
Spikenard	10 drops	Rose Maroc	10 drops
Chamomile Roman	10 drops	Chamomile Roman	2 drops
Bergamot	10 drops	Linden Blossom	10 drops

ESSENTIAL OILS TO HELP RELEASE UNEXPRESSED ANGER

Tuberose, Black Pepper, Ginger, Ormenis Flower, Cedarwood, Patchouli, Clove

RELEASING UNEXPRESSED ANGER

BLEND 1		BLEND 2	
Ormenis Flower	*15 drops*	*Patchouli*	*15 drops*
Ginger	*5 drops*	*Tuberose*	*5 drops*
Black Pepper	*5 drops*	*Clove*	*1 drop*

ANXIETY

Anxiety is, in a sense, the heightened awareness of things that can go wrong. It is a normal component of the human being and serves to keep us on our toes. But for whatever reason, and there may be more than one, our sense of impending doom balloons out, so to speak, inside us, filling us with unease, and even fear. In some instances the impending doom is a real event – a forthcoming exam, driving test or, for authors, deadline! For others, it's just a daily generalized feeling of unease – mild to intense – about everything – the safety of the family, the state of everyone's health, financial problems or whatever – brought on by years of actual hard life experience. We can only take so much.

You can guess you're pretty anxious if you find yourself sighing a lot, gasping for breath or needing to take in large chunks of air. It might even be that you're running to the toilet all the time, getting headaches or back pain, or just can't relax. A sense of tiredness is common, as is restlessness, even tremors. Anxiety can make you dizzy, perspire or blush, and it can raise your blood pressure. One can feel dry in the mouth, or belch a lot, feel nauseous, get diarrhoea, vomit. The stomach muscles can tighten up in a spasm, causing terrible pain. Anxiety causes stabbing pains in the chest, and stronger, faster heartbeats. It can make a person feel so unwell they seriously wonder if there isn't something physical wrong – which causes more anxiety, of course. So then you can't sleep well at night. And these are just some of the symptoms!

The real cure for anxiety is to win the lottery, get a guarantee from an angel that no member of your family will have an accident or get ill ever again, and hear on the news that all wars have stopped. But frankly, I don't think it's going to happen. Somehow we'll just have to continue coping as best we can. Fortunately, however, nature's little helpmates, the essential oils, can do a lot to help.

Because there are so many symptoms of anxiety, I am breaking this section into four different types, with blends for each. But we start with a general list of essential oils that can deflate the anxiety, and bring it down to a normal level.

Bergamot

ESSENTIAL OILS TO HELP RELIEVE GENERAL ANXIETY

*Bergamot, Lavender, Mandarin, Sandalwood, Chamomile Roman,
Vetiver, Cedarwood, Neroli, Rose Otto, Melissa, Geranium,
Juniper, Frankincense, Patchouli, Clary Sage*

TENSE ANXIETY – TYPE 1

Symptoms: bodily tension, muscle pain, aches, sore body

Essential oils: Sandalwood, Lavender, Clary Sage,
Chamomile Roman, Patchouli

RESTLESS ANXIETY – TYPE 2

*Symptoms: over activity, sweating, palpitations, dizziness, lump in
throat, frequent urination or diarrhoea (over activity of the
autonomic nervous system), upset stomach*

Essential oils: Vetiver, Cedarwood, Juniper, Chamomile Roman,
Frankincense

APPREHENSIVE ANXIETY – TYPE 3

*Symptoms: unease, apprehension, worrying, brooding, over-
anxious, paranoia, sense of foreboding*

Essential oils: Bergamot, Lavender, Neroli, Rose Otto, Melissa,
Geranium

REPRESSED ANXIETY – TYPE 4

*Symptoms: feeling on edge, irritable, difficulty in concentrating,
insomnia, feeling exhausted all the time*

Essential oils: Bergamot, Melissa, Neroli, Rose Otto, Sandalwood,
Vetiver, Cedarwood

The following blends relate to the four anxiety types above.
The quantities given here could be blended with 30 ml base oil

to make a massage oil, or use these proportions to make a synergistic blend, which can be used in the bath, or in a diffuser or other room method, or inhaled from a tissue. See Chart 5.1 for quantities to use.

TENSE ANXIETY – TYPE 1		RESTLESS ANXIETY – TYPE 2	
Clary Sage	10 drops	Vetiver	5 drops
Lavender	15 drops	Juniper	10 drops
Chamomile Roman	5 drops	Cedarwood	15 drops

APPREHENSIVE ANXIETY – TYPE 3		REPRESSED ANXIETY – TYPE 4	
Bergamot	15 drops	Neroli	10 drops
Lavender	5 drops	Rose Otto	10 drops
Geranium	10 drops	Bergamot	10 drops

APATHY

The word 'apathy' derives from the Greek word for feeling, '*pathos*', and means to be without feeling – without joy, passion, excitement, and without sadness, hurt and pain. It can be brought on by various emotional situations including romantic heartache, depression, worthlessness and guilt, as well as by illness and pain. Apathetic people are difficult to get motivated, and they watch the news and say 'so what?' Nothing moves them. They don't care about their appearance, or whether they're going to lose their job, or what they're going to eat tonight. Apathetic people slump around the place, with an air of weariness and listlessness around them, like a little grey fog. Worse than this, they're like emotional zombies – scaringly half-dead!

Essential oils can certainly help in cases of apathy, but the person needs to examine why they are feeling so isolated, and ask what could have caused it in the first place. Counselling may be required, or a physical examination because apathy can have an underlying physical cause.

ESSENTIAL OILS TO HELP FIGHT APATHY

Cardamon, Lemon, Ginger, Black Pepper, Bergamot, Orange, Jasmine, Rose Otto, Rose Maroc, Ormenis Flower, Basil, Peppermint

Choose from the following blends which most seems appropriate and use these quantities diluted with a base oil to make a massage oil, or make up a synergistic blend using these proportions and use it diffused in the atmosphere, at home or at work, or sniffed from a tissue.

GENERAL APATHY		APATHY WITH EXTRA INDIFFERENCE	
Basil	5 drops	*Cardamon*	15 drops
Bergamot	10 drops	*Ginger*	10 drops
Cardamon	15 drops	*Orange*	5 drops

APATHY WITH DEPRESSION	
Black Pepper	15 drops
Basil	5 drops
Bergamot	10 drops

BEREAVEMENT

The people we love are our only true security in this life and it is they who make life loving and worth living, and help it make sense. When they go, a part of us goes too – perhaps a very large part, but all the structures of our life go as well – the security, the love and the sense of it all. Whatever the circumstances of the death, bereavement is the most profound loss, a wrenching away of a part of us, and of course it hurts terribly.

I can't imagine the pain of losing a child, but thousands of parents must go through this ghastly fate each year, while tens of thousands of us will lose a parent, our anchor in life. As each death is such an individual experience, no person can be expected to react in a predictable way. I've known people throw themselves into work trying to blank out the pain, and others who sit in a chair for months not saying a word. Everyone has to work it through in their own way. Sometimes bereavement counselling can help and in the addresses section you can find the contact addresses for the National Associations of Widows, Stillbirth and Neonatal Death Society and Age Concern, who may all be able to put people in touch with services in their area. Perhaps the worst experience is for those who have unfinished emotional business with the deceased, and who never had the chance to say 'goodbye' and 'I love you'. For sure, around the experience of death there are many emotions aside from sheer, awful empty grief – there could be guilt and remorse too.

Clearly, essential oils can only soften the terrible blow of bereavement and they cannot fill the gap. But many people have found them a tremendous support and comfort during these terrible times, and through the lonely times ahead. They are particularly effective in baths or massage oils. Also, gently diffused in a room, they can help provide a calm and comforting atmosphere in which the mourning process can take place.

ESSENTIAL OILS TO USE IN BEREAVEMENT

Benzoin, Rose Otto, Neroli, Linden Blossom, Lavender, Melissa, Mandarin, Chamomile Roman, Vetiver, Patchouli, Cypress, Rose Maroc, Geranium

You can make up individual blends from the above list, or by choosing oils from other sections in this chapter – such as those in *Grief, Loss, Sorrow, Depression, Anger, Anxiety* and *Insomnia*, depending on the emotions you are going through at any particular time, which are probably going to change with the process of mourning. Alternatively, use one of the comforting ones below. Blend these quantities with 30 ml base oil to make a massage oil, or use these proportions to make a synergistic blend of oils, which can be used in any of the other methods. See Chart 5.1 for quantities to use.

COMFORTING BLEND 1		COMFORTING BLEND 2	
Benzoin	*5 drops*	*Mandarin*	*15 drops*
Rose Otto	*12 drops*	*Geranium*	*8 drops*
Chamomile Roman	*2 drops*	*Patchouli*	*7 drops*
Mandarin	*2 drops*		

COMFORTING BLEND 3		COMFORTING BLEND 4	
Neroli	*12 drops*	*Vetiver*	*5 drops*
Linden Blossom	*5 drops*	*Geranium*	*20 drops*
Melissa	*8 drops*	*Patchouli*	*5 drops*

BREAKDOWN

If you haven't suffered a breakdown it can be very difficult to understand just how that person might feel, and identify with the torment they are going through. They, meanwhile, may not be able to express all the fears and emotions they are feeling. For the sufferer, it is a very lonely business, and for the family a very bewildering one. Breakdowns happen to all kinds of people – smart and stupid, old and young, fat and thin. I heard of a woman recently – a head of department at a university, juggling her work with two children – who recently had a breakdown. She seemed to be fine and was calmly going about her job with her usual efficiency and good-natured outlook but at home she was building huge edifices on the kitchen table, out of anything and everything, and taking it all rather too seriously – as if this were her *real* job. She had cracked, but it took her family a few days fully to realize what was going on. Eventually, after some high trauma, she was led away, as they say, by the men in white coats, with her husband pleading with her to sign the paper saying she was booking herself in for treatment, not being sectioned under the Mental Health Act. This dramatic scene would have been quite unthinkable to the family just a short week earlier. The woman *seemed* to be coping. She was her usual laid-back, smiling self, a master at covering up what anguish was going on beneath – like so many of us. In fact, this breakdown will probably force her to face the real problem in her life.

'Nervous breakdown' is a vague, non-medical term for the onset of a wide variety of problems usually related to our situation and circumstances, and our ability to cope with them. With the vast majority of people, the breakdown is just a hiccup in an otherwise normal life – a break caused by mental stress that can in time heal. 'Mental breakdown', on the other hand, can take away all mental reasoning, all sense of self, of the world and reality and, sadly, some people never really recover. Many others, of course, do.

Any kind of breakdown requires professional help, comfort, care and attention. Gentleness and compassion are the order of the day. Once the crisis is over and the recovery period has begun, essential oils can be used in a massage oil for use on the hands, feet and, possibly, neck, shoulders and forearms, using gentle stroking movements known to masseurs as 'effleurage'. Essential oil baths are particularly welcoming and help the person tremendously in the return to full mental health. Also, diffusing essential oils in the atmosphere is very beneficial.

Psychiatric units and hospitals are often unwelcoming places, certainly the ones I have visited, and if the management budget can't stretch to a lick of paint, a pleasant ambience can be created quite cheaply by using essential oils. Ideally, commercial size diffusers could be installed, but if not, use the Landel diffuser – one that involves no fire or electricity. See Appendix III, for the supplier.

People who have undergone a breakdown often experience a heightened sense of smell, or have smell hallucinations. These effects may sometimes be related to the drugs being used. Clearly then, using aroma in these circumstances has to be done with sensitivity, and consultation with the patient(s). Essential oils can be chosen from appropriate lists, according to the symptoms, or taken from the following lists:

ESSENTIAL OILS FOR USE IN CASES OF GENERAL BREAKDOWN

Lavender, Clary Sage, Lemon, Orange, Chamomile Roman, Geranium, Neroli, Helichrysum

ESSENTIAL OILS FOR USE IN CASES OF EMOTIONAL BREAKDOWN

Lavender, Cypress, Geranium, Sandalwood, Rose Otto, Mandarin, Benzoin, Neroli, Chamomile Roman

For quantities to use, and methods, see Chart 5.1.

BURN-OUT

Burn-out is usually thought of as a physical thing, but burn-out can relate to the emotional and mental processes, which then affect the physical. You can get burn-out when there are no more tears to cry, no feelings any more, just emotional exhaustion. And the thing is, when the emotions shut down, so does the body!

Someone could get burn-out, for example, after caring for a sick partner or relative with a terminal illness, perhaps over a long time. This can use up all one's reserves of compassion in coping with the person's needs, plus there is the distressing experience of watching the loved one die. After this, emotional burn-out is, understandably, quite common. But there are many other situations which might cause emotional burn-out, after a lost love perhaps, or even during particularly deep times of self-examination or thinking emotionally about close family members. We are emotional beings, and sometimes our emotions come in for excessive use, leaving a state of emptiness or numbness.

Burn-out can paralyse a person, leaving them a dead-weight in a chair, or simply feeling exhausted and depressed – to greater or lesser degree. All the feelings that go to make up a human personality seem missing, disappeared somewhere.

Also, people can have a sense of being in a vacuum, or a glass bubble – unable, as the song goes, to reach out and touch somebody's hand. The feelings are there, of course, but the emotional side has closed down for a while, to recharge the batteries. The following essential oils would be a good choice for those with all types of emotional burn-out, including that experienced by carers of the terminally ill.

ESSENTIAL OILS TO HELP LESSEN THE EFFECT OF EMOTIONAL BURN-OUT

Vetiver, Bergamot, Rose Otto, Neroli, Linden Blossom, Melissa, Patchouli, Sandalwood, Hyacinth, Marjoram, Lavender, Benzoin, Clary Sage, Helichrysum, Lemon, Frankincense, Chamomile Roman, Petitgrain, Ginger, Jasmine

The following two blends are for general emotional burn-out and they are half measures because, with burn-out, it is better to start softly, using only 15 drops of essential oil to the usual 30 ml base vegetable oil for a massage oil, and if you make a synergistic blend, only use 1–2 drops in the bath or 1–2 drops diffused in the atmosphere.

BURN-OUT 1		BURN-OUT 2	
Vetiver	*2 drops*	*Lavender*	*3 drops*
Bergamot	*10 drops*	*Clary Sage*	*2 drops*
Lavender	*3 drops*	*Marjoram*	*3 drops*
		Lemon	*7 drops*

As time goes on you can add to the number of drops of essential oils in the blend, up to the usual 30 drops of essential oil to 30 ml base oil – which is a general rule of 1:1 (1 drop essential oil to 1 ml vegetable oil). You can refer to other sections in this book and choose which essential oils to add, those which seem appropriate for you, or look at the chart at the back of the book.

CONFUSION

The symptoms of confusion are not remembering places, being unable to finish or even start simple tasks, giving the wrong or inappropriate answers to questions, and feeling in a muddle and not being able to make sense out of anything. Confusion can be caused by stress, overwork, physical or mental illness, by head injury or senile dementia. The morphine given for pain relief sometimes can produce confusion, while certain medical conditions may lead into confusion and then dementia. Confusion can also be caused by epileptic fits, drug overdose, drug addiction, depression and schizophrenia. Sometimes loss of memory and confusion go together, but not always.

If the confusion has been caused by something physical there is often an associated high temperature and a general feeling of being unwell. Although such confusion can come on rapidly and be alarming, it might last only a few days. However, it might indicate a developing serious condition and medical attention should be sought immediately.

If there is a high temperature you can help to bring it down by removing the clothing and sponging the body down with a solution of 2 drops of essential oil of eucalyptus in 1 litre of cool water. If the confusion has been caused by a head injury, drug overdose, or insulin deficiency, again the doctor should be called immediately. Clearly, however, in the elderly, senile dementia might be progressive.

The essential oils are, here, being recommended for situations in which there is no clinical reason for the confusion, when they can help us focus and concentrate.

ESSENTIAL OILS THAT MAY HELP WITH CONFUSION

Cardamon, Ginger, Black Pepper, Bergamot, Geranium, Petitgrain, Helichrysum, Grapefruit, Ormenis Flower, Basil, Rosemary, Peppermint, Cypress, Juniper, Pine, Thyme Linalol, Lavender

For the kind of confusion that hits us all at some point in our lives, perhaps as a result of overwork, or of stress and anxiety, the following blend should help. These quantities can be added to 30 ml base oil to make a massage oil, or make a synergistic blend using these proportions for use in the diffuser or inhalation methods. See Chart 5.1 for quantities to use. Do not use these synergistic blends or basil or peppermint in the bath.

CONFUSION BLEND 1		CONFUSION BLEND 2	
Cardamon	13 drops	Basil	7 drops
Black Pepper	5 drops	Helichrysum	5 drops
Ginger	4 drops	Grapefruit	10 drops
Grapefruit	8 drops	Ginger	8 drops

DEJECTION

To be dejected is to feel disheartened and dispirited, possibly as a result of being rejected in some sense – not appreciated at work, cast away by a lover, even perhaps profoundly disappointed by the negativity one experiences in life in general. Dejected people are weakened by their experience and seem to have had the sparkle taken out of them – a result of the spirit and emotional-heart being damaged. People can have an 'air of dejection' about them which seems to permeate the things they do, objects they make and even meals they cook. One can practically taste the dejection in the food!

One of the best things for dejection is sunshine – lots of it! Also, bright colours really help – so pull out those old Hawaiian shirts! Or if that's too much, at least wear a bright, colourful scarf or tie. These are the essential oils that can help, use them in all the usual ways:

ESSENTIAL OILS THAT CAN HELP DISPEL FEELINGS OF DEJECTION

Bergamot, Frankincense, Grapefruit, Mandarin, Geranium, Nutmeg, Mimosa, Linden Blossom, Orange, Rose Maroc, Jasmine, Petitgrain, Neroli, Ylang Ylang

DELIRIUM

Delirium is a state of acute mental confusion and to suggest it can be controlled with essential oils would be totally wrong. However, essential oils can help bring down the temperature often associated with it, and reduce the restlessness, and so it has been included here. Delirium can be precipitated by the use of alcohol over long periods, and by drugs and certain poisons; it can also develop after major surgery – notably in children and the elderly. Most importantly, it can give evidence of serious physical disorder and a doctor must be called straight away. Shortage of oxygen and brain damage can both cause delirium, while many elderly people also sometimes get delirious as a consequence of dementia.

In delirium, all normal conscious thought is disrupted, there is memory loss and mental confusion. Disorientation and restlessness are classic symptoms, anxiety and mood swings are common, shakes and tremors a possibility. In severe cases, there could be illusions or hallucinations, which are often monstrous and terrifying. Panic and shouting are not uncommon.

After calling a doctor, take the temperature. If it is too high, try to help bring it down by sponging the person with 2 drops of eucalyptus mixed in with 1 litre of cool water. You could also diffuse a cooling essential oil in the atmosphere – such as peppermint or eucalyptus. If there is no temperature and the person is restless, diffuse lavender essential oil in the room as this may have a calming effect.

ESSENTIAL OILS TO USE IN CASES OF DELIRIUM

Peppermint, Eucalyptus Globulus, Eucalyptus Radiata, Lavender, Marjoram

Delirium Tremens

The 'DTs', as they're known, affect those going through drug withdrawal and chronic alcoholics – especially after a period of abstinence. The classic picture of DTs is of someone brushing imaginary insects off their sleeves, terrified. The DT sufferer is in a frightening world of confusion, and they're shaking. Disorientation, sleeplessness, restlessness and agitation is usual, as is fever, sweating, and a faster heartbeat. Vivid visual and sometimes auditory hallucinations make life a nightmare. Not surprisingly, the person sometimes gets aggressive.

Dehydration is a problem, and an attack of the DTs might require a stay in hospital to rehydrate, as well as to sedate and rest. If someone suffers an attack, the doctor must be called immediately. Giving soothing hand and foot massages might help overcome the effects of withdrawal; or for the person to use essential oils in the bath. Alcoholics have a severe shortage of thiamine, which is helped by giving vitamin B complex. Calming essential oils can be diffused in the atmosphere, used in a bath, or in a massage oil, or a drop can be placed on a pillow or cushion. Use the essential oils singly, on their own, not in mixes, and make sure the person with delirium tremens likes the fragrance. Lavender and lemon have been found particularly useful in cases of alcohol withdrawal (see *Addiction*) and the DTs, but all the following oils are useful:

ESSENTIAL OILS TO USE IN CASES OF DELIRIUM TREMENS

Lavender, Petitgrain, Lemon, Chamomile Roman, Marjoram, Valerian, Geranium

DEMENTIA AND ALZHEIMER'S DISEASE

Dementia used to be thought of as a disease of old age but, because of the HIV virus, many young people are now experiencing dementia – which perhaps fills them with more dread than any other symptom of their illness. To slowly lose one's mental capacity is bad enough at an old age, but when a person is in their thirties, it is really tragic. Dementia can also affect people who have suffered strokes, both young and old, and those who have Alzheimer's. For anyone looking after a loved one with dementia, the whole experience is terribly upsetting as the person becomes a shadow of their former selves – not remembering recent events, getting lost in familiar surroundings, losing sense of time, and not even recognizing the caring family and friends who are offering their support. It is appalling to watch a loved one literally lose their mind, slowly day by day, but for the person suffering from dementia, who must be at least occasionally aware of slipping mentally away, it must be horrific, like slipping into a black hole.

Unfortunately, there is no cure for dementia unless it is caused by encephalitis, syphilis, anaemia, or several other conditions which can be treated. Most cases get worse. The best we can do for them is care in a practical sense, by way of feeding, cleaning and so forth. Because of the powerful olfactory link with memory, aromas might be the last link between the real experienced world, and the mind which is now hidden within. Aroma may be the last thing the sufferer can hold on to. Plus essential oils have other benefits too. However, aroma preference is a very powerful thing, and the person should be consulted if essential oils are to be used. A choice of aromas could be offered – if they sniff in deeply and nod their head, you can guess they like it, but if they turn up their nose and grimace, they don't.

Essential oils can be used diffused in the atmosphere, dropped in warm baths, or made into a massage oil, which is very effective in hand and foot massages. There is no need to do a body massage and if you are a carer, perhaps temporary, you are a stranger, essentially, and a body massage could be seen as invasion. But a regular hand massage from a caring person would be very welcome, and the aroma would provide a continuity link with regular care, which would be beneficial. What I mean by that is that the person suffering from dementia will come to associate the aroma with a particular person – the carer – and 'recognize' them by smell, if not by face. Choose oils from the *Concentration, Confusion*, and *Memory* sections, or from the lists below. We start with a general list for oils that are helpful:

ESSENTIAL OILS TO HELP IN CASES OF DEMENTIA

Basil, Cardamon, Ginger, Black Pepper, Rosemary, Rose Otto

The following floral oils are particularly appreciated by women and they are generally good in massage oils for restlessness and tremors.

GENTLE ESSENTIAL OILS TO HELP IN CASES OF RESTLESSNESS AND TREMORS

Rose Otto, Neroli, Lavender, Geranium, Jasmine, Chamomile Roman

Appetite can be stimulated by diffusing the following fruit and spice essential oils in the atmosphere, and these aromas tend to bring back memories, which is a good thing. These oils are listed here:

APPETITE STIMULANT AND MEMORY-EVOKING ESSENTIAL OILS

Lemon, Orange, Lime, Grapefruit, Nutmeg, Cinnamon, Clove, Ginger, Coriander, Cardamon, Black Pepper

ADDITIONAL MEMORY-EVOKING ESSENTIAL OILS

Basil, Rosemary

One thing which might be helpful in the fight to hold off dementia is ginkgo biloba, a plant widely used by naturopaths all over the world, and available from health food shops. An excellent review of ginkgo's effectiveness against 'cerebral insufficiency' appeared in *The Lancet*[2] and should be referred to by all who care for those suffering with dementia. 'Cerebral insufficiency' is defined as 'absentmindedness, anxiety, confusion, decreased physical performance, depressive mood, difficulty in concentrating, difficulty in remembering, dizziness, headache, lack of energy, tinnitus and tiredness'. A great deal of research has now been carried out on ginkgo, all over the world, and its benefits are well established. Also, there have been no reports of any side-effects. It's said that the ginkgo biloba tree is the oldest tree known (possibly 160 million years old!), and clearly it still has much to offer mankind. Vitamin supplements are also useful, such as a vitamin B complex, vitamins C and E, plus a multi-mineral.

Dementia – The Carers

Carers of people with dementia often have to endure a great deal. Aside from the physical work, there is the fact that it can make the person uncharacteristically difficult – they can make unreasonable demands, and accusations. The carer is tormented by the sadness of watching and feeling the loved one slowly lose touch, and on top of that, they may feel guilty – probably for no good reason.

Choose gentle oils that help deal with the anxiety, stresses and strains of coping with delirium on a regular basis; and those which help with the sadness inevitably felt as someone experiences a loved one mentally and emotionally drifting away. Use the oils in all the usual methods. The following quantities can be blended with 30 ml base oil, or make a synergistic blend using these proportions. For quantities to use, see Chart 5.1.

CARERS' GENTLE COMFORT			
BLEND 1		BLEND 2	
Geranium	7 drops	Benzoin	10 drops
Patchouli	5 drops	Rose Maroc	7 drops
Bergamot	8 drops	Orange	6 drops
Rose Maroc	10 drops	Jasmine	7 drops

DEPRESSION

The 'Black Dog', as Winston Churchill called it, hits between 5–15 per cent of people in Britain at some time in their lives according to various estimates, although the figure may be higher than this because it's thought that men don't always go to the doctor and report their symptoms, i.e. *feelings* – perhaps turning to drink or violence instead. Some 1–2 per cent of depressed persons are classified as bi-polar or manic depressive because they have sharp mood and activity swings.

The main symptoms of depression are as you would expect – feelings of sadness, hopelessness and pessimism. Another classic symptom is no longer having a positive interest in life's pleasures, including sex. Sufferers may additionally experience the slowing down of physical or mental actions, tiredness, loss of concentration, indecision, and impaired memory. Sometimes the depressed person finds themselves crying for no apparent reason, and unable to control the tears. Worthlessness and guilt – excessive and/or inappropriate – often accompany depression, making it easy for someone to say to themselves, 'Oh, they'd be better off without me', and this is the biggest danger of depression – suicide – which is why it must be taken seriously, and why help must be sought.

We all get depressed sometimes but we can usually be brought out of it by a holiday or even a good evening out with friends. These measures don't help the depressive at all – and is further evidence that they need help. People do react to depression in different ways, particularly in their eating and sleep patterns – which can be either to overeat or not to eat, and either to oversleep or not be able to sleep.

In 1989 clinicians in America carried out a survey amongst 1,800 managers and engineers at the huge Westinghouse Electric corporation, to try and establish the degree of depression experienced by them. Psychiatry professor Evelyn Bromet of New York University, who carried out the research, found that 23 per cent of people interviewed had experienced an episode of major depression in their life, a result she called 'astounding'. Depression often hits people who are particularly ambitious or hardworking, both young and old. In an article about depression among executives, the American magazine *Fortune* included an interview with one man who had been at the top of his career, who had never been ill but who suddenly couldn't eat or sleep. He said, 'I could barely think. I'd stare at six pairs of identical white underwear in the morning and couldn't decide which pair to put on.' For him, and for many others, the depression came on without apparent cause. This is known as endogenous depression, while depression that results from an identifiable event is called exogenous depression. Strangely perhaps, depression can stem from both good and bad life-changes, from a promotion or a redundancy, and from a birth as well as a death. However, depression usually has no one identifiable cause and just comes, appropriately, 'from the blue', because that's what it is – a major case of the blues.

Anyone who feels depressed, for whatever apparent reason, should certainly seek medical advice because there is a chance that there is an underlying physical disorder at fault, possibly involving the thyroid gland, and making depression a form of hormonal imbalance (of which we are also aware in post-natal depression). In one unconfirmed report in the American press I saw that a study by the University of Miami School of Medicine has shown that nearly half the people in their sample diagnosed as having severe depression actually had thyroid problems. They were treated with thyroid hormones for two months, and their depression began to lift after the fourth week. Another interesting study by psychologists David Roth and David Holmes at the University of Kansas showed that students suffering from the blues were not helped by relaxation training but were helped by aerobic exercise, so if you're too depressed to get up and go to aerobic classes, buy a workout video for home.

However, this might sound like too much effort for most depressives, who can get so low they can hardly get out of bed. As one sufferer so eloquently put it: 'Depression should have a blacker name. It is a disease which shrinks the spirit and sucks the colour from life.'[3] How do you get out of that? The man who wrote that was helped by anti-depressants, as many people have been. There does, however, seem to be some disagreement over how long the drugs should be used, and at what dose. And although the dosage doesn't have to be increased over time to achieve the same effectiveness, they are still addictive, and one has to come off them very slowly. (See *Addiction.*) The old generation of anti-depressants, the tricyclics and enzymatic MAO (monoamine oxidase) inhibitors have been put in the shadow recently by the new generation of 'selective serotonin re-uptake inhibitors'. Since the introduction in America of the first of these drugs, Prozac in 1988, at least seven separate serotonin receptors have been identified by scientists. This illustrates that this whole area of neuro-transmitter research is extremely new, and as I discussed earlier, we have much to learn.

As for the natural pharmacopoeia, some interesting research comes from Dr Tanaka *et al.* at Kyoto University, Japan. They found that the root of *Glycyrrhiza uralensis*, a species of liquorice widely used in Chinese medicine, has MAO inhibiting effects. One derivative of the plant extract is 450 times as effective as a standard MAO inhibitor.[4] Another natural anti-depressant is the amino acid tryptophan, which is converted into an intermediate product known as 5-HTP, from which it becomes serotonin. Studies of dieters have shown them to have lower levels of tryptophan, which may explain why dieters get depressed. In some countries tryptophan can be bought over the counter as a food supplement, but it was taken off the market in Britain in 1990 for some unknown reason, which the regulatory bodies may be able to explain. If it's any consolation, bananas are packed with tryptophan.

Depression, then, might be caused by tryptophan deficiency (probably not treatable with a bunch of bananas), by thyroid problems, by a genetic factor, by problems in life – either specific or cumulative, by changes in life – either good or bad, or for no apparent reason at all. Probably, not all these people can be helped by psychotherapy, but certainly some can, especially if they've been through a bad life experience. Drugs clearly have a place in the treatment of depression, and the first point here is to make sure the doctor doesn't give you tranquillizers, which are likely to slow you down further. At least, there have been many reports in the press about misdiagnosis in depression. You know your feelings best; refer to the *Anxiety* section, and see the difference in symptoms.

Anti-depressants don't have a street value as illicit drugs because they don't do anything to you unless the body needs it – *that's the theory anyway* – so they are being recommended as a diagnostic tool. If the person responds favourably to the serotonin uptake inhibitor, they were depressed and needed it. If they were 'normal', they wouldn't need it and the drug will do nothing for them. What all the anti-depressants do is alter the uptake of a variety of brain chemicals.

The 'tricyclics', which have a common core chemical structure, work in different ways: one drug will block the re-uptake of norepinephrine and serotonin, but not dopamine; another blocks the re-uptake of serotonin; while another has an effect on the uptake of norepinephrine, and so on. We're talking about a lot of fine-tuning going on here, and it helps to have a doctor who knows the ins and outs of antidepressant drugs (and advises on their side effects!). Balance is all. There are now a dozen serotonin-related drugs available, some increasing the level of it – sometimes at specific receptor sites, and others lowering the level at specific receptors. With all these options, it is possible there's a drug which can suit a depressive's requirements, the trick is finding it and staying on it only as long as absolutely required. Addiction can become a problem and the new drugs are by definition untested by time and may hold some surprises in terms of long-term effect. We just don't know. Having said that, I would not recommend anyone to stop taking anti-depressant medication without medical advice.

If you can as a therapy complementary to medical care, I recommend you visit an aromatherapist who can offer support and encouragement, as well as the benefits of therapeutic touch and essential oils. As depressives often have trouble receiving loving touch, an aromatherapy treatment can be a great help in overcoming that barrier. Also, friends of depressives should seek them out and lend a listening ear. Time and love are the greatest gifts and although the depressive will not be able to express their thanks, your concern will be a vital component in their recovery.

Essential oils can help in cases of depression brought about by trauma – reactive or exogenous depression as it used to be called, although there are usually many different elements to depression and each case should be treated differently. The symptoms can also be cross-referenced with the charts on pages 309–32 and 530–49. Following this general section there are additional recommendations for types of depression classified as W*eepy*, *Agitated* or *Anxious*, *Lethargic* and *Hysterical* – please refer to them also. *Manic Depressive*

Psychosis is another type of depression altogether and is discussed page on 214. However, there follows here a list of essential oils which could be called 'General' oils for depression, which have been traditionally shown in aromatherapy to be effective in the treatment of depression. They will not provide a magic cure but will definitely support and complement any other therapy or help in which the depressed person may be engaged:

ESSENTIAL OILS USED TRADITIONALLY IN AROMATHERAPY FOR DEPRESSION

Mandarin, Chamomile Roman, Lemon, Bergamot, Grapefruit, Orange, Jasmine, Ylang Ylang, Rose Otto, Rose Maroc, Neroli, Geranium, Petitgrain, Helichrysum, Eucalyptus Citrodora, Sandalwood, Clary Sage, Marjoram, Lavender, Frankincense

The quantities in the following blends can be diluted with 30 ml of base oil to make a massage oil to use on yourself, or make a synergistic blend of oils using these proportions and use the synergistic blend in room methods and inhalation methods, using the quantities recommended in Chart 5.1 *Methods of Use*. Blends 2, 3 and 4 can be used in baths.

CLASSIC BLENDS OF ESSENTIAL OILS TO USE IN CASES OF DEPRESSION

BLEND 1

Benzoin	10 drops
Black Pepper	5 drops
Geranium	15 drops

BLEND 2

Clary Sage	15 drops
Lavender	5 drops
Bergamot	10 drops

BLEND 3

Rose Otto	10 drops
Sandalwood	15 drops
Lemon	5 drops

BLEND 4

Ylang Ylang	5 drops
Nutmeg	10 drops
Coriander	15 drops

BLEND 5

Neroli	*20 drops*
Petitgrain	*10 drops*

Weepy Depression

The weepy depressive will appear normal, carry out their work as usual, function at home, tend to everyone's needs, and then burst into tears. Out and about in the street, this type of depressive can be set off into a tearful episode by the words in a song played through the musak system of a supermarket, or the sight of a couple in loving embrace in the park, or by a child trustfully grasping its mother's hand – anything, in fact, can spark off the tear response, even the smallest gesture of concern or thanks. This tearful response might not be classified as 'depression', but something is clearly wrong, and the person involved often feels desperate – they don't smile as much, they feel unwanted, and often wonder 'why bother living?' Because they usually function so well on a superficial level, few people around them realize what agony they're going through until suddenly they snap and end up in hospital (because they were found cuddling a lost kitten in the gutter, crying their eyes out). Worse still, they might try to kill themselves. Although this person feels depressed all the time they may not visit a doctor, and may shrug off the crying episodes as being 'out of sorts', not telling those around them how often they occur. Because they may seem to cope with life's stresses and strains so well, unless one actually witnesses these crying episodes, it's quite easy not to suspect that the person is really very depressed. Obviously, some people cry more easily than others, and we all occasionally cry with pain, rage, temper, frustration and sadness, but the weepy depressive finds that crying is the only way they can react, and that is a different thing altogether. Quite often, the weepy depressive person has been through an emotional trauma, or a series of traumas, and nobody, including themselves, has realized just how deeply it has affected them. Essential oils which may comfort and bring a sense of relief should be used.

ESSENTIAL OILS TO HELP IN CASES OF WEEPY DEPRESSION

Rose Otto, Neroli, Chamomile Roman, Sandalwood, Patchouli, Geranium, Ylang Ylang, Benzoin

Whatever the degree of weepy depression, start with the 'Light' blend. If things don't improve after three days, progress to the 'Moderate' blend. If things improve, stay on the 'Moderate' blend until you feel better, and then slowly return to the 'Light' blend. (When using the 'Moderate' blend, you can substitute 2 drops of an essential oil of your choice, relative to your condition, for the chamomile roman.) If, after a week on the 'Moderate' blend things do not improve, go on to the 'Deep' blend.

WEEPY DEPRESSION: 'LIGHT'		WEEPY DEPRESSION: 'MODERATE'	
Sandalwood	15 drops	Geranium	24 drops
Geranium	10 drops	Chamomile Roman*	2 drops
Ylang Ylang	5 drops	Benzoin	5 drops
		* This chamomile can be substituted with an oil suitable for the person.	

WEEPY DEPRESSION: 'DEEP'	
Rose Otto	10 drops
Neroli	2 drops
Sandalwood	3 drops

The quantities in the above blends can be diluted with 30 ml of base oil to make a massage oil, or make a synergistic blend of oils using these proportions and use a quantity of it in room methods, in baths and inhalation methods, using the quantities guidelines in Chart 5.1 *Methods of Use*.

Agitated or Anxious Depression

The agitated depressive can never sit still for long. They're constantly moving, fidgeting or twiddling with something –

with their hair, or fingers, pens on the desk ... anything. Although they're very busy, they're not really bothered whether a job has been done properly, so long as it's been done and they can move on to the next job. They'll have long faces, tired and drawn, but their minds will be racing ahead to all the plans and jobs they've got to get through. This type of depression causes symptoms such as pressure headaches, eye problems, twitches, ticks, jumping muscles and a feeling as if a tight band was being gripped around the skull. The head may feel like it's about to explode.

Agitated or anxious depression causes deep anguish which expresses itself as anger over the slightest thing. The person will despair if a little mark has been made on the furniture, as if it were the end of the world, and there could be rapid mood swings. The constant fretting will be covering up deep feelings of worthlessness and fear. There may be palpitations, and unexplained tears, and thoughts of suicide – 'just to get some peace'. The person suffering this type of depression usually throws themselves into work, as a means of covering up the underlying feeling of inadequacy.

ESSENTIAL OILS TO USE IN CASES OF AGITATED OR ANXIOUS DEPRESSION

Melissa, Cedarwood, Lavender, Chamomile Roman, Bergamot, Marjoram, Nutmeg, Ormenis Flower, Valerian, Lemon, Orange

Whatever the degree of agitated depression, start with the 'Light' blend. If things don't improve after three days, progress to the 'Moderate' blend. If things improve, stay on the 'Moderate' blend until you feel better, and then slowly return to the 'Light' blend. If, after a week on the 'Moderate' blend things do not improve, go on to the 'Deep' blend.

AGITATED DEPRESSION 'LIGHT'		AGITATED DEPRESSION 'MODERATE'	
Lavender	15 drops	Cedarwood	20 drops
Ormenis Flower	5 drops	Orange	10 drops
Bergamot	10 drops		

AGITATED DEPRESSION 'DEEP'	
Cedarwood	5 drops
Lemon	15 drops
Ormenis Flower	5 drops
Nutmeg	5 drops

The quantities in the above blends can be diluted with 30 ml of base oil to make a massage oil or make a synergistic blend of oils using these proportions and use in room methods, in baths and inhalation methods, using the quantity guidelines in Chart 5.1 *Methods of Use*.

Lethargic Depression

A lot of people have been struck with the depression that basically makes them want to stay in bed all day, with their head under the pillow. The lethargic depressive doesn't want to go anywhere or do anything. Everything is an effort, even switching on the TV. It's difficult to concentrate on books and papers. It can get very difficult to get out of bed in the morning, wash, and get dressed. Sleep beckons like welcoming arms. Important phone calls are ignored, vital letters never get written. Everything is overwhelming, including washing the hair. The sleeping causes more tiredness, more sleep, more tiredness, and when they're awake, they're asking everyone else to do things for them.

Lethargic depressives are not friendly – not at the moment anyway. Aside from the fact that they won't meet you in town for a social engagement, when you go to visit they're so unpleasant, you'd think they were trying to drive you away;

Helichrysum

which they are, of course, but it isn't personal. Anyone can get depressed like this. It might be a creative person being too critical of themselves, or a timid person who has been deeply hurt and emotionally wounded, even a selfish, dominating person – now criticizing everyone for not being able to do things properly, but having no energy for doing it themselves. However, many people have been diagnosed with (a lethargic form of) depression when they in fact had ME – myalgic encephalomyelitis, and vice versa, people with depression are diagnosed as having ME. The difference between them can be detected in the depressive's hopelessness and overwhelming desolation.

ESSENTIAL OILS TO USE IN CASES OF LETHARGIC DEPRESSION

Grapefruit, Cypress, Rosemary, Melissa, Helichrysum, Peppermint, Clary Sage, Eucalyptus Citriodora, Eucalyptus Piperita

Whatever the degree of lethargic depression, start with the 'Light' blend. If things don't improve after three days, progress to the 'Moderate' blend. If things improve, stay on the 'Moderate' blend until you feel better, and then slowly return to the 'Light' blend. If, after a week on the 'Moderate' blend things do not improve, go on to the 'Deep' blend.

LETHARGIC DEPRESSION 'LIGHT'		LETHARGIC DEPRESSION 'MODERATE'	
Grapefruit	*5 drops*	*Cypress*	*15 drops*
Rosemary	*10 drops*	*Eucalyptus Citriodora*	*15 drops*
Eucalyptus Citriodora	*15 drops*		

In the 'Moderate' blend, you can substitute another essential oil, relevant to the situations and difficulties that led to the depression. If you do substitute, reduce the cypress and eucalyptus citriodora to 10 drops each, and add another 10 drops of your chosen essential oil, making the usual total of 30 drops to 30ml base oil.

LETHARGIC DEPRESSION 'DEEP'	
Helichrysum	*15 drops*
Clary Sage	*5 drops*
Eucalyptus Citriodora	*10 drops*

The quantities in the above blends can be diluted with 30 ml of base oil to make a massage oil, or make a synergistic blend of oils using these proportions and use in room methods, bath and inhalation methods, using the quantities recommended in Chart 5.1 *Methods of Use*.

Hysterical Depression

It's sometimes difficult to know whether someone is suffering hysterical depression or having a bout of bad moods and temper. The hysterical depressive will exaggerate everything, want to be noticed, and will let everyone know they are suffering. They will heave great sighs, shout, scream and cry. They might be vivacious one minute and suicidal the next. Nobody will be able to do anything right. If you tread quietly, you'll be 'creeping about', and if you carry on normally, you'll be told you don't care, especially if you're cheerful.

Shy, introverted people can become hysterical depressives, just as the naturally exuberant personality can. It often affects people who have become depressed through circumstances such as job loss, bereavement, financial problems, relationship failure, misunderstandings and loneliness. The person may start having nightmares, and/or may become paranoid, talking of evil spirits and the like. Their rapid mood changes make one wonder if they aren't two people in one skin. They often become suspicious and jealous, and are constantly moaning, and feeling miserable – to the point of crying. Shaking and trembling can be signs of hysterical depression – which is a most unpleasant state to be in. These are some of the essential oils that may help:

ESSENTIAL OILS TO USE IN CASES OF HYSTERICAL DEPRESSION
Mandarin, Chamomile Roman, Linden Blossom, Vetiver, Bergamot, Neroli, Narcissus, Lavender, Marjoram, Valerian, Spikenard

Whatever the degree of hysterical depression, start with the 'Light' blend. If things don't improve after three days, progress to the 'Moderate' blend. If things improve, stay on the 'Moderate' blend until you feel better, and then slowly return to the 'Light' blend. If, after a week on the 'Moderate' blend things do not improve, go on to the 'Deep' blend.

HYSTERICAL DEPRESSION 'LIGHT'		HYSTERICAL DEPRESSION 'MODERATE'	
Lavender	10 drops	Neroli	15 drops
Chamomile Roman	15 drops	Mandarin	15 drops
Mandarin	5 drops		

HYSTERICAL DEPRESSION 'DEEP'	
Vetiver	15 drops
Bergamot	10 drops
Chamomile Roman	5 drops

The quantities in the above blends can be diluted with 30 ml of base oil to make a massage oil or make a synergistic blend of oils using these proportions and use in room methods, baths and inhalation methods, using the quantities recommended in Chart 5.1 *Methods of Use*.

Manic Depressive Psychosis

Extreme mood swings and behaviour patterns mark manic depressive psychosis, which is much rarer than the other forms of depression. During the 'mania' stage, a person will be at the peak of positivity – more talkative, their thoughts will be racing, they'll get involved in many projects, take on too much work – with unrealistic projections, and too many commitments all round. At this stage, the person often has an inflated self-esteem (which is why they think they can do so much), but they lose their power of judgement and even self-control. It is not unusual to find a manic depressive drinking to excess or spending money like it was going out of style. If they don't have money to spend, the manic depressive will use their credit cards, or borrow. They appear bright and cheerful, although perhaps laughing a little too loud or playing a little too hard. Anger can be quick to surface if the person is wronged, and even when they are not. They can become violent if denied something they want.

Then, as if by magic overnight, the manic depressive cannot get out of bed. They feel miserable, wretched, guilt-ridden, shameful, worthless and full of despair. Self-esteem is extremely low, and they blame themselves for everyone's troubles, and the world's troubles too. During this depressive stage of sadness and self-hatred, the sufferer also has a variety of physical symptoms, including insomnia or strange sleeping patterns, weight loss or gain, no appetite or constipation. Because of the risk of suicide, if this depressive stage continues for a long time, the person is often hospitalized and put on lithium salts or other drugs (which may have severe side effects during the manic stage).

Then, just as suddenly, the pendulum swings, and the person is rushing through life at a speed it's hard to catch up with. It's not known why these mood swings should happen, or be so severe, and many theories have been put forward. In some people, the condition may be caused by a defective gene (on chromosome 11), and changes in the level of the brain chemical dopamine may be involved. Intolerance to certain chemicals in modern life has also been suggested as a cause.

Complementary to medication, aromatherapy has helped many people through this condition, and in others, made life more tolerable. If the manic depressive is on any type of drug therapy, the usual number of essential oils used should be reduced by half – i.e. use a maximum of 15 drops of essential oil in 30 ml base oil for massage oils, and no more than 4–6 drops of a synergistic blend of oils in a bath. In a sense it's difficult for a manic depressive to treat themselves because they don't recognize that they need help when in the manic stage, and can't be bothered to do anything when in the depressive stage. However, if something can be done, start off with chamomile roman, lavender, geranium, mandarin, rose otto and neroli. They are included in this larger list of useful oils for this condition:

ESSENTIAL OILS IN CASES OF MANIC DEPRESSION

Chamomile Roman, Chamomile German, Frankincense, Geranium, Grapefruit, Mandarin, Rose Otto, Lavender, Lemon, Neroli, Patchouli, Sandalwood

During the manic stage, it's best to use a single oil – a maximum of 15 drops to 30 ml base oil for a massage oil, or 4 drops in a bath. Use lavender, chamomile roman, neroli or rose – alone. Rose is also helpful during the depressive stage – use 10 drops to 30 ml base oil. Alternatively, try one of these blends:

DEPRESSIVE STAGE 1		DEPRESSIVE STAGE 2	
Mandarin	*5 drops*	*Chamomile Roman*	*2 drops*
Geranium	*4 drops*	*Lavender*	*6 drops*
Lavender	*6 drops*	*Frankincense*	*4 drops*
		Geranium	*3 drops*

The quantities in the above blends can be diluted with 30 ml of base oil to make a massage oil, or make a synergistic blend of oils using these proportions and use in room methods, in the bath and inhalation methods, using half the quantities recommended in Chart 5.1 *Methods of Use*.

The essential oils can be varied, choosing from the list above, but cross-referencing with the symptoms mentioned throughout this book, and pages 309–32 and pages 530–49. For example, for the feeling of unworthiness or self-hatred, choose rose otto or geranium.

Vitamins are useful in this condition – especially those in the B Group, 1, 3 and 6, vitamins C and E, and also zinc, magnesium and calcium – which help sleep.

DOUBT

Doubt is a useful feeling, part of intuition. Being doubtful may prevent us entering a disastrous business deal, or prevent us making a mistake that could affect our future, or our relationships. When someone says, 'I have my doubts' about something, they are usually right to steer clear away. However, doubt can flood over into inappropriate areas so a person is in a state of uncertainty as to the truth or reality of anything. Trust, of course, goes out the window. Although it may be hard not to doubt people if you have been crossed or put at a disadvantage by someone, this only blanks out your intuition, of which doubt is but a part.

Diffuse the essential oils gently in the room, use them in the bath or give yourself a massage. Also see Chapter 7, *Emotional Healing – Confidence.*

ESSENTIAL OILS TO HELP BALANCE DOUBTFULNESS

Coriander, Basil, Frankincense, Benzoin, Angelica Seed,
Ylang Ylang, Litsea Cubeba*

* Should not be used in baths

The quantities in the following blends can be diluted with 30 ml of base oil to make a massage oil, or make a synergistic blend of oils using these proportions and use in room methods and inhalation methods. See Chart 5.1 for quantities to use.

FEELING DOUBTFUL 1		FEELING DOUBTFUL 2	
Frankincense	*15 drops*	*Coriander*	*20 drops*
Benzoin	*5 drops*	*Basil*	*5 drops*
Ylang Ylang	*10 drops*	*Angelica Seed*	*5 drops*

EMOTIONAL VIOLENCE

Emotional violence is probably far more widespread than anyone realizes. It can happen in the home, at school, at work, and can even come from so-called friends. Some people suffer emotional violence every minute of their lives, growing up in a house with antagonistic parents, perhaps, and then marrying someone with the same disposition – when if the verbal abuse isn't constant, the dread and anxiety of knowing it will start again is.

Emotional violence is not simply verbal abuse, but also malicious, purposeful violation of the emotional state. It is when someone knows our most vulnerable and sensitive emotional points and goes for them, viciously trying to put us down or hurt us. It could come in the form of words that cut through to the very soul, or a look that says 'you are dirt'. Emotional violence is the tool of the tyrant. And the sad thing is, it is usually perpetrated by the very people we love – our parents, partners, siblings, even children. So-called 'friends' are good at this too – especially if they know your secrets (and are threatening to tell your entire world).

Emotional violence is invisible – there are no black eyes or bruises to tell the tale – but it hurts far more and lasts much longer. The end result can be hopeless despair, anxiety, tension, and a lifetime of terror. The simple answer to the problem is to get away from the person who is doing it, but that is more easily said than done, especially if they are a parent, the mother or father of your children, or the girl you've been sitting next to in school. Counselling can help, as can classes in being assertive, but the real solution is to get out of the person's orbit ... to 'Tipp-Ex them out of your life', as one friend puts it. But this isn't always possible, and for every person day-dreaming about winning the lottery, I bet there is another planning their escape from some perpetrator of emotional violence!

Essential oils appear to help by cushioning the emotions, and the bathroom could become your refuge – particularly if you use the correct essential oils. Use the oils in the bath, lock the door, breathe the aroma in deeply, and practise a relaxation exercise. This escape may help you cope, and perhaps give you confidence to remove yourself from the emotional violator.

ESSENTIAL OILS TO HELP THOSE SUFFERING FROM EMOTIONAL VIOLENCE

Frankincense, Juniper, Carnation, Geranium, Rose Otto, Neroli, Chamomile Roman, Jasmine, Hyacinth, Benzoin, Melissa, Lavender

The essential oils can be used in all the usual methods but it is a good idea to make up a synergistic blend of oils which you can carry with you everywhere. Get a small bottle from the chemist and make up one of the following synergistic blends, using these proportions, or make up your own from the list above. Then sniff from the bottle whenever you feel the need, or put a couple of drops from the bottle onto a tissue and carry that in your pocket, and sniff from it when required.

EMOTIONAL VIOLENCE 1		EMOTIONAL VIOLENCE 2	
Frankincense	*10 drops*	*Chamomile Roman*	*5 drops*
Jasmine	*5 drops*	*Carnation*	*5 drops*
Melissa	*5 drops*	*Neroli*	*10 drops*

EMOTIONAL VIOLENCE 3	
Frankincense	*5 drops*
Juniper	*10 drops*
Geranium	*5 drops*

The above blends can each be diluted with 30 ml base oil for a massage oil. Also use in the room methods, in baths, and the inhalation methods.

FACING DEATH

In recent years there has been a growing awareness of 'near-death experiences', when people invariably talk about a tunnel of light and being met on the other side by dear departed friends and relatives, all of whom are extremely happy. Other people are convinced there is an after-life because of their religious beliefs. Scientists even talk of a 'holographic universe' in which death doesn't happen, you move on. This is reassuring, but not all beliefs make facing death so acceptable.

I can think of one eighty-five-year-old lady, who had spent her entire life doing voluntary work for the church, and who strongly believed in heaven and hell, lying fearful in her hospital bed at the thought of going to hell. One might think she had nothing to worry about, but that's old-fashioned indoctrination for you.

On the other hand, one hears stories about small children who are dying and seem well-adjusted to the idea, philosophical even, and who give counselling and support to their parents, who are of course devastated by the situation in which they find themselves. These remarkable children may not have had the time to comprehend death and they have no trouble believing that Jesus, the angels or Mohammed will meet them and take care of them until they can see mummy and daddy again. Telling a child they are dying is not an easy thing to do. One woman told me she had said to her son 'perhaps you will get well, miracles do happen', but he didn't, and later sadly said, 'I guess God doesn't love me enough for a miracle.' What can one say to that? And children, simply by watching a certain amount of TV, see death associated with gory blood, and boxes being put in the cold earth. For many children, teenagers and adults, death can be an unknown, frightening experience, however brave a face one puts on it.

It must be very irritating to be facing death and have people say things to you like 'we all have to go through it', or 'it'll happen to me too some day' or 'now you can have some rest', or some such thing which somehow aims to negate the experience. Death is the biggest transition we make in this life, it's not like moving house! Let's not belittle the experience.

I would certainly recommend books on near-death experiences to anyone who is facing death, as well as the relatives. They are very reassuring. However, giving them to someone facing death and saying, 'Here, look, it's not so bad, what are you so worried about?' can be in danger of minimizing what they are going through. Death is not a minimal thing to experience. To grieving parents I would particularly recommend *Children of the Light* (Bantam) which documents the near-death experiences of children. It may also be that at this time books about religion and philosophy can offer a new insight into the subject of life, death and the meaning of it all.

If we could think of death as a life cycle completed, rather than a life cycle cut short, the anguish may be easier to bear because a long list could be drawn up of accomplishments including, perhaps, children. But what does one tell a teenager who is too old to believe in Father Christmas, but too young to have had a working, exploring, life of their own? Standing on the threshold of a whole new life, the loss must be particularly great for them to bear. Why shouldn't they ask 'why me?' and rant and rave in anger? Let them do it, and give plenty of time to listen, in great compassion, because they are right – it isn't fair. If they want to revert to childhood as a means of avoiding their present condition, let them, and if they say 'no, I won't let it happen to me', support them because with mind over matter being the powerful thing it is, they might just pull off a miracle!

Because dying is a lonely experience, having people around you who are loving and caring must be the greatest comfort of all. To pass over to the other side holding the hand of someone you love, or with their arms around you, must be the gentlest way to leave this world. It is this, love, which is the greatest gift we can receive at this time, and to die pain-free in dignity and peace.

Throughout known time people have been burning incense around the dying in the belief that the aroma will take the soul as it rises to heaven. The word 'perfume' comes from *per fumin* – by fire. We also give flowers at funerals, and it was once traditional to give strong-smelling flowers, herbs and spices, so the aroma could lift the spirit to the other side. Essential oils carry on this tradition.

The best essential oils now are the ones that you love, the ones that give you a lift and make you feel good about yourself. And use them for any state of mind or emotion that you may be feeling. A collection of essential oils seems to be commonly chosen when facing death, but that might only be because they are easily available. These are listed below, and may not include your personal favourite oils, and if so, just choose other oils that appeal to you.

ESSENTIAL OILS USED WHEN FACING DEATH

Rose Otto, Jasmine, Linden Blossom, Frankincense, Neroli, Chamomile Roman, Geranium, Benzoin, Bay, Carnation, Sandalwood, Cedarwood, Bergamot, Juniper, Hyacinth, Rose Maroc, Tuberose, Narcissus, Lemon

All the oils above blend well with each other and can be made into combinations. Use however many drops of each essential oil you want, up to 30 drops of essential oil to 30 ml base vegetable oil, is the general rule. Just as the life cycle is individual, so is the journey ahead, so be as individualistic as you like, or not. Essential oils are pure pleasure, and now is a good time to explore them. Life is for living, now more than ever, and the fragrances of essential oils are fabulous additions to any life and are there to be enjoyed. Use them in all the usual methods.

Some people ask for fragrance to be used at the funeral ceremony, to comfort the mourners and also give them an aromatic signature to remember them by. Then, as they go about their lives later, they'll smell that same aroma on the airwaves and say, 'Oh, yes, so-and-so, I wonder where they are now?' – gone but not forgotten. And it is the good things we remember about people, especially the people we love.

FATIGUE, TIREDNESS AND EXHAUSTION

You may not be surprised to see the headlines in the papers saying 'Nearly half the population suffer from unexplained exhaustion. . .'[5] You may feel exhausted yourself. A new term has appeared, TATT – tired all the time, to identify the thing, which is the biggest complaint doctors hear. There may be some underlying physiological reason, including low blood pressure, hypothyroidism – an underactive thyroid gland, and thyrotoxicosism – an overactive one, anaemia or iron-deficiency, rheumatoid arthritis and the totally debilitating myalgic encephalomyelitis (ME) and many other things. You need to establish that you're not just tired from overwork, depression, drinking too much or insomnia, and that you're not in the recovery period from a viral or bacteriological infection, which would inevitably leave you tired.

It's estimated that about 40 per cent of tiredness cases are caused by psychological or life style reasons which, if they were recognized, could be worked on. The working environment is a good place to start – are you sitting too close to photocopiers, fax machines, computers or air-vents for the air-conditioning system? Or are you hunched over in a taut position all day on a factory assembly line, with noise banging in your ear? The answer to this is a nice long holiday in the sun, but unfortunately we can't go for fifty-two weeks of the year!

Essential oils have a long tradition of helping in the many different kinds of tiredness, fatigue or exhaustion there are. This section has been arranged under the headings of *Exhaustion, Nervous Exhaustion, General Mental Fatigue, Intellectual Fatigue* and *Mental Tiredness*, each of which has suggested oils and one or two blends. Use the oils in all the usual ways, adding the quantities given in the blends to 30 ml base oil to make a massage oil, or mix the essential oils into a synergistic blend. See Chart 5.1 for quantities to use and methods.

Eucalyptus

ESSENTIAL OILS TO HELP IN CASES OF EXHAUSTION

Chamomile Roman, Cypress, Bergamot, Marjoram, Rosemary, Eucalyptus Radiata, Frankincense, Litsea Cubeba, Black Pepper, Cardamon, Eucalyptus Radiata, Ginger, Lemon, Pine, Grapefruit

EXHAUSTION 1		EXHAUSTION 2	
Lemon	*10 drops*	*Eucalyptus Globulus*	*15 drops*
Frankincense	*5 drops*	*Rosemary*	*10 drops*
Pine	*15 drops*	*Grapefruit*	*5 drops*

ESSENTIAL OILS TO HELP IN CASES OF NERVOUS EXHAUSTION

Rosemary, Petitgrain, Juniper, Neroli, Lavender, Orange, Chamomile Roman, Marjoram, Clary Sage

NERVOUS EXHAUSTION 1		NERVOUS EXHAUSTION 2	
Petitgrain	*18 drops*	*Juniper*	*10 drops*
Neroli	*10 drops*	*Lavender*	*15 drops*
Lavender	*2 drops*	*Rosemary*	*5 drops*

ESSENTIAL OILS TO HELP IN CASES OF GENERAL MENTAL FATIGUE

*Lemon, Petitgrain, *Basil, *Peppermint, Rosemary, *Eucalyptus Piperita, Eucalyptus Citriodora*

GENERAL MENTAL FATIGUE	
Basil	*15 drops*
Lemon	*15 drops*

ESSENTIAL OILS FOR INTELLECTUAL FATIGUE

*Ginger, Black Pepper, Rosemary, Lemon, *Basil, Cypress, Grapefruit, *Peppermint*

*Should not be used in baths.

INTELLECTUAL FATIGUE 1		INTELLECTUAL FATIGUE 2	
*Ginger	14 drops	Rosemary	15 drops
Black Pepper	15 drops	Black Pepper	10 drops
*Basil	1 drop	*Peppermint	5 drops

ESSENTIAL OILS TO HELP IN CASES OF MENTAL TIREDNESS

*Clary Sage, Lavender, Marjoram, Rosemary, Litsea Cubeba, Grapefruit, *Peppermint*

TIREDNESS BLEND

Marjoram	10 drops
Litsea Cubeba	15 drops
*Peppermint	5 drops

*Should not be used in baths.

It may seem strange to use essential oils that are traditionally used to calm, but in tiredness, to overstimulate can sometimes result in increased tiredness, not relief from it.

FEAR

Fear is a life-saver – it puts us on alert so the 'flight-fight' hormones can swing into action and give us that extra impetus we need to get out of a fix. It's fear of a large, crazed dog that'll make you leap a ten-foot wall to escape – and on a normal day you couldn't jump a three-foot wall! That's fear for you. It gives you extra strength, sharpens the senses, makes reactions quicker, and makes your body do things you didn't know it could do.

Fear makes the adrenal glands release adrenalin which stimulates the sympathetic nervous system, causing a speeding up of heart rate, an increase in perspiration, the drying up of the saliva glands (making the mouth dry), and stopping the digestive system working. There are of course degrees of fear and it's quite common for people exposed to a sudden terrifying experience to urinate or defecate without control. Soldiers, exposed to fearful situations day after day, can become suddenly paralysed, unable to move a muscle.

There's plenty to be frightened about. Burglars and rapists can break into the house at night and the streets are full of people who act in strange, unpredictable ways. In America, according to a report in the *Los Angeles Times*,[6] one person in seventy-five suffers from fear attacks of sufficient severity to make them think they're having a heart attack or about to go mad, and the attacks don't relate to actual frightening experiences but to the *possibility* that something could go seriously wrong in their lives – as a result of financial troubles, work or relationship problems, for example. And I don't suppose the fear quotient in that country is helped by the violent crime statistics, which are high enough to put anyone into a permanent state of fear.

There is so much fear about, we now have a wide vocabulary to deal with it. The generalized fear talked about above is known in America as 'panic disorder', then there's 'stropophobia' – the fear of moving or making changes, 'gamophobia' – the fear of marriage, 'decidophobia' – the fear of making decisions, 'sciophobia' – the fear of shadows, and, among other phobias, 'triskaidekaphobia' – fear of the number thirteen! (See *Phobias*.)

'Topophobia' is better known as stage fright and it even affected that best known of actors, Laurence Olivier, who suffered with sweating, trembling and a constricted throat before each performance. Another well-known actor avoided live performances for fourteen years and a famous singer was kept away from the stage for eight years. Birmingham University's Neuropsychiatry clinic is now advising actors to use aromatherapy to dispel the fear, by choosing a relaxing essential oil, having a massage with it while a hypnotist suggests the actor feels relaxed, then sniffing that same aroma before going on stage. It's certainly a better option than giving up your profession or lying down on the stage to do relaxation exercises during a performance!

Normal fear is the reaction you feel when threatened, while

abnormal fear is fear out of all proportion to the scary object or event. Pathological fear, however, is a permanent state of mind that continues long after the fearful event has passed. Fear is accompanied by an intense feeling of apprehension or dread and is often felt in the 'pit of the stomach', and frequently accompanied by nausea and cold sweats. Outside the normal circumstances where one would expect a person to feel fear, exaggerated fear or chronic fear have no benefits whatsoever. It is an incapacitating and limiting feeling, that essential oils can help dispel. As there are so many types of fear, this section is arranged under several specific headings. However, we start with the essential oils that can help in cases of fearfulness and dread with no apparent cause (apart from life itself!).

ESSENTIAL OILS FOR USE IN CASES OF FEAR

Sandalwood, Chamomile Roman, Cypress, Vetiver, Lemon, Bergamot, Orange, Cedarwood, Neroli, Ormenis Flower, *Basil, Frankincense, Clary Sage, Lavender, Galbanham

*Should not be used in baths.

In addition to these oils there are those which are very appropriate for particular types of fear, as follows:

FEAR OF FAILURE

Fennel, Coriander, *Basil, Ylang Ylang, Frankincense,

FEAR OF MADNESS

Fennel, Cedarwood, Ylang Ylang, Frankincense

FEAR OF CHANGE

Ylang Ylang, Frankincense, Lavender, Ormenis Flower

FEAR OF GOSSIP

Cypress

FEAR OF FEELINGS

Fennel, Frankincense, Neroli, Sandalwood

FEAR OF SEXUALITY

Rose Maroc, Ylang Ylang, Patchouli, Vetiver, Galbanham

FEAR OF LOVE	FEAR OF LOVING
Rose Maroc, Neroli, Carnation, Hyacinth, Benzoin	Neroli, Ylang Ylang, Carnation, Benzoin, Rose Maroc

FEAR OF BEING UNLOVED	FEAR OF LETTING GO
Rose Otto	Rose Maroc, Frankincense, Galbanham, Cypress

*Should not be used in baths.

The essential oils can be used either singly or made into blends and used in baths, diffusers and other room methods, inhaled from a tissue or direct from the bottle, or inhaled as a steam vapour. The quantities of the following blends should either be diluted with 30 ml base oil, or made into a synergistic blend using these proportions. For quantities to use see Chart 5.1.

FEAR OF CHANGE

Lavender	5 drops
Ylang Ylang	15 drops
Frankincense	5 drops

FEAR OF FEELINGS

Sandalwood	20 drops
Fennel	3 drops
Frankincense	7 drops

FEAR OF SEXUALITY

Rose Maroc	16 drops
Ylang Ylang	10 drops
Patchouli	2 drops
Galbanham	2 drops

FEAR OF LOVE

Benzoin	10 drops
Carnation	5 drops

FEAR OF LOVING

Neroli	15 drops
Benzoin	10 drops
Ylang Ylang	5 drops

FEAR OF BEING UNLOVED		FEAR OF LETTING GO	
Rose Otto	*30 drops*	*Cypress*	*10 drops*
		Galbanham	*5 drops*
		Rose Maroc	*15 drops*

FITS (EMOTIONAL) OR OUTBURSTS

In psychological terms, fits are thought of as outbursts – like 'a fit of jealousy' or 'a fit of anger', something that comes on suddenly. Someone who is prone to explosions of emotions could consider counselling or see an aromatherapist who can both offer support and use the oils to help diffuse the build-up of tension. Essential oils can be diffused in the room, inhaled from a tissue, used 8 drops in a bath, or made into a massage oil. Consider the essential oils which have a calming and soothing effect but look at the situation holistically and refer to other sections in the book.

ESSENTIAL OILS FOR THOSE PRONE TO FITS AND OUTBURSTS

Lavender, Marjoram, Eucalyptus Citriodora, Litsea Cubeba, Chamomile Roman

EMOTIONAL FITS OR OUTBURSTS 1		EMOTIONAL FITS OR OUTBURSTS 2	
Lavender	*10 drops*	*Chamomile Roman*	*8 drops*
Marjoram	*5 drops*	*Eucalyptus Citriodora*	*14 drops*
Litsea Cubeba	*15 drops*	*Lavender*	*8 drops*

FORGETFULNESS

Forgetfulness can happen to us all, and sometimes it doesn't matter and at other times it matters a lot. To try not to forget things we need concentration and focus, which essential oils may help with. Gently diffuse them in the atmosphere during the time you are trying to collect your thoughts, or sniff them from a handkerchief.

ESSENTIAL OILS TO CHALLENGE FORGETFULNESS

Cypress, Lemon, *Ginger, Black Pepper, Cistus, Frankincense, Rosemary, *Peppermint, *Basil

FORGETFULNESS 1		FORGETFULNESS 2	
Rosemary	*15 drops*	*Black Pepper*	*10 drops*
*Peppermint	*5 drops*	*Frankincense*	*5 drops*
Lemon	*10 drops*	*Cypress*	*10 drops*

*Should not be used in baths.

GRIEF (Intense Sorrow)

Although the word 'grief' is usually associated with bereavement, it encompasses all kinds of intense sorrow which may include the death of a loved one, but may equally include the sorrow one feels when a loving relationship breaks down and the loved one leaves not the world in general, but you in particular. The grieving that takes place after such a loss can be intense, and last for years. One can grieve for pets, as well as people, and for objects too. People have been made intensely sad when, for example, an object of deep sentimental value is lost or stolen, or when the family's collection of photographs is destroyed in a fire. Some people may grieve the loss of a job, or home, or lifestyle while others may even grieve the loss of a much-loved car. Many women grieve in silence over a miscarriage, abortion or hysterectomy, sometimes for the rest of their lives. Others may be grieving the loss of a limb. Poets have eloquently grieved for the fate of a nation, and spiritual masters have long grieved for the sad state of the human race.

Grieving goes beyond sadness or sorrow – etching itself on to every cell of our body and making a deep impression on our soul. It's felt as a deep sinking feeling in what's called 'the pit of the stomach', a feeling that never seems to go away. Immediately after the loss, one can feel numb and disbelieving, hoping it's all been a bad dream. This is a form of shock and the sufferer may experience uncontrollable shaking and have nausea and an overwhelming sense of hopelessness. Often it's accompanied by feelings of loneliness and isolation. Then comes a preoccupation with how you feel, as the sadness fills your mind and your time. Despondency and despair set in, as we feel we shall never be able to experience happiness again.

Then comes the anger and guilt: 'if only I'd done this' (or that); 'I should have said this' (or that). You may have vivid memories of the good times and the bad times, and find yourself running over in your mind the good times that will never be, making you irritable. If the loss is of a person, there is often rage or jealousy, regret, blame and lots of tears. You can lie in bed, tossing and turning, churning over every detail of the loss, over and over again. Aches and pains are common with grief, as is stress and anxiety, loss of appetite or overeating.

Grief can last a few weeks or for years on end – when it is called atopic grief. It's often accompanied by a sense of failure or worthlessness and, if the emotional pain becomes too great to bear, it can lead to suicide. Perhaps the only way to avoid grief is never to become involved with another person ever again, or so attached to a thing, but to be alive is to feel love, and to feel love is sometimes to feel the pain of loss. Grieving is, then, an inevitable part of life which we must all, at some time, try to get through as best we can. To deny it is potentially dangerous, both psychologically and physiologically and so grief must be allowed to take its course. If you feel rage, beat the walls, if you feel like screaming, do it, if you feel like crying, let those tears roll. We all have our own ways of coping. One friend, after a broken relationship, locked herself away at home where she sobbed uncontrollably as she listened to love songs and watched sad love movies all day and all night for months on end. People said to her 'snap out of it, there's plenty of fish in the sea', which didn't help at all and, had this advice been taken up, it could have been dangerous in the long run because she *needed* to express her sorrow. Eventually, she emerged, weak and listless, and slowly picked up the pieces of her life. Now she's fine!

Grieving is a process that has to be gone through, no matter how long it takes. If you don't feel you can unload your problems onto a friend, seek out some counselling or even phone the Samaritans, and talk it over with them. If you can, visit an aromatherapist as the gentle massage combined with the essential oils, chosen individually for you, will certainly help release some of the grief.

Essential oils have long been used to comfort and console but they will *not* stop the grieving process. That is not what they are there for. What they can do, however, is help you express the grief and come to terms with it. Choose an essential oil from the lists below, or choose several to make into a blend. Use them in the bath, diffused in the atmosphere, inhaled as a vapour, sniffed from a tissue or straight from the bottle, or made into a massage oil. See Chart 5.1 for quantities to use.

ESSENTIAL OILS TO HELP EXPRESS GRIEF

Hyacinth, Rose Maroc, Rose Otto, Neroli, Melissa, Helichrysum, Benzoin, Mimosa, Vetiver

ESSENTIAL OILS TO HELP DISSIPATE GRIEF

Cypress, Chamomile Roman, Rose Maroc, Rose Otto, Helichrysum, Ormenis Flower, Frankincense, Narcissus, Bergamot, Carnation, Vanilla, Nutmeg, Spikenard

The following blends can each be diluted with 30 ml base oil to make a massage oil, or you can make up a synergistic blend using these proportions and use that blend in all the methods mentioned above.

GRIEF-INDUCED NUMBNESS, SHOCK AND DISBELIEF		GRIEF-INDUCED STRESS	
Cypress	5 drops	Carnation	5 drops
Helichrysum	5 drops	Rose Maroc	4 drops
Frankincense	10 drops	Chamomile Roman	1 drop
Bergamot	5 drops		

GRIEF-INDUCED DEPRESSION		CONTINUED DEEP SADNESS	
Ormenis Flower	10 drops	Cypress	5 drops
Benzoin	10 drops	Rose Maroc	15 drops
Nutmeg	10 drops	Hyacinth	5 drops

Also, please see the *Bereavement* section.

GUILT

There is so much to be guilty about. There are the library books that haven't been taken back, the 'thank-yous' that haven't been said, the sick relatives we haven't visited, the money we shouldn't have spent, the bills we are ignoring, and the jobs that haven't been done. We've all felt guilty eating chocolate bars, and some of us feel guilty for buying books when the teenager wants a new pair of trainers. Some people are guilty because they have hurt someone, or lied, cheated or stolen. People with children have a whole stack of more guilt: leaving a child with a babysitter or taking it to piano lessons it hates. Everyone has some kind of guilt or other, we just don't go around talking about it all the time. If you are feeling guilty . . . shhhh . . . you are not alone!

Aside from the guilt we devise for ourselves there is the guilt we inflict on other people – particularly children – and on this subject I recommend *Cutting the Ties That Bind* by Phyllis Krystal. Then there is the guilt other people put on *us*, in the form of a parent who says 'you never phone', for example, a teenager who says 'you never buy me smart clothes', or the partner who says 'you never dress up any more'. All the little bits of guilt can add up . . . those little jobs you forgot to do for someone; the time you can't spend with the children. These outside demands can create a general atmosphere of guilt, but if there is someone close constructing their sentences so they instil you with guilt, that is a more gruelling experience with which to deal. Many partners use illness, unhappiness or financial issues to make the other feel guilty, it's like you can't do a thing right. However, none of this inflicted guilt is as bad as the guilt of having killed someone, perhaps as a soldier, and deep guilt such as this should be discussed with a counsellor, to try to come to terms with it.

For normal, everyday guilt that gets out of hand, strange as it may seem, essential oils and aromatherapy may be able to help. Aromatherapy treatments are also helpful in all kinds of guilt because the massage techniques allow emotional release. As you will see from the *Massage* section in Chapter 9, deep-seated emotions are often felt in our bodies and are effectively released by trained therapists. As not everyone can afford professional help, guidance can be sought from the illustrations on pages 286 and 287 which show which areas of the body tend to hold emotional tension. Relaxation exercises will be able to help further.

For normal, everyday use choose essential oils from other sections of this book which seem relevant to you. The following list is of oils which have traditionally been used for guilt. Use them in a massage oil, in the bath, or diffused or inhaled.

ESSENTIAL OILS TO HELP COPE WITH GUILT

Linden Blossom, Vetiver, Jasmine, Pine, Rose Otto, Juniper, Clary Sage, Ylang Ylang, Nutmeg

The quantities in the following blends can be diluted with 30 ml of base oil to make a massage oil, or make a synergistic blend of oils using these proportions and use in baths, room methods and inhalation methods. For quantities to use see Chart 5.1.

EVERYDAY GUILT		DEEP-ROOTED GUILT	
Ylang Ylang	12 drops	Juniper	15 drops
Nutmeg	10 drops	Clary Sage	5 drops
Vetiver	8 drops	Pine	10 drops

If you feel guilty about indulging yourself, this blend will help you enjoy your guilt!

INDULGENCE GUILT	
Linden Blossom	5 drops
Jasmine	5 drops
Rose Otto	5 drops

HYPOCHONDRIA

If a hypochondriac has palpitations, they think they have heart disease, if they get a twinge or cramp in their bottom, they've got bowel cancer, if they have a bout of indigestion, they've got angina, and the bad back they got gardening will be kidney trouble. Hypochondriacs have fixations about their bodies, and a real fear of illness or dying (although there is another type of hypochondriac who uses potential ill health to gain sympathy, visits or attention, who usually reports vague feelings of being unwell). All this is to be distinguished from *psychosomatic illness*, in which there are real physical disorders brought on by certain mental activity.

Not all hypochondriacs are well. Doctors undoubtedly sometimes diagnose 'hypochondria' in the person sitting in front of them, just because they can't find what is wrong – which may be depression or some other mental illness. Unfortunately, once you admit to being even mildly depressed, there's a good chance that henceforth everything physical you complain of will be dismissed as hypochondria!

Sometimes nothing can be done for the hypochondriac, no matter how many times the doctor is visited. Therapists can help as they have more time to give, and can listen to the

troubles. Reflexologists often have success with hypochondriacs because they can give the equivalent of an 'X-ray'
diagnosis on each visit, and reassure the person. (Reflexology
is the manipulation of the soles of the feet, in which all the
functions of the body are supposed to be mirrored.) Essential
oils may help, as can homeopathy, and they are usually harmless when administering treatment to oneself on a first-aid
basis, but if the hypochondriac recognizes they have a
problem, counselling may be an answer.

If you have a hypochondriac in the family, buy them *The
Fragrant Pharmacy* – my book on using essential oils on
physical problems – and a family treatment book for homeopathy, and another on Bach flower remedies, and any other
books you can find on self-help, plus a set of essential oils, and
the person might become so busy looking up the various treatments, they'll forget they had a problem! Often, when a
hypochondriac uses essential oils and starts administering to
themselves it deflects the dependency on others and shifts
responsibility to themselves, thereby often clearing up the
problem.

ESSENTIAL OILS FOR HYPOCHONDRIACS

*Marjoram, Rosemary, Valerian, Hops, *Basil, *Peppermint, *Thyme,
Ormenis Flower, Tea Tree, Manuka, *Oregano, Galbanham*

*Should not be used in baths.

Use the oils singly or in blends – in all the usual methods.

HYSTERIA

Although as a word 'hysteria' is becoming less used by the
medical profession in favour of a variety of terms which more
accurately describe the range of emotional problems people
have to deal with, we all know what it is for someone to be
'hysterical' – to display unusual, emotionally excited behaviour, such as screaming and shouting loudly, with perhaps crying, sighing, temper, or rage. It is often the way a person finds
they can attract attention to themselves, to a problem they face,

Marjoram

or a situation in which they find themselves, and hysteria also releases some pent-up anxiety. Hysteria is medically classified as a neurotic behaviour disturbance, and immortalized on film by the black and white images of hysterical actresses getting a slap across the face.

Mass hysteria is when a group of people all get hysterical together, setting each other off – as among a large group of young women at a rock or pop concert, for example. Clever individuals can set off group hysteria at business meetings, for example, disrupting the proceedings.

If a person is known to have hysterical tendencies they could carry a bottle of essential oil to use when the anxiety starts. The oils will help to calm them down. But each case is different and some people get hysterical because they think they can make an advantage out of it, and in this case nothing will stop the hysteria starting. After an hysterical outburst, when things have calmed down, essential oils are very good in a bath or massage oil. They can also be used on a more regular basis, in all the usual ways.

ESSENTIAL OILS TO USE IN CASES OF HYSTERIA

Mandarin, Chamomile Roman, Linden Blossom, Vetiver, Bergamot, Rosemary, Neroli, *Peppermint, Narcissus, Lavender, Marjoram, Valerian, Spikenard, Hops

The quantities in the following blends can be diluted with 30 ml of base oil to make a massage oil, or make a synergistic blend of oils using these proportions and use in all room methods and inhalation methods. See Chart 5.1 for quantities to use.

HYSTERIA 1		HYSTERIA 2	
Marjoram	*8 drops*	*Spikenard*	*8 drops*
Lavender	*14 drops*	*Chamomile Roman*	*17 drops*
Valerian	*8 drops*	*Bergamot*	*5 drops*

SHOCK-HYSTERIA	
*Peppermint	*10 drops*
Rosemary	*15 drops*
Lavender	*5 drops*

*Should not be used in baths.

INSOMNIA

We've all had the occasional night when we couldn't sleep. We go to bed and shut our eyes, but nothing. We don't drift off, we're awake. So we toss and turn for an hour, then sit up and read a book. An hour later we turn off the light and try again. Again, nothing. We're beginning to feel very heavy and agitated. We try relaxation techniques and counting sheep, plump up the pillow, get into a comfortable position . . . but nothing. We begin to think of all the things we've got to do tomorrow and for which we are going to be too exhausted. Time passes. The birds begin to sing. By now we feel like lead. The sun rises, the alarm clock goes, another day begins. And for the insomniac, the day begins like that almost every day.

It's estimated that five to ten million people in Britain have a sleep problem and that one in three adults will get insomnia at some time in their lives. In England and Wales, doctors write out twenty million prescriptions for sleeping pills (hypnotics) each year. In the financial year 1992–3, the NHS spent £24 million on hypnotics but the Audit Commission (a regulatory body, responsible for overseeing the finances of the NHS, and other public funds) would like to see this figure reduced by £14 million. They quote a report by the *British National Formulary*, a joint publication from the British Medical Association and the Royal Pharmaceutical Society of Great Britain: 'Prescribing . . . is widespread but dependence and tolerance to their effects occurs. [They] should not be prescribed indiscriminately and should be reserved for short courses to alleviate acute conditions after causal factors have been established.'[7]

Insomnia is caused by worry, anxiety, tension, stress, pain, fear, overtiredness, caffeine, eating late at night, shift-work, stimulants, excitability and noise, among other things. Certain mental states also affect the sleeping pattern – depressives tend to have trouble getting to sleep and wake early; people with dementia are afraid of the dark and that makes them confused, restless and noisy; schizophrenics can be tortured by voices and pace up and down all night, while people with mania are hyperactive and don't sleep much at all. Apparently there are as many as eighty classifications of sleep disorder, and new scientific fields are being created to deal with them all, including somnologists – sleep experts, and chronobiology – the science linking natural body rhythms with physiology and psychology.

During a good night's sleep, research shows we go through periods of non-rapid eye movement (NREM) interrupted by about five episodes of rapid eye movement (REM), presumably indicating dreaming. There is 'delta sleep', which is more refreshing, and 'alpha sleep', which is lighter and can be easily interrupted. During sleep, our temperature fluctuates. Some researchers think our natural pattern of sleep would be to have a short nap in the afternoon, and a sleep at night. Apparently, our body rhythms are at their slowest between three and six o'clock in the morning.

Nobody really knows why we sleep but it's during this time that the body shuts down functions such as digestion, and concentrates on repair and healing. Missed sleep can affect concentration and efficiency and bring on irritability, nervousness, sleepiness, tiredness, exhaustion and aches and pains of which we would not normally be aware. I've known women become insomniac after having their sleep pattern interrupted by babies and worry about the children, and men who could never return to a normal sleeping pattern after spending years on shift work. DJs and other night workers have a very difficult time finding a good, long sleep, let alone on a regular basis. Essential oils can help all these situations, and please refer to the blends to see which seems most appropriate to you.

Warm baths, relaxation exercises and hypnotherapy tapes could all help with insomnia, as could switching to decaffeinated coffee or tea. Have a night-time routine, use a comfortable bed, shut out noise and read a book or have sex. Warm calcium drinks or malt drinks can help. The homeopathic tablets arnica, aconitum, ignatia, kali-phosphoricum or coffea might be useful too, or herbal tablets such as valerian. If nothing works, just get up and read *The Mind-Map Book* by Tony Buzan,[8] and draw yourself a mind-map and see what's keeping you awake!

Any of the following oils can be used singly or in combinations. Use 10 drops in a warm bath before bed. A massage oil also helps to calm and relax. Gently diffuse the essential oils in the room, or place the essential oils on a tissue or cotton wool ball and place under the pillow:

ESSENTIAL OILS TO HELP IN CASES OF INSOMNIA

Lavender, Mandarin, Linden Blossom, Clary Sage, Marjoram, Cistus, Valerian, Hops, Vetiver, Chamomile Roman, Sandalwood, Lemon

The quantities in the following blends can be diluted with 30 ml of base oil to make a massage oil, or make a synergistic blend of oils using these proportions and use in baths, and all room and inhalation methods.

INSOMNIA NIGHTMARES WAKE YOU		INSOMNIA NOISE WAKES YOU	
Lavender	15 drops	Lavender	10 drops
Chamomile Roman	5 drops	Lemon	15 drops
Mandarin	10 drops	Vetiver	5 drops

INSOMNIA RESTLESSNESS		INSOMNIA FITFULNESS	
Vetiver	10 drops	Marjoram	5 drops
Clary Sage	10 drops	Lavender	15 drops
Lemon	10 drops	Lemon	10 drops

INSOMNIA ANXIETY		INSOMNIA WORRY	
Chamomile Roman	10 drops	Cistus	5 drops
Sandalwood	15 drops	Lavender	15 drops
Lemon	5 drops		

INSOMNIA EXHAUSTION	
Valerian	5 drops
Lemon	10 drops
Mandarin	10 drops

IRRITABILITY

We all get irritable sometimes, at various stages of our life or just during some stage of a normal day. There are possible underlying factors which should be addressed because irritability can be caused by an illness or by an emotion, such as unhappiness, sadness, worry, stress and tension. Pre-menstrual tension (PMT) also causes irritability.

Irritability is enshrined in the expression 'I got out of the bed on the wrong side today', and it's definitely within the normal range of human emotions. It may have a place as a means of expressing dissatisfaction – of which, let's face it, there is plenty in this life – so it is expressed outwards rather than inwards. But, as ever, it is a question of degree. It's one thing to get irritated listening to a politician being interviewed, but another thing to want to actually kill the person. Children can get irritable if they are tired, but if it happens on a regular basis, they should be checked over by a doctor. Rational people will recognize that one day a thing that would normally pass unremarked can the next become an irritation, and it all depends on our mood. But when we're getting irritated or 'ratty' over everyday events on a regular basis, flying off the handle over minor problems, sensitive to suggestions, remarks and even touch, then it is time to do something about it.

Clearly, if there is something to be said and the irritability is just covering up that fact, then say what it is you have to say. It is not the job of essential oils to 'cover up' what underlies irritability – you must express yourself and let the cause of irritability pass, not linger. Having said that, the essential oils can certainly help reduce irritability. Use them singly, or in blends, cross-referencing with the lists elsewhere in this book.

ESSENTIAL OILS TO USE IN CASES OF IRRITABILITY

Cypress, Chamomile Roman, Chamomile German, Coriander, Litsea Cubeba, Neroli, Ylang Ylang, Melissa, Narcissus, Lavender

The quantities in the following blends can be diluted with 30 ml of base oil to make a massage oil, or make a synergistic blend of oils using these proportions and use in all the usual methods – particularly in baths. See Chart 5.1 for quantities to use.

IRRITABILITY 1		IRRITABILITY 2	
Cypress	10 drops	Ylang Ylang	15 drops
Coriander	10 drops	Coriander	10 drops
Lavender	10 drops	Chamomile Roman	5 drops

LONELINESS AND ALONENESS

People who are alone are often thought by other people to be depressed or lonely. This isn't always the case. Sometimes people yearn for aloneness and even devise daily stratagems so they can get a bit of it. Being alone can be an energizing, fortifying experience, drawing on the peace within, but it can also mean feeling isolated and out of touch with other people, especially people you love.

Essential oils can help in both extremes, strange as that may seem. When you've been working with essential oils as long as I have you can practically see the loneliness cloud lift from people after their regular use of them. It is not simply the 'you are never alone with essential oils' factor, which all users appreciate, but something else, as if something has been added, making the person complete, and strong – alone or in a crowd.

The very fact that someone can feel alone in a crowd illustrates that the problem is not to do with physically having people around, as such, but with how a person feels about themselves in relation to other people. In a sense then, advice about going out and meeting people or getting a new hobby is not going to help – all it means is one will be lonely in a crowd instead of lonely alone at home. More is required to shift the consciousness, away from non-peace to peace. When we are at peace, people are much easier to handle and they do not have to be shunned.

There is nothing wrong with being alone. When alone we

can re-orientate ourselves and go forward, or come to terms with particular feelings or actions. And the views can be amazing when one wanders lonely as a cloud, exhilarating even, untouched by other people's wants, needs and expectations. Being alone only becomes a problem when one feels loneliness, and then essential oils can help by giving comfort, the ability to cope, and enjoyment. Use the oils singly or in blends, in all the usual methods:

ESSENTIAL OILS TO USE WHEN FEELING (NEGATIVE) LONELINESS

Bergamot, Helichrysum, Narcissus, Chamomile Roman, Neroli, Benzoin

ESSENTIAL OILS FOR (POSITIVE) ALONENESS

Orange, Neroli, Rose Otto, Rose Maroc, Jasmine, Melissa, Frankincense, Chamomile Roman

The quantities in the following blends can be diluted with 30 ml of base oil to make a massage oil, or make a synergistic blend of oils using these proportions and use in baths, and all room and inhalation methods. For quantities to use see Chart 5.1.

MELANCHOLIC LONELINESS		PEACEFUL ALONENESS	
Benzoin	*10 drops*	*Neroli*	*10 drops*
Helichrysum	*5 drops*	*Orange*	*5 drops*
Bergamot	*10 drops*	*Rose Otto*	*10 drops*
Chamomile Roman	*5 drops*		

MISERY

We all feel miserable at times, but some people feel more misery than others. I have a friend who once shared a flat with a woman, Betty, who came back from work each evening and complained about the journey, about her workmates, the poor quality of the food in the shop she stopped off at, her lack of money, the fact that the laundry needed doing, the fact that nothing was on TV, the fact that there was nowhere to go and so on. My friend tells me that she used to hear the key go in the lock, look at the clock and time how long it would take Betty to make the first complaint about her (inevitably) miserable day. It was usually in under two minutes . . . and went on all evening! Betty was the flatmate we all dread having!

People who are miserable usually know they are miserable, even if they don't put their plethora of complaints down to it. They would dearly like to shake their misery off, but just can't. The unhappiness and wretchedness just cloaks them, like a second skin. It is distressing to be miserable, because it is not the intended human state, and it can lead to serious emotional discomfort and, ultimately, depression. Therefore, help should be sought before things get too bad. If the feelings of misery only come during the autumn and winter months it could indicate a degree of seasonal affective disorder (SAD), which affects, to some extent, as many as one person in twenty and is caused by a lack of light. Help is available for this disorder in the form of a light-box.

Using essential oils will not magically dissolve the problems which caused the misery, but they may alleviate the negative feelings which have arisen as a consequence of them, which ultimately leaves the person free to deal with those problems.

ESSENTIAL OILS TO USE WHEN FEELING MISERABLE

Narcissus, Petitgrain, Benzoin, Orange, Neroli, Rose Maroc, Jasmine, Clove, Cinnamon, Ginger, Carnation, Pimento Berry

The quantities in the following blends can be diluted with 30 ml of base oil to make a massage oil, or make a synergistic blend of oils using these proportions and use in all room and inhalation methods. For quantities to use see Chart 5.1.

WARMING AND COMFORTING		CUSHIONING	
*Clove	5 drops	Benzoin	10 drops
Pimento Berry	10 drops	*Cinnamon	5 drops
Orange	15 drops	Rose Maroc	15 drops

*Should not be used in baths.

MOODINESS AND MOOD SWINGS

Moods can swing *real* fast. We can feel all bright and happy and then the final demand arrives from the mortgage company and, bang, our mood is foul; then the doorbell rings and a delivery man is standing there holding a big bunch of flowers; 'Oooh,' we say, excitedly, 'I wonder who they're from?'

Like most other things in this world, moods are under the scrutiny of scientists, who are coming to the conclusion that moods are catching. In one piece of research tiny electrodes were attached to different facial muscles of the subjects, who were shown pictures of people in different moods – happy, sad, angry and so on. The subjects responded to the photos by subtly moving their muscles to mimic the expressions of the faces in the pictures. We seem to have an innate ability to harmonize our moods with other human beings – which is a strong force for social cohesion. Mood synchronization can also be seen as a form of communication. Some people are particularly responsive to 'emotional contagion', as psychologists now call it. These are the 'good listeners' who have great empathy with other people and pick up on all their moods, often not expressing their own.

Moodiness is not uncommon in teenagers, and during the premenstrual days of a woman's cycle, and there may well be a hormonal factor involved. More generally, moodiness is brought on by particular events during the day, or by life in general. Moody people can be fed up, or frustrated, bored, isolated, repressed, irritable or bad tempered, and usually think nobody understands them. (Well, in this frame of mind, who would want to?)

The essential oils can be used in all the usual methods:

ESSENTIAL OILS TO USE WHEN FEELING MOODY

Lemon, Geranium, Eucalyptus Citriodora, Neroli, Lavender, Ylang Ylang, Ormenis Flower, Patchouli

ESSENTIAL OILS TO HELP BALANCE MOOD SWINGS

Geranium, Cardamon, Lavender, Coriander, Angelica Seed, Cypress, Cedarwood, Linden Blossom, Helichrysum

The quantities in the following blends can be diluted with 30 ml of base oil to make a massage oil, or make a synergistic blend of oils using these proportions and use in baths, and all room and inhalation methods. For quantities to use see Chart 5.1.

MOODINESS		MOOD SWINGS	
Eucalyptus Citriodora	*12 drops*	*Cedarwood*	*15 drops*
Ormenis Flower	*8 drops*	*Helichrysum*	*5 drops*
Geranium	*10 drops*	*Cypress*	*15 drops*

OBSESSIONS AND COMPULSIONS

This is a true story; only the names have been changed. A man called George went with his friend, David, to visit David's mother. The house was spotless. David's mother went out and George and David went into the kitchen to make coffee. In the cupboard George noticed some home-made mincemeat waiting to be put in the Christmas pies and, being a gourmet and cook, he took half a teaspoonful out of the jar and ate it. David went mad saying 'If Mother sees that. . .!' and got a clean spoon and started rearranging the top layer of mincemeat in the jar so it wouldn't look as if it had been touched. Obviously, Mother didn't miss a trick. George went to the toilet and, standing there, he had a thought. He flushed the toilet, put the seat down, stood on the toilet seat and ran his finger across the top of the cistern. He couldn't believe it – not a speck of dust!

Some people are just obsessive about a particular thing – washing hands, checking doors, dressing in a certain way and so on. In a sense, these are just sensible things done to extreme – washing hands is hygienic, checking locks is a protective measure, and dressing in a certain way can even be thought practical. But when a person washes their hands five times, or checks the locks five times, that is orderliness gone to extreme.

Anxiety and fear are usually at the root of obsessions. It could be that the obsession keeps the person so busy, and that helps them shut out what the anxiety is about. Psychotherapy often helps, as do such things as art therapy, behavioural therapy and autogenic training. Certainly, help must be sought from a professional because the obsession can easily lead to depression, as well as a disrupted life. Obsessions very often lead to being unable to function well with other people because they can never come up to the obsessive's standards of orderliness (unless they become obsessive themselves!). The family, of course, suffers most.

Essential oils are no substitute for therapy, but they can have a beneficial role in managing obsessions. The obsessive could choose an essential oil, or make a blend, from the anxiety-relieving essential oils, or the list below (or any other favourite and relevant oil) and sniff from the bottle, or tissue, each time they felt the obsessive behaviour coming on. They should sit down, close their eyes, breathe the aroma deeply and let the thought pass. This approach has one advantage in that it provides an alternative ritual (which can be dealt with later), and another advantage in that it relieves the anxiety which can often be the cause of the obsessive behaviour (which, hopefully, won't be around later to have to deal with). These diversionary aroma tactics would work best with people who are committed to changing their behaviour. Many people, of course, do not accept they are obsessed.

Treatments from an aromatherapist who has also trained as a counsellor would be particularly helpful, although the essential oils can also be used at home in all the usual methods – massage oils, baths, diffused in the atmosphere or inhaled from a tissue. Use the oils singly, or in blends:

ESSENTIAL OILS TO USE IN CASES OF OBSESSION

*Sandalwood, Vetiver, Cedarwood, Narcissus, Clary Sage,
Orange, Lemon*

OBSESSIONS RELAXING		OBSESSIONS ANXIETY RELIEVING	
Clary Sage	5 drops	Lavender	5 drops
Orange	15 drops	Orange	10 drops
Cedarwood	10 drops	Sandalwood	15 drops

Compulsions are more or less the same as obsessions, although they are rather more related to unhappiness than anxiety. Anorexia and bulimia develop from compulsions, as can overeating. Anorexia, refusing to eat food, is said to be the expression of the unconscious desire to be childlike, so not having to take responsibility. It usually affects teenage girls, with only 1 in 15 anorexics being male. Anorexia is life-threatening and help must be sought. Bulimia is the compulsion to binge on food, which is vomited up to prevent weight gain. It also gives the feeling of being in control. Bulimia is often associated with deep unhappiness and guilt.

Compulsions sprout from a thousand scenarios, all true and heartfelt. There's Joanne who overeats because she wants to punish her husband for having an affair, and subconsciously refuses to be attractive to him; and Denise, who had to look after her elderly mother who sabotaged her romantic connections, so made herself feel unattractive by getting overweight and settled the dilemma that way . . . and resolved to look after manipulating mother. Then there's Rachel who found being overweight put her in a non-woman category, which helped in the sexist business world; and Annette, who got overweight to stop herself having affairs – not because she was worried about losing the husband she didn't love, but because she didn't want to lose the children; while Lisa, constantly chided as a child, became overweight because she didn't think she deserved to be happy. All these women are unhappy – about the faithless husband; the manipulative mother; the sexist environment; the loveless marriage; and the negative parents. But their stories show that overeating is more than oral gratification or 'comfort eating'. It is a strategy of life, and for the compulsion to change, the circumstances of the life have to change too. At least, they should be discussed, and dealt with, perhaps in therapy – with or without other family members, or partner.

Essential oils can help compulsive behaviour in the areas of *Self-Esteem, Self-Blame* and *Confidence*, among others, and they are discussed elsewhere. Coriander, geranium and lemon are three oils which people have said they find most helpful, and they would work very well in a blend.

PAIN

Wouldn't it be nice to be a baby again and able to cry out loud with pain? We could open our mouths wide and wail and howl, tears rolling down our faces, and everyone would run towards us, concerned. When you're a grown-up, though, you're expected to deal with the pain without making too much fuss. This can be a bit difficult, especially when it sucks up all your energy, so you can't even think. People don't understand that, inside, you are fighting a violent battle with a monster that threatens to leave you with nothing left.

The pain of toothache which we all get sometimes is like a pebble compared to the mountain of pain some people have to deal with each and every day, and night. The amount of pain going on in the world is mind-boggling, and a constant reminder to those of us not in pain how lucky we are. Yet we never see pain so, actually, don't often think about it. Unless, of course, we have it and then we think about it all the time. Even when we're not in pain, we wonder when it will come again.

Pain can be caused by disease, accident, swelling, inflammation or degeneration. It affects people with arthritis, osteoporosis, cancer, lower back pain, pain in the neck and shoulders, tension headaches and many other conditions. Childbirth is a painful experience, but people do experience it differently. I remember one midwife telling me that when she worked in the north of a particular African country she found the women went through childbirth with hardly a word – still and quiet, yet in the south of the country the women went wild – throwing themselves around the walls of the room (along with their many loud and supportive female friends and relatives), wailing and screaming at the tops of their voices. To a certain extent then, the experience of pain is cultural. Presumably their potential for pain was the same, the women just approached it differently. As to which group felt the least pain, I'm afraid I do not know.

It is well known that feeling happier and better in yourself can reduce the *experience* of pain, if not the pain itself. This link between emotion and pain occurs in endorphins – morphine-like substances produced by the human body which also play a part in determining mood; and in enkephalins, protein molecules with an analgesic (painkilling) effect which also have sedative and mood-changing effects. The action of these chemicals may explain why the mood can affect the pain.

Certainly the mood affected the pain of Bert Trautmann, goalkeeper for Manchester City football team in the 1950s, when he broke his neck during a cup final at Wembley but played on, not realizing what damage had been done. The excitement of playing on such an important occasion had clearly dulled the pain. Unfortunately, life is not usually so exciting for people with chronic pain when there is no mood-altering event to alleviate that pain. Indeed, their pain is liable to become worse because they get so fed up with it, and exhausted, they lose confidence and get depressed – their mood alters into the negative, painful range.

The ability of the human mind to lessen the experience of pain is now well documented, especially due to the good work of the pain-relief clinics which have been set up around the country. By counselling, teaching relaxation techniques and encouraging an outgoing attitude, the person coping with pain can certainly learn to manage the pain better. Everything is worth trying. Acupuncture has been extremely effective for many people, as have hypnotherapy and healing. Tension headaches happen to twice as many women as men because, it is thought, they have the extra and conflicting demands of family as well as work. For them, a possible re-arrangement of lifestyle is the only answer. At the end of this chapter I briefly explain some techniques which may help the relief of pain, including *Visualization* and *Relaxation*.

Essential oils may help ease the tension and stress that comes with pain, and so bring relief. They can be used in all the usual ways and it would be particularly useful to diffuse them in the atmosphere when doing relaxation exercises. A massage oil will help relieve the tension and a warm bath at night will aid sleep. Some essential oils do have analgesic value but it takes a skilled therapist to help in this area as it is so individualistic. Choose from the following list of oils classically used in the area of pain relief:

ESSENTIAL OILS USED FOR PAIN RELIEF

Betula Alba (Birch), Nutmeg, *Clove, Rosemary, Lavender, Chamomile Roman, Sage, Clary Sage, Helichrysum, *Peppermint, *Basil

*Should not be used in baths.

If the pain is associated with inflammation, use Chamomile Roman. The tension-relieving oils include marjoram, lavender, clary sage and vetiver. To relax, use lavender or neroli. Also check the lists elsewhere in this book and choose oils that suit you best.

PANIC AND PANIC ATTACKS

Panic sometimes follows on from trauma of some sort – such as accident or bereavement – or is brought on by fear, anxiety or phobias. In some cases the panic is expressed as panic attacks, which reinforces the fears of phobics. *Phobias* are discussed in a later section because not everyone who has a panic attack has a phobia.

The mind-body connection is very obvious in the case of panic attacks – a thought in the mind can set off a whole range of physical sensations such as hyperventilation, perspiration, dizziness, faints, nausea, shaking, trembling and feelings of being very hot or cold. The heart can start to race, the breath can be difficult to catch, there may be choking, and pains in the chest. Not surprisingly, people sometimes think they are dying. This thought is heightened by the terror of some imaginary impending disaster. Another symptom is to have feelings of stepping outside oneself, depersonalization, and feelings of being in a state of perceptual distortion, like in a dream, known as derealization. If someone has four or more of these symptoms, it is classified as a panic attack, although many people have these symptoms with more long-lasting generalized feelings of panic unrelated to any particular thing, person or environment.

Panic attacks can cause hyperventilation in some people and the best remedy I know for this is to breathe into a brown paper bag. This was one of the first things I learned as a student in Switzerland. It ensures the intake of carbon monoxide, which is lost during the process of overbreathing. Over the years the paper bag trick has come in very handy. I remember once on a transatlantic flight the call went out for a doctor because a passenger seated nearby had started hyperventilating, sweating and trembling. He was refusing oxygen from the crew and was clearly distressed. His girlfriend said he was frightened of flying. The doctor who had come forward from among the passengers had no remedy and immediately agreed that we should try the paper bag method for the hyperventilation, and lavender oil to relax. The man was perfectly fine after five minutes, and continued the flight panic-free.

It is essential for anyone prone to panic attacks to learn deep breathing techniques which can be utilized immediately the sensations begin. Use deep, slow breaths from the abdomen. This technique works wonderfully well to relax in times of stress. It would also be sensible to learn a relaxation technique for regular practice at home.

Luckily, panic attacks do not last too long and gradually the body's metabolism adjusts to withstand the onslaught, and the blood and hormone levels return to normal. However, they can be socially debilitating, and physically very unpleasant and worrying.

ESSENTIAL OILS FOR USE IN PANIC ATTACKS

Lavender, Frankincense, Helichrysum, Marjoram

The oils above are among the best that someone can use if having a panic attack which, if severe, might require medical help. If you feel a panic attack coming on, use lavender essential oil neat (undiluted) on the chest and neck area, and in view of this effective remedy it would be worth carrying a bottle around with you. After an attack, a warm relaxing bath will be helpful – add 8 drops of lavender. Also, add 5 drops of lavender to a teaspoon of vegetable oil, mix well, and massage across your abdomen, shoulders and neck. If you are prone to attacks, make up a panic-attack blend using the proportions given below. For quantities to use see Chart 5.1.

PANIC ATTACK CALMING BLEND

Lavender	*5 drops*
Frankincense	*5 drops*
Helichrysum	*5 drops*
Marjoram	*5 drops*

Add the quantities above to 30 ml base oil to make a massage oil or blend the essential oils together in these proportions and make a synergistic blend of oils which can be used in baths, and in all room and inhalation methods. For a synergistic blend, multiply the quantities of the formula above by three and put those undiluted essential oils in a small bottle to carry around with you at all times. You can simply sniff from the bottle, or put a drop on a tissue and inhale from that.

PASSIVITY

If you feel you cannot complain to the chef when he prepares you a terrible meal, or feel that you shouldn't bother the shopkeeper who sold you faulty goods, or if you get pushed around by other people, you may be too passive for your own good.

Pine

Passive people hang around on the fringes of conversations, feeling unable to join in. They might even pretend to agree with people, so they are liked, and keep their own opinions to themselves, so there isn't an argument. Passivity can even extend to feelings of love, worth, caring and sharing, so one finds oneself 'accidentally' involved with someone romantically, almost by default.

It is inviting to think that passivity is always good in so much as it doesn't cause much harm. Pacifists, after all, don't start wars. But passivity is not innocent. By *allowing* things to happen, by not interrupting the course of events, one *is* involved. And if it is in something you don't like – change it! These days passivity is not encouraged in the work situation, managers want pro-active people around them, and many people are going to assertion classes to address that issue. Women too have traditionally been encouraged to be passive (which has got them into all kinds of trouble) and there are many classes available for them to change that attitude. Passivity can cause frustration, stress, tension, feelings of worthlessness, helplessness, loneliness, anger and depression. All of which is bottled up, of course, and then eats away inside. Clearly, it takes time to shake the passivity off and come into one's own, but it is well worth the try and it gets easier by the day. The essential oils can help overcome passivity and encourage you to become more assertive, used in all the usual ways:

ESSENTIAL OILS TO HELP COUNTERACT PASSIVITY

Rose Maroc, Ylang Ylang, Cedarwood, Pine, Jasmine, Tuberose, Orange, Patchouli, Bay

The quantities in the following blends can be diluted with 30 ml of base oil to make a massage oil, or make a synergistic blend of oils using these proportions and use in baths, and all room and inhalation methods. For quantities to use see Chart 5.1.

PASSIVITY FORMULA 1		PASSIVITY FORMULA 2	
Rose Maroc	*10 drops*	*Jasmine*	*8 drops*
Orange	*10 drops*	*Cedarwood*	*5 drops*
Patchouli	*5 drops*	*Ylang Ylang*	*7 drops*
Tuberose	*5 drops*	*Bay*	*5 drops*

Both the above blends are, unfortunately, rather expensive, but the following would be less so:

PASSIVITY FORMULA 3	
Patchouli	*10 drops*
Ylang Ylang	*5 drops*
Bay	*5 drops*
Orange	*5 drops*

PHOBIAS

To have a phobia is to have an ongoing, irrational fear of a particular object or situation. The most common fear is of open spaces or public places – agoraphobia, and people are also afraid of heights, flying, or enclosed spaces – claustrophobia. The most common so-called 'specific' phobias are the fear of dogs, snakes, spiders and mice. 'Social' phobias, which are much rarer, are concerned with interactions with other people in some way, so a person may be generally frightened of people and excessively shy, fearful of eating in front of other people, or speaking, fearful of using cups and cutlery in restaurants, or using public toilets, or fearful of getting crushed and stamped on.

Phobias have been described as a fear which is out of all proportion to the situation, which logic and discussion cannot dispel, is not under voluntary control, and leads to avoiding the feared situation. This makes phobias a psychological reaction, an emotional reaction, a behavioural reaction and, if panic attacks are involved, a physiological reaction. The whole person is involved, and their lifestyle, and, possibly, the lifestyle of their family and friends.

Phobias may be related to a major change in life earlier – perhaps a house move, or a traumatic incident, bereavement, or accident – or they may have developed from a particular incident – in the case of being bitten by a dog as a child, for example. Some kind of therapy is probably needed to work through the phobia, and success rates at specialist clinics are good. It is even possible that the phobia will resolve itself. Mary was an animal lover with many pets, but *terrified* of spiders. A group of her young friends decided to go on a camping holiday in Greece. Everyone was going but Mary immediately thought about the spiders, which might be crawling in the tent. It was a very tough decision, but her friends insisted she came. The amazing thing was, when they got there, there *weren't* any spiders. Mary slowly relaxed and by the end of the first week she was wondering where all the spiders had gone. By the end of the second week she was *looking* for them. She never found one. But, when she got back home, she looked for a spider again, and found one, which she put in a box . . . and looked at occasionally. They became friends, then she let him go, to roam her house again.

Further information about phobias can be obtained from the Phobics Society and Phobic Action (see Appendix IV), and there is specialist help. There is even a company which takes people afraid of flying up in the air. I would suggest reading *Living With Fear* by Professor Isaac Marks or some other literature on the subject. Phobias can be overcome. If you have a phobia it is wise to seek professional help in the form of counselling, psychotherapy or whatever. Relaxation exercise (see pages 291–2) can also be of use, as can aromatherapy treatments. Behavioural therapy will encourage you to recognize the fear and may help you to face the fear in a controlled way. Hypnotherapy can help too, as can homeopathy. If you have therapeutic treatments, ask your therapist if he or she would mind diffusing an oil while they give the positive messages of reassurance. This same aroma can then be taken out, on a handkerchief for example, and sniffed whenever required. Diffusing the oils while doing relaxation exercises would be helpful too, and the same essential oil can be used in the same way later, sniffed for reassurance when feeling phobic, so possibly bringing relief. Choose an oil you really like the smell of, from the list of calming and relaxing oils. Then carry that same oil with you, especially when possibly facing the feared object or situation. The oil can be put on a tissue or handkerchief and just sniffed, and there are even necklaces being sold with little bottles for a pendant, which can hold essential oils, and of course bottles of essential oils are tiny enough to fit into even the smallest evening handbag. There is no need to be without nature's helpmates. If you're not worried about the material, a few drops of essential oil could even be put on a jacket or shirt sleeve and sniffed when required. Just by running your fingers through your hair, reassuring aroma molecules will waft into your nose. The memories of the therapy may flood back, the fear will hopefully dissipate – and nobody need ever know.

Used in phobias, essential oils can help in panic attacks, build up confidence, allay anxiety, help a person come to terms with the phobia and also develop the balance needed when, for example, having to face up to the problem. Plus, the essential oils can help overlay good memory patterns over bad. Some people might say it's bad to encourage a dependency on something, an oil in this case, but smell/memory/behaviour patterns can easily be overlaid. If there is a psychologist or psychotherapist involved, it will help them do their job better if you are relaxed, perhaps by the anxiety-relieving essential oils – which are listed on page 313. Also, looking at the chart section will help you decide what your symptoms are and which oils are best suited to your situation. There are of course many more calming and relaxing essential oils than those listed below, but these have been reported as being the most useful for this situation:

CALMING, RELAXING ESSENTIAL OILS

Lavender, Linden Blossom, Clary Sage, Neroli, Ylang Ylang, Marjoram, Ormenis Flower, Chamomile Roman, Sandalwood

There are no general blends that help with phobias as so many systems are involved and the phobia expresses itself so differently in different people. It is best to write a list of all your symptoms and make up your own personal oil.

PSYCHOSOMATIC ILLNESS

Psychosomatic illnesses *feel* real but aren't. The symptoms are real enough, but they are not caused by anything, other than the mind. It's all very confusing – to the patient and doctor alike. Headaches, nausea, irritable bowel syndrome, peptic ulcer and asthma sometimes have a psychosomatic cause, or are made worse by psychosomatic factors. This connection between the mind and body is well known but difficult to diagnose and treat. No doubt there are many people going to their doctor and being treated for something which could be better treated by counselling, and no doubt there are people diagnosed by their doctor as having psychosomatic illness when they do not. Those of us in the complementary fields have seen many such patients over the years, and often a problem is found and the person is told to go back to their doctor again. Clearly, the biggest danger is to miss an actual symptom of real disease because the psychosomatic factor makes diagnosis a problem. It's the old 'crying wolf' syndrome – it can get one into trouble.

There are no specific oils for this problem. As the symptoms are real – the pain is actually felt, there is no reason not to treat them with essential oils, and I refer you to my book *The Fragrant Pharmacy*. Please also refer to other sections of this book which may be relevant, including *Anxiety*.

QUARRELSOMENESS

Quarrelsome people are difficult to be with because everything you say, every opinion you have, is twisted and turned around into an argument. If you have a quarrelsome person in your family it can make life unbearable. Some people react by saying nothing. I know of at least one woman who has learned to skip over any event she knows may provoke her partner, who must watch her tone of voice, who looks at everything in a split second, evaluating the trouble it could cause, and arranging things so it doesn't. But of course, her quarrelsome partner still finds things to set him off.

Trying to change somebody else's attitude isn't really what *The Fragrant Mind* is about but if you yourself feel that you are perhaps overdoing the way you get your point across, maybe it's time to look at things from a different perspective. (If you really enjoy being antagonistic that is a different matter, and perhaps you should join a debating club . . . and give the family some peace.) Use the essential oils in all the usual methods:

ESSENTIAL OILS FOR QUARRELSOMENESS

*Clary Sage, Lavender, Lemon, Sandalwood, Patchouli, Cistus, *Clove*

*Should not be used in baths.

The quantities in the following blends can be diluted with 30 ml of base oil to make a massage oil, or make a synergistic blend of oils using these proportions and use in all room and inhalation methods.

QUARRELSOMENESS 1		QUARRELSOMENESS 2	
Lemon	20 drops	Sandalwood	10 drops
Clove	8 drops	Patchouli	5 drops
Cistus	2 drops	Lemon	15 drops

RAGE

Unlike normal anger, rage is a violent form of intensive anger, often completely uncontrollable. People can go 'blind with rage' and become violent, even kill, giving loss of reason as a defence. Rage is an outburst that wells up from somewhere deep inside, usually in response to an intensely provoking incident.

There are no specific essential oils for rage but some people could undoubtedly benefit from them by using oils for aggression, stress and tension. However, in rage type of personalities the stress and tension does not easily dissipate but remains lodged in the muscles and it would be best to visit an aromatherapy practitioner who can, through specialist techniques, release the tension.

Choose essential oils from the stress and tension lists or from the one below; use in all the usual methods. For quantities to use see Chart 5.1.

ESSENTIAL OILS TO HELP LESSEN RAGE
Chamomile Roman, Ylang Ylang, Ormenis Flower, Vetiver, Clary Sage, Lavender, Marjoram, Galbanham

RAGE BLEND 1		RAGE BLEND 2	
Vetiver	8 drops	Ylang Ylang	8 drops
Chamomile Roman	10 drops	Ormenis Flower	12 drops
Lavender	12 drops	Galbanham	10 drops

REGRET

It is amazing how many people say they don't have any regrets, despite the fact that they may be terminally ill or have had, to the outside eye, a pretty miserable life. Edith Piaf sung the immortal song 'Je ne regrette rien', and her life was no picnic. We seem instinctively to realize that in bad experiences there are lessons to be learnt, and that, in fact, we gain insight from bad experiences. How can one regret that? Even so, we probably all have one or two regrets kicking about somewhere which, with the benefit of hindsight, we can identify. But we don't dwell on them. The thing we regret just flickers quickly through the mind occasionally, perhaps when things are particularly bad, and then is forgotten. At least, it should be. However, there are some people who cannot rid themselves of thoughts of regret and who let it overcome their life so they are no longer living present day life to the full. If this is you, use the following essential oils singly or in blends in all the usual methods:

ESSENTIAL OILS FOR REGRET

Hyacinth, Cypress, Pine, Rose Maroc, Rose Otto, Mimosa

The quantities in the following blends can be diluted with 30 ml of base oil to make a massage oil, or make a synergistic blend of oils using these proportions and use it in baths, and in all room and inhalation methods.

REGRET 1		REGRET 2	
Rose Maroc	*5 drops*	*Rose Otto*	*10 drops*
Hyacinth	*5 drops*	*Cypress*	*2 drops*
Mimosa	*3 drops*	*Mimosa*	*4 drops*

REGRET 3	
Cypress	*20 drops*
Pine	*10 drops*

REJECTION

The dictionary definition of 'to reject' is 'to throw away as useless or worthless' – and that's just about how it feels. To feel rejected in love is perhaps an essential requirement in the 'to have experienced life' department and I doubt that one could claim to be an artist until you could identify with the depths of that despair. Or perhaps that is being dramatic and it would be fabulous to be the 'golden' boy or girl who manages to go through life getting everything and everyone they want. For most of us, however, it isn't like that. It isn't a question of *if* rejection will come but a question of how much and in what form.

Professionally, the recessions bring a trail of rejections in the form of people who have been told they've lost their job. Employment adverts for architects routinely say, 'don't bother if you're over 40', perhaps not in so many words, and when you go for the interview, they talk to you as though you were grandpa, somehow out of place. People over forty are expected to be partners in their own firms, or directors. And the crazy thing is, *logic* would tell you that an architect over forty was the better candidate because they had the experience. But logic doesn't always come into rejection.

Some very sensitive souls often feel rejected because they can 'sense' the underlying rejection of one of their ideals, or the unwillingness of someone else to accept a situation, a kind of rejection of their plans and desires. This is hurtful because it is disrespectful, as if we were useless and worthless. But also, some people feel rejected when it is not actually the case, they are misreading the situation – are being too sensitive.

I can think of dozens of people who have rejected tricky or uncomfortable changes, usually by doing and saying nothing – playing dead, refusing to accept that a situation has changed, that they are being asked to move on. This is rejection of reality and it can have a profound effect on us and even lead to depression and stress. The only answer is to come to terms with the truth and the inevitability of the situation.

Rejection needs comfort and understanding. Try to talk your situation through with someone, perhaps an outsider.

Rejection is definitely distressing, but it doesn't last for ever, or doesn't have to. These would be the essential oils to try, either singly or in blends, in all the usual methods:

ESSENTIAL OILS TO USE IF FEELING REJECTED

Pine, Cypress, Sandalwood, Benzoin, Chamomile Roman, Neroli, Rose Otto, Ylang Ylang, Hyacinth, Tuberose, Carnation

The quantities in the following blends can be diluted with 30 ml of base oil to make a massage oil, or make a synergistic blend of oils using these proportions and use in baths, and in all room and inhalation methods. For quantities to use see Chart 5.1.

REJECTION BLEND 1		REJECTION BLEND 2	
Carnation	*5 drops*	*Tuberose*	*5 drops*
Ylang Ylang	*5 drops*	*Benzoin*	*15 drops*
Sandalwood	*15 drops*	*Cypress*	*2 drops*

REPRESSION

Just as repression can stunt the growth of a people or nation, repression can stunt the growth of individuals. Repression by a person or situation can often be dealt with by becoming assertive, although this is easier said than done, especially in the home or workplace. We may feel unable to speak out, tell our truths, be who we are. There is repression too in feeling unable to fight against injustice, as if our views were ineffectual because of the largeness of 'the system', and our feelings of anger and dismay can never be heard where they are intended. It isn't *everyone* who gets a private conversation with the Prime Minister.

Once you can shake off the feelings of repression it will be as if a heavy winter coat and hat have been lifted from you. Again, talking helps. Many writers took up the pen as a way of being able to speak out and break free of repression, and you can do it too. Keep a diary, make lists, draw up brain maps –

anything to express what you are feeling inside.

Watch out too for self-repression – keeping uncomfortable feelings, actions or situations away from our conscious mind. It is a safety mechanism to protect our emotional state, but it is of limited value. There should come a time when it is no longer required.

To help shake off repression, use the following essential oils in all the usual methods, especially in baths, diffused around the home, or in a massage oil.

ESSENTIAL OILS FOR REPRESSION

Hyacinth, Jasmine, Frankincense, Ylang Ylang, Cedarwood, Pine, Patchouli, Vetiver, Juniper

The quantities in the following blends can be diluted with 30 ml of base oil to make a massage oil, or make a synergistic blend of oils using these proportions and use in the bath, and in all room and inhalation methods. For quantities to use see Chart 5.1.

REPRESSION 1		REPRESSION 2	
Patchouli	*5 drops*	*Cedarwood*	*14 drops*
Frankincense	*15 drops*	*Pine*	*8 drops*
Jasmine	*10 drops*	*Juniper*	*8 drops*

SCHIZOPHRENIA

The word 'schizophrenia' conjures up images of 'mad' behaviour, like hearing voices, talking nonsense and jumping into the lion's den. Symptoms include having incorrect beliefs, for example that people are conspiring against you, or believing that you are another person, perhaps a dead one, or being controlled. The senses are very much affected in that voices can be heard, and tastes, smells or sights imagined. Schizophrenics also tend to have confused thinking, a loss of interest in and affection of other people – even to the point of laughing at their misfortunes – self-absorption and self-neglect.

But these are generalizations because each schizophrenic experiences the illness in a different way. Schizophrenics do *not* have a split personality. They are suffering changes in perception which are affecting their thinking, behaviour and feelings.

One young man described the nightmare thus: 'I had never felt so terrified. I was confused and helpless, trapped in a menacing world where everyone and everything conspired against me.'[9] And this is a nightmare one in every hundred people in Britain will suffer before they reach forty-five, perhaps as a one-off incident or as a series throughout life. Each attack might last a few weeks or longer and in-between times, the person appears perfectly normal. Usually, schizophrenia develops for the first time when people are in their twenties.

Why it should do this is a mystery. Certainly the chemical messenger dopamine is involved and by regulating it more effectively the new generation of drugs is having tremendous impact on treatment, which is much improved (unless you are one of the unlucky few who develop agranulocytosis, a serious condition of the bone marrow).

Bearing in mind the drug treatment schizophrenics should be on and should continue to take, they should reduce by half the usual number of essential oils used, in massage oils, baths, diffusers, inhaled or whatever, or use less still. Only use these gentle oils:

ESSENTIAL OILS TO USE IN CASES OF SCHIZOPHRENIA
Lavender, Mandarin, Geranium, Chamomile Roman, Lemon, Rose Otto

When choosing your essential oils, bear in mind your condition at the time which may vary. The two blends below, for example, are more appropriate for different times of the day. For quantities to use see Chart 5.1.

DAY TIME		NIGHT TIME	
Geranium	5 drops	Lavender	8 drops
Lavender	5 drops	Lemon	4 drops
Lemon	5 drops	Chamomile Roman	3 drops

To make a massage oil, blend either of the above with 30 ml vegetable oil, or make a synergistic blend by mixing the essential oils in these proportions. Use a maximum of 4 drops in a bath – geranium is particularly useful. Lavender is excellent in diffusers – use 4 drops, three times a day, with 2 drops of lemon also each time. If the feel of oil on the skin is unpleasant, benefit can still be obtained by applying the massage oil and showering or bathing a short time later. The oils could also be diffused during any therapy sessions.

It is well worth exploring the link between allergies and schizophrenia, and it may be worth keeping a diary of what was eaten and drunk, and when the attacks occurred. There may be no link, but it's worth a look. Allergy tests are available and a nutritionist may also be able to give advice as to which foods may cause an allergic reaction, such as glucose and gluten for example. A high-protein, low-carbohydrate diet is often recommended, along with no caffeine. Vitamins which might be taken are those of the B group – B12, B3, B6, along with vitamins C and E; also thiamine, biotin, folic acid, zinc or PABA (para aminobenzoin acid). A group of psychiatrists called orthomoleculists use vitamins as part of the treatment, along with conventional methods. Homeopathy may be able to help too.

SELF-BLAME

We all blame ourselves at some time for things we should have done, situations that shouldn't have been. They can range from the minor, as when we knock over an ornament and say, 'Oh, I am stupid,' for example, to the major, as when we drive carelessly and harm someone. Self-blame is occasionally justified and shows that we are human, compassionate and aware. But sometimes it goes too far and people blame themselves for everything – including the weather. 'Sorry', 'sorry', 'sorry', 'sorry', they say, rather like a crowd of English people bumping into each other on a pavement.

Self-blame can develop if a child is made to feel that everything is their fault, and the guilt gets carried forward into adulthood. This is particularly sad because children do in any case blame themselves for all sorts of things that are not their fault, including domestic strife or divorce and shortage of money. Their little shoulders carry all sorts of self-blame that we can probably not imagine, but it pops out occasionally and makes us aware.

For young and old alike, it is very helpful to discuss self-blame, to try and get a realistic perspective on the subject. Words are powerful things and if you can just hear the sentence which self-blames, and reword it in your head, things might start to be different. Having the courage to say they are different would be even better. The crucial thing with essential oils is to choose those that make you feel good about yourself. You might find them on lists in other sections of this book or among those below. Use in all the usual methods.

ESSENTIAL OILS TO USE WHEN FEELING SELF-BLAME

Rose Otto, Lemon, Geranium, Chamomile Roman, Bergamot, Orange, Ylang Ylang, Carnation, Tuberose, Benzoin, Melissa, Eucalyptus Citriodora, Ormenis Flower

---

The quantities in the following blends can be diluted with 30 ml of base oil to make a massage oil, or make a synergistic blend of oils using these proportions and use in the bath, and in all room and inhalation methods. For quantities to use see Chart 5.1.

SELF-BLAME 1		SELF-BLAME 2	
Lemon	*10 drops*	*Eucalyptus Citriodora*	*15 drops*
Bergamot	*10 drops*	*Chamomile Roman*	*5 drops*
Orange	*8 drops*	*Ylang Ylang*	*10 drops*
Ormenis Flower	*2 drops*		

SORROW

Deep sadness can be caused by grief, loss, disappointment, suffering and regret. It can last a long time depending on the person and the cause. Some people never get over sorrow and carry it with them always. See also *Bereavement* and *Grief*. The following oils have been found to be helpful; use in all the usual methods:

ESSENTIAL OILS FOR SORROW

Cypress, Hyacinth, Melissa, Benzoin, Frankincense, Sandalwood, Rose Otto

The quantities in the following blends can be diluted with 30 ml of base oil to make a massage oil, or make a synergistic blend of oils using these proportions and use in the bath, and in all room and inhalation methods.

SORROW 1		SORROW 2	
Sandalwood	*15 drops*	*Hyacinth*	*5 drops*
Frankincense	*10 drops*	*Sandalwood*	*10 drops*
Benzoin	*5 drops*		

STRESS

Psychologists talk about three types of stress: *Normal Stress, Distress and Eustress*. *Normal Stress* is what one would feel after narrowly escaping a car accident – short of breath and with a racing heart. This physical reaction is caused by the release of chemicals from the adrenal 'gland', which has two distinct parts – the central *adrenal medulla* and an outer *adrenal cortex*. This is a mechanism for survival, a sudden and immediate shot in the arm, so to speak, to get us out of a fix, to sharpen reactions so we can move faster and use all our wits. It may be that we have to decide which way to turn the car steering wheel to best avoid an accident, or which way to jump in front of an oncoming herd of buffalo – it's all stress. This emergency system is chemical and involves *epinephrine* and a smaller amount of *norepinephrine*, which are released directly into the bloodstream. The heart begins to pound immediately. Metabolic changes take place which cause energy immediately to be supplied where required, especially to the brain. The adrenal cortex releases the stress-related hormone *cortisol* which, among other things, increases the level of glucose in the blood and redirects it to the brain and causes hypertension – which are handy physiological back-ups when looking a tiger in the eye.

Stress isn't meant to be an everyday occurrence. What happens is that we get overloaded on the natural chemicals because we're stimulated by stressful situations too much and it gets bottled up. This chronic situation is called, appropriately, *Distress*. It is dangerous because it can lead to a hardening of the arteries, heart attacks and strokes, and lesser problems. One way people find to off-load their stress is to work it off with exercise and I know several New York high-flyers who say they simply wouldn't *survive* without their hour's workout at the gym each day. Another answer is to rearrange your life or job so there isn't so much stress to deal with. Most especially, look at the degree of control in your life. An American study found that the people who suffered most stress were those who had high demands made of them, but little control – such as waiters, cooks, firemen and cashiers. Another interesting piece of research from Sweden tested commuters at journey's end for their level of stress and found that those who boarded early, and had choice in where to sit, were less stressed – control again. Working mothers of young children are a group who are particularly prone to stress because they have all the pressures but little control – if little Billy wets his bed in the middle of the night, you get up, you have no choice. *Eustress* is the ideal state – buzzed up over some exciting project which is under our control, the energy flowing and the work going great.

You know you've got distress if you 'blow a fuse' or have a 'hair trigger' as far as everyday annoyances go – like getting het up in a traffic jam or shouting at the kids for the smallest thing. You may have persistent doubts about being able to cope, or feel helpless and out of control. Stress can arise from mental causes – such as exam or office pressure; from emotional problems – such as a relationship break-up; from physical pressures – such as too much driving, squash or gardening; from chemical sources – such as too much caffeine or drugs; and from environmental pressures – such as persistent noise on the factory floor. Symptoms of the mind include irritability, loss of sense of humour, difficulty in making decisions or concentrating, or doing jobs in logical order, feeling defensive, angry inside and disinterested in large areas of life. Physical symptoms include insomnia, sweating, breathlessness, faints, loss of appetite and bingeing, indigestion, constipation or diarrhoea, headaches, cramps, muscle spasms, eczema and sexual disinterest, but of course the biggest symptom is heart attack or stroke, by which time stress-management will be too late.

Until relatively recently 'stress' wasn't taken very seriously and was pigeon-holed as a thing which only affected powerful executives with a thousand telephone calls to make. We now know that isn't true. It's as likely to be the poor secretary being ordered around by her tyrannical boss that has the stress, especially if she's juggling with child care arrangements as well as her job. The government certainly takes stress seriously, with an estimated 100 million days lost each year through it, to the cost of £1.5 billion a year. This is a massive financial loss to the nation and an inestimable loss in terms of human happiness.

Essential Oils and Stress

Potentially, all essential oils can help combat stress because they are used in massage and baths, which are themselves therapeutic procedures. Of course, essential oils go much deeper than this, and some essential oils work particularly well on stress. Indeed, so effective are they that essential oils may provide the most successful way of coping with the problems associated with and caused by stress. They certainly strengthen the immune system, which gets considerably weaker during stressful periods, whereas people who lead stress-free lives have a better ability to fight off disease.

Each aromatherapist has their own favourite oils to use in the fight against stress and the ones listed below consist of

those in common use and easily available. They all blend
well with each other and can be successfully interchanged,
each having medical properties that are useful in treating
stress.

ESSENTIAL OILS TO HELP ALLEVIATE STRESS

*Bergamot, Chamomile Roman, Ormenis Flower, Frankincense,
Geranium, Grapefruit, Lavender, Lemon, Mandarin, Marjoram,
Melissa, Neroli, Rose Otto, Sandalwood, Vetiver, Clary Sage,
Ylang Ylang, Bay, Jasmine, Benzoin, Eucalyptus Citriodora,
Osmanthus, Tuberose, Hyacinth, Narcissus, Linden Blossom,
Nutmeg, Hops, Spikenard, Valerian, Yarrow, Litsea Cubeba*

Of the above, one of my favourites is the much-neglected
eucalyptus citriodora (eucalyptus lemon). Not only does it
have antibiotic, antifungal and slightly antiviral properties, it

Neroli

appears to boost the immune system, has electrical properties akin to our own energetic force, and is adaptogenic, which basically means it's subtle and bends to our needs. All these properties make it a must for anyone who is dealing with stress and its harmful effects.

The following oils could be considered the 'essential stress kit' oils because various combinations of them would be suitable in most situations. They have been selected from the recommended lists drawn up by aromatherapy organizations, and they are reasonably priced. All will work well, singly or in combinations, and have been the basis for aromatherapy relaxation and stress-relief treatments for a considerable length of time.

THE ESSENTIAL STRESS KIT

Eucalyptus Citriodora, Lavender, Geranium, Clary Sage, Ormenis Flower, Chamomile Roman, Ylang Ylang, Sandalwood, Petitgrain, Mandarin

If resources were unlimited, I would include in my personal stress kit the essential oils of rose otto, rose maroc, hyacinth, carnation, linden blossom, neroli and jasmine, each of which has proven its worth in the treatment of stressful disorders time and time again. These highly emotional essential oils can be added to your personal stress kit, as and when funds allow. By choosing your additions to the essential stress kit carefully you can build up a set of oils that will suit all types of stress and problems that are incurred because of it. However, using only the original stress kit oils, many formulations can be made, as can be seen below.

The following blends have been designed for general use with stress. The quantities can be diluted with 30 ml of base oil to make a massage oil, or make a synergistic blend of oils using these proportions and use in the bath, and in all room and inhalation methods.

STRESS LEVEL ONE: tiredness, irritability, aches and pains, occasional depression

STRESS LEVEL ONE: BLEND 1		STRESS LEVEL ONE: BLEND 2	
Eucalyptus Citriodora	10 drops	Mandarin	15 drops
Geranium	15 drops	Ylang Ylang	5 drops
Lavender	5 drops	Petitgrain	10 drops

STRESS LEVEL TWO: anxiety/depression, food allergies, persistent infection, sub-acute disease, hidden weaknesses (such as otherwise dormant viral infections)

STRESS LEVEL TWO: BLEND 1		STRESS LEVEL TWO: BLEND 2	
Clary Sage	10 drops	Ormenis Flower	10 drops
Chamomile Roman	5 drops	Ylang Ylang	5 drops
Lavender	5 drops	Petitgrain	5 drops
Geranium	10 drops	Sandalwood	10 drops

STRESS LEVEL THREE: complex pattern of symptoms (anything from suicidal tendencies to stomach pain), fear, withdrawal from society, despair

STRESS LEVEL THREE: BLEND 1		STRESS LEVEL THREE: BLEND 2	
Chamomile Roman	5 drops	Geranium	6 drops
Clary Sage	15 drops	Eucalyptus Citriodora	14 drops
Ormenis Flower	5 drops	Mandarin	10 drops

Stress Management

Write up a list of all the activities you have in your life and order them in terms of priorities. Get rid of those things which come at the bottom of your list, the non-essentials, by delegating responsibility for them to someone else or simply deleting them from your life. Ask yourself, as you look at your list, who am I doing this for – me or someone else? Then re-evaluate them again – are they really necessary? Make time for yourself, so you can do something you enjoy in peace. Talk to people about your problems and see what solutions they can come up with. Think laterally – do you enjoy your job, and are you good at it? – if not, change it. Do ten minutes' relaxation each and every day. Take vitamins, cut caffeine, get some exercise, laugh, cry and then go out and *enjoy* yourself!

TRAUMA

Many emotional problems start during a traumatic situation, whether this is a crisis or a tragedy that changes a whole life, or a deeply personal event. Many therapists believe that a traumatic birth can lead to emotional wounding later in life, particularly if the following events of life give no comfort. We know that physical and environmental trauma – caused by accidents, having an illness or being in an earthquake and so on – affects the body's structure, causing blockages and stresses and tensions in the way the body functions. Emotional trauma – such as leaving home, changing a job or losing a loved one – can do the same thing. Vibrational trauma can come when the electromagnetic patterning around us, our aura, gets disturbed by outside factors. Our etheric state can also have an effect on our mind and body.

Clearly, trauma is an intensely personal thing, with many sources, and how much it affects us depends on how we view them. But traumas do have an effect on us all in some way, whether we like it or not. Human beings are mind/body/spirit complexes, walking, talking electrical energy, and we cannot separate these three, especially in the case of trauma. Therefore all three must be considered when using essential oils for this condition.

ESSENTIAL OILS TO USE IN CASES OF TRAUMA

Thyme Linalol, Lavender, Geranium, Lemon, Marjoram, Petitgrain, Clary Sage, Chamomile Roman

If you have suffered from trauma look at the lists and charts throughout this book to find your symptoms and choose oils from there. Trauma victims need to release the tension and stress to stop further complications happening. If you can, visit an aromatherapist who may be able to help you further.

WITHDRAWAL FROM LIFE

Withdrawal from life is very common. People hide themselves away or seem to be withdrawn inside themselves. This may happen gradually in a series of small steps towards solitude, such as not going out any more, not making phone calls, or visiting friends and not buying clothes and paying attention to themselves.

Withdrawal from life may follow a trauma or deeply felt emotion or event, but it is not normal and most people are dreadfully unhappy with the situation in which they find themselves. Withdrawal of emotional feelings is another aspect of withdrawal, for example, no longer to give freely of love, compassion, understanding and even anger. Again, this is not right and often goes hand in hand with withdrawal from life.

Another kind of withdrawal is the kind yogis do, sometimes for years in a cave – contemplative withdrawal. This is the kind of withdrawal that gives us insight, peace and strength. Some people withdraw for periods of meditation, to feel near God, to look deep inside themselves or perhaps to create a masterpiece.

WITHDRAWAL FROM LIFE

Narcissus, Orange

WITHDRAWAL OF EMOTIONS

Bergamot, Rose Otto, Hyacinth, Chamomile Roman, Neroli, Mandarin, Geranium

WITHDRAWAL FOR PEACE

Rose Otto, Chamomile Roman, Neroli, Carnation, Bergamot, Frankincense, Geranium, Cypress, Cedarwood, Juniper

The quantities in the following blends can be diluted with 30 ml of base oil to make a massage oil, or make a synergistic blend of oils using these proportions and use in the bath, and in all room and inhalation methods. For quantities to use see Chart 5.1.

EMOTIONAL WITHDRAWAL 1		EMOTIONAL WITHDRAWAL 2	
Chamomile Roman	*1 drop*	*Bergamot*	*15 drops*
Neroli	*10 drops*	*Hyacinth*	*5 drops*
Geranium	*1 drop*		

WITHDRAWAL FOR PEACE

Frankincense	*5 drops*
Juniper	*5 drops*
Bergamot	*5 drops*

To the above blends you could add another 15 drops of essential oil. Use essential oils that you feel particularly attuned to. Spend some time meditating and then use your intuition to guide you to the right ones for you.

WORTHLESSNESS

Feeling that you have no worth or are without value, that you are despicable, and not fit to walk this planet, may seem alien to some. But many people have to live with these feelings every day. It is crucial to talk these feelings through, if only with yourself. Write down *who* said you were worthless, *when* and *why*, *what* are you worthless at exactly, and what are you good at? Try to trace *when* you began to feel worthless, and write down *what* was going on at the time. If you can't figure out where these feelings of worthlessness came from, take your notes to a counsellor or psychotherapist and see if they can figure it out. Perhaps hypnotherapy can reveal a cause you hadn't thought of. At least find a friend to talk to, even a stranger. A professional aromatherapist will be able to tell a great deal from seeing which muscles tense and stress as you speak and will be bound by ethics never to repeat your most inner thoughts. Also, relaxation techniques can help to clear your mind, and as that happens, you might just find the answer to it all. Essential oils can help you to sort out your feelings by working on the limbic system, helping you focus your thoughts. Use in all the usual ways:

ESSENTIAL OILS TO HELP ALLEVIATE FEELINGS OF WORTHLESSNESS

Frankincense, Sandalwood, Cedarwood, Clove, Ormenis Flower, Neroli, Juniper, Chamomile Roman, Geranium

The quantities in the following blends can be diluted with 30 ml of base oil to make a massage oil, or make a synergistic blend of oils using these proportions and use in all room and inhalation methods. For quantities to use see Chart 5.1.

WORTHLESSNESS 1.		WORTHLESSNESS 2	
Juniper	*10 drops*	*Clove*	*5 drops*
Cedarwood	*10 drops*	*Sandalwood*	*15 drops*
Frankincense	*5 drops*	*Chamomile Roman*	*5 drops*
Geranium	*5 drops*	*Ormenis Flower*	*5 drops*

Chapter Nine

TAKING CONTROL

AUTOGENIC TRAINING

IN THE LATE 1920S A GERMAN NEUROLOGIST CALLED DR JOHANES Schultz became intrigued by the possibility that the healing benefits of hypnotism could be reproduced without actually putting the patient into a trance. He developed autogenic training which basically consists of a series of six mental exercises which can be done in one of three positions – lying on one's back, sitting upright on a chair, or sitting on the edge of a chair with the head and shoulders slumped forward. The technique is used not only to reduce anxiety, stress or depression and induce relaxation but, by allowing the body's natural healing mechanisms to work effectively, has a beneficial impact on many physical disorders including bronchitis, colitis, irritable bowl syndrome, high blood pressure, migraine and ulcers.

The tremendous success of autogenic training has spawned over 3,000 pieces of research, which can prove its effectiveness but not explain why it works so well. That secret is still tied up with the mystery of the mind-body connection. It is possible to get autogenic training on the NHS as many therapists are also trained health workers such as doctors, psychologists and nurses.[1] Almost anyone can benefit from autogenic training, from businessmen who want to operate at their peak of efficiency, and sportspersons who want to improve their performance and stimulate the body's healing mechanisms so injuries can heal faster, to people trying to cut down or come off drugs.

Taking whichever of the three positions mentioned above is the most comfortable (or appropriate given the time of day because this technique can also be practised while sitting on a commuter train, for example), the person can go through one or more of the six mental exercises, each of which are accompanied by a phrase which is silently repeated. During the first exercise, which focuses the thoughts on *heaviness* of the arms, legs, neck and shoulders, the phrase might be 'my left arm is heavy'. The *warmth* exercise involves concentrating on the warmth felt in the arms and legs. The *heartbeat* exercise is simply to focus on the heartbeat. The fourth exercise is to focus on *breathing*; the fifth is to focus on a feeling of warmth in the *stomach;* and the sixth is to concentrate on a feeling of coolness on the *forehead*.

Ideally, the technique should be taught by a trained therapist, a process which takes eight to ten sessions of one hour each – probably within a group setting. You may be able to find books on the subject, or try it yourself. In the 'slumped' position, sit on the edge of the chair with your hands on your thighs and feet about 12 inches (30 cm) apart. In the 'reclining' position, lie flat on your back with a pillow under your head and another under your knees, arms resting to the side. Breathe deeply and slowly from the abdomen. To begin with, just do the heaviness exercise, concentrating on heaviness in the arms, legs, neck and shoulders, then progress to the other exercises, adding them as you become more adept at concentrating. For each exercise, repeat a phrase which helps focus your mind on what you are doing – such as, for number six, 'my forehead is cool, my forehead is cool'. People do autogenic training every day, from as little as two minutes three times a day, to twenty minutes three times a day. If you have any physical area that is causing problems, mentally direct your healing energy to that region. One interesting aspect of autogenic training is 'autogenic discharges' – fleeting but often powerful impressions of aromas, tastes, touch and so on, which are related to events that happened in the past. This release of trapped energy causes a flow or rush of energy.

The 'autogenic discharges' are perhaps a strange phenomenon, but one sees the same thing happening during aromatherapy treatments when emotions such as anger and grief are dislodged from the musculature, and many other therapies report the same releasing dynamic at work. If essential oils are to be diffused while doing the exercises, choose an oil from the relaxing list, or one that is particularly relevant to your requirements.

BREATHING

Learning to breathe properly is essential to health. When we breathe in, oxygen is absorbed into the blood and circulated to all organs and when we breathe out, waste gases are expelled. As we all know, breathing rates change to suit the situation. If we're building a house of cards we hold our breath; and if we're anxious, we can find ourselves gasping for breath. Fear and excitement tend to make people breathe from the chest, as does aerobic exercise.

The kind of breathing that is done for relaxation and health is diaphragmatic breathing. Basically, it is a controlled and slightly prolonged variation on the old advice to 'take a couple of deep breaths' before stressful situations. This uses the diaphragm muscle which separates the chest and abdominal cavities. When you breathe from here, the ribs expand as the lungs are filled with air and the abdominal organs can actually be massaged by the diaphragm muscles as they rhythmically move. In very stressful situations one of the easiest and quickest ways of relieving tension or coping with the nerves, before public speaking for example, is a few deep, controlled diaphragmatic breaths.

Using essential oils while doing breathing can make the exercise even more effective. Essential oils are reported to help oxygenate the blood and as they may also work directly on the nervous system, the combination can help all manner of problems. Deep breathing should be used during all relaxation exercises and is an integral part of yoga, for example. Clients are also often asked to breathe deeply several times before and after an aromatherapy massage or reflexology treatment, first, to help the energy flow and, second, to help expel any gases that may have been released from the muscles and organs during treatment.

MASSAGE

All over the world, and for as long as we know, people have massaged each other. They do it on Pacific Islands, in Moroccan bath houses, in Chinese shops, everywhere, in fact, where there are people. Many systems of massage have developed and they have different intents and purposes. Some are simply about relaxation, some are therapeutic, and some are designed to release blockages which might be called 'mental' because they originated in the mind, but which are actually physical, because they are lodged in the body itself. The simplest form of massage is the kind done to young children who have bumped themselves. We 'rub it better', not simply by giving attention and showing love, but by stimulating the area so more blood comes there, and healing can progress.

On a simple level, we can see from someone's hunched up shoulders that they are carrying tension. It doesn't stop there though. The human body holds all the traumas, pain, distress, tension and emotional crisis within its muscular structure. Every thought and feeling we have is etched in our body, the map of our experiences. Some people can read the maps better than others and know which areas to work with specialist techniques to relieve some of the tension. We are not here concerned with those techniques but with safe and efficient massage that can be carried out at home. One very important benefit of massage is that it increases blood circulation which enables the body to get rid of the waste products produced by all our cells and organs. The oxygenation of massage, combined with the detoxifying, stimulating and healing properties of essential oils is extremely effective, but is even more so in the hands of a trained aromatherapist using specialist massage techniques which also release the emotional blockages in the body itself.

Consider for a moment what happens when you hear a loud bang in the street. We are 'startled' – our eyes blink; our body can 'jump out of its skin' or at least the muscles in the head, neck, shoulders, arms, legs and abdomen become taut; our nerves get tense; our hearts race; while the mind is calculating the danger and figuring out whether a car is out of control and we should prepare to jump out of the way. All this happens instantaneously, but the effects linger on. Some events linger longer than others, lodged in the body until something releases them. Fear, pain, anxiety, fatigue, stress and depression can all be locked in the body which, like the face, has a story to tell. Negative emotions tend to shorten the neck muscles, which then displaces the head and back muscles, putting more stress on the body.

Swedish Massage

The system known as 'Swedish massage' was developed by Per Henrikling as part of a medical programme designed to assist in the eradication of disease. People who are bedridden are particularly disadvantaged because they don't get the exercise that allows oxygenation and the elimination of cellular waste products, and they were of particular concern to Henrikling. Some of the massage strokes were designed to be more stimulating, some more relaxing, but all strokes went towards the heart to stimulate the circulation as well as lymphatic flow. (The lymphatic system of vessels extends through the entire body and is part of the immune system; the lymph nodes are filters that trap unwanted micro-organisms and destroys them with lymphocytes, white blood cells.) There are five basic strokes to Swedish massage, only two of which are required for home use:

Effleurage movements are strokes – which can be long or short, gentle or hard. Do them in an unhurried way, simply stroking in long, smooth movements.

Petrissage movements are more like the action of kneading dough. Although the whole hand is involved, the two thumbs work in a circular movement (right, clockwise; left, anticlockwise) and a fair amount of pressure is exerted – but not so much that any pain is felt. The movement is like a squeezing, rolling action, involving the thumbs and fingers more than anything else, but also the flat of the hand as it comes into contact with the skin.

The other movements are *Vibrations, Frictions* and *Tapotement*, which should not be done without further information or instruction as they're not that easy to perform correctly and may cause harm to the underlying organs. But using effleurage – stroking – and petrissage – the rolling, squeezing, kneading movement, carried out only on the muscles, is not harmful and can be done to anyone – even to oneself, to promote health and well-being.

Massage is a wonderful therapy because it relaxes, heals, and involves touch – itself a healing tool. However, there is one problem with it – it can be an excuse for people to exert power over others. Never jump up and say, 'Oh, you're so tense, I'm going to give you a shoulder massage' and impose your will on another person in this way. OK, they may be tense, but this isn't the approach to take. In a way, you're saying, 'Oh, you're so tense and I'm not, I'm better at coping than you are, here let me show you what a selfless, caring, giving person I am.' All of which can make the person feel worse than they did to begin with! I can't remember the number of times I have seen some poor person attacked by another in this way, imposing their will. The person being massaged sits there, even more tense, as the imposer pushes and pummels their already strained muscles, with the person (trying to be polite) saying, 'Yes, that's lovely, fine, yes, that's it, now I'm OK, can you stop please,' just wishing the thing were over. Please make sure you do not fall into the category of imposer, and get *permission* to massage, and make sure your intent is pure (and not intended to show how great you are), thoughtful and respectful. Only then will it be a pleasure, and help, to both receiver and giver.

The diagrams on pp. 286–7 show which parts of the body

are liable to hold emotional tension, both past and present. These areas can be worked on using gentle effleurage or petrissage movements, although if you find sore areas (which is not unusual and does not necessarily mean something is wrong) they should not be overworked. Throughout this book I have referred to 'massage oils' and while, certainly, these can be put on the body as part of a massage, they could also simply be *put* on the body and rubbed into the skin in the same way that you apply body lotions, but particularly on those areas of the body that, you can see from the illustrations, might be holding the particular tensions you have.

We also carry tension in our faces, and this can be helped with essential oils. Use 30ml of a good skin oil, such as macadamia, hazelnut or sweet almond and a maximum of 30 drops of a single essential oil – either lavender, geranium, chamomile roman, rose otto, or ylang ylang – or blend these according to your needs. Recipes for skin care can be found in *The Fragrant Pharmacy*.

Other Therapies

There are a great number of therapies which involve some form of massage or body-work and the sheer number of them is confusing. Instead of asking, 'which is the best?' it may be better to consider the fact that 'there are many routes to the same place' – they may all be 'best', but one route may suit you better. One major step forward in recent years, however, is that there is a growing appreciation of the mind-body connection and body-work is becoming more commonly used as an integral part of talking-therapy. These days, psychologists study body-work and body-workers study psychology.

Humanistic Psychology is a new discipline that utilizes body-work and, through talking, encourages the release of emotions in a safe setting. *Psychiatric Orgone Therapy* combines the techniques of psychoanalysis and character analysis with body-work principles established by Wilhelm Reich. *Reichian Therapy* aims to make the client aware of how their posture, breathing and muscular tension – called 'body armouring' – reflect their emotions. Physical manipulation is

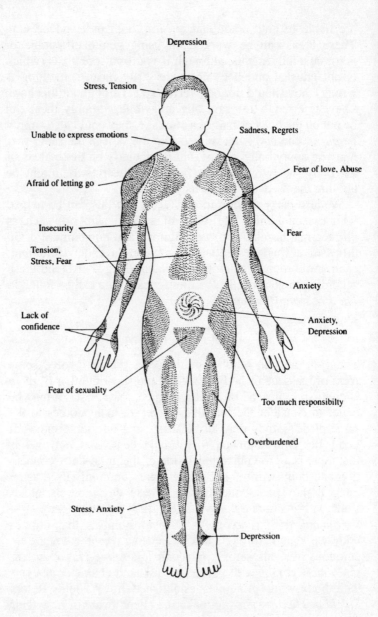

Emotional Muscular Sites
Front of Body

Emotional Muscular Sites
Back of Body

used to release physical/emotional tension, after which clients often report a feeling of energetic 'streaming' – energy flowing through the body. Reich had a student called Alexander Lowen who took aspects of Reich's body-work theories and developed *Bioenergetics*. Again, therapists aim to make the client aware of the way their body is holding emotions and to unlock the 'character armouring' so that the body is able to function freely, and healthily.

For Professional Therapists

There has been a tendency in the past for therapists to ask their clients to 'keep silent and relax' during treatment but this is, in a sense, a contradiction in terms. Relaxing is about 'letting it all out' and you can't do that if you've been asked to keep quiet! Therapy is a time for releasing the bottled-up emotions, and that involves talk, so encourage the client to chat about themselves. Don't chat about yourself and your lovely holiday or whatever – *you* are not the one who needs to talk, but be sensitive to the client's need to express themselves as you work on the body and release emotionally congested areas of it.

MEDITATION

Meditation used to be the preserve of New-Agers and, before them, the hippy generation. Now everybody does it, and you can even get transcendental meditation on the NHS because it is recognized as a useful tool in the drive to curb pain or disease. Meditation is an exercise of the mind designed to calm and connect the mind, body and spirit. Yogis have been teaching the benefits of meditation for thousands of years and now we have machines which can actually record these benefits. For example, machines which record the electrical impulses sent out by muscles show that while meditating, muscular tension drops to almost zero. Circulation is also improved, and EEG (electroencephalograph) readings have shown that brain activity during meditation is almost the same as we have while asleep – which explains perhaps why meditation is so relaxing and refreshing.

People who have practised meditation for some time can do it anywhere, any time. When starting out, however, find a quiet room, take the phone off the hook and get yourself into a comfortable position. It is preferable not to have eaten or drunk anything for half an hour beforehand. Some people like to lie down but teachers do not approve of this as a rule because there's a chance the person might fall asleep. Keeping the back straight is important, whether you sit in an upright chair, or with a cushion under your bottom. Some people meditate with their eyes open, others with their eyes closed. People with their eyes open might be concentrating on a particular image – a candle, for example, or a picture of a flower, or a yantra – an abstract picture with metaphysical meaning. People with their eyes closed might be visualizing an image. These images are for a purpose – to give you something to focus on so that when distracting thoughts come into your mind they can be replaced with the meditative image, so the distracting thoughts can float away. Whether with eyes open or closed, some people have a mantra – a word or few words – which they repeat over and over again, to block out distracting thoughts and also to set up a vibration conducive to meditation. Others concentrate on their breathing. In any case, breathe deeply through the nose, expelling the breath through the mouth if you wish. Also try relaxing – mentally say to your forehead 'relax', to your clenched teeth, 'relax', and so on. There are many classes, books, audiotapes and videos available, all of which can be very useful.

Even ten minutes' meditation each day is extremely beneficial. The essential oils are helpful in that they help to focus the mind and their aroma can even become the thing on which you concentrate as a means of blocking out unwanted thoughts. The list below shows the oils which are most popular for meditation but you may prefer to use one of your personal choice, or one that will help with any particular problem you have, chosen from the lists throughout this book. If you have high blood pressure, tension and stress, lavender would be a good oil to choose. Also see *Focus* and *Concentration* in Chapter 7. You can use essential oils singly or in blends.

Oils should be used to help the atmosphere and set the scene. *Do not* wear them in the form of perfume or massage oil because this combination of essential oils and meditation may be too much and you don't really need it. Simply use a room method, 4–6 drops at the most. Many people make their own formulations exclusively for use in meditation. Using essential oils can also contribute to the ritualistic element involved, which helps to focus the mind on the meditation to come. Calm the mind as you go about preparing the room, lighting a candle perhaps, or putting on a music tape, and preparing your diffuser.

Juniper

POPULAR ESSENTIAL OILS FOR MEDITATION

Lavender, Neroli, Lemon, Juniper, Frankincense, Sandalwood, Jasmine, Rose Maroc, Rose Otto, Chamomile Roman, Carnation, Hyacinth, Geranium, Bergamot, Cedarwood, Cypress, Ylang Ylang

MEDITATION BLEND 1		MEDITATION BLEND 2	
Lavender	5 drops	Neroli	16 drops
Lemon	15 drops	Ylang Ylang	2 drops
Juniper	5 drops	Bergamot	10 drops
Geranium	5 drop	Frankincense	2 drops

RELAXATION

Relaxation is recognized as an integral part of physical and mental health but stress and tension prevent the type of relaxation needed for health of mind and body. Relaxation depends on good breathing techniques (see *Breathing*), among other things. A good exercise to help you recognize areas in your body where you may be carrying tension and stress is the 'tense and release' exercise, a classic relaxation technique used in hospitals and by various therapists, and I have personally taught this version to many patients and people in workshops.

First of all make sure you have time to do the exercise with no interruptions. Turn off the radio, although you may play some relaxing music you particularly enjoy. Turn down any bright light and get yourself comfortable in a chair that supports your back. We start the exercise with the feet:

Tense and Relax Exercise

Feet: Some people prefer to concentrate on one foot at a time, some concentrate on both at the same time:

(a) Concentrate on your feet; totally think yourself into the feet; consciously focus on the toes, and then the toenails; feel the skin on your feet; and the soles. Now feel the feet becoming very heavy.

(b) Now tense the feet as hard as you can, pointing the toes and pushing the feet away from you. Hold the tension, count to five and relax. Make a point of noticing how you feel about the feet – are there any tense areas when you relax them?

Legs: Again, some people may prefer to concentrate on one leg, some do both at the same time:

(a) Focus on your calf muscles and clench them tightly; you may want to stretch out your legs to do this more effectively.
(b) Then relax them, noticing if there are any areas that feel tense or uncomfortable. If so, tense those areas again and relax them.

Thighs: One or both:

(a) Focus on the thigh muscles; relax them by making them feel heavy; then tense them as tightly as possible, pushing them into the seat of the chair.
(b) Now relax them, focusing on any areas that feel tense and uncomfortable; if so, tense them again, and relax.

Bottom: Tense the muscles in the cheeks of your bottom as tight as you can, clenching them together (which will also help you notice any tight areas that are retained in your thighs); then relax. This is an area that often holds tension, surprisingly to many people.

Abdomen:

(a) Tense the muscles of the abdomen by pulling them in really tightly, and gripping them there.
(b) Then relax them, and notice if there are any areas of discomfort; if so, repeat the exercise.

Back:

(a) Tense the muscles of the back by pushing the lower back hard against the back of the chair.
(b) Relax. We all carry tension in this area and it really feels good to tense and relax here. Again, notice any discomfort or any tense areas and repeat the exercise once more.

Hands: One at a time or both together:

   (a) Tense the hands by making fists as tight as you possibly can.

   (b) And then let them go. Some people like to imagine they are gripping on to something – money (greed), pain, fear or guilt, for example – and then, just let it go as you release the hand muscles.

Arms: One or both:

   (a) Tense the muscles as hard as possible by pushing the arm downward as far as you can.

   (b) Release, noticing any areas of discomfort and, as before, repeating the exercise with them.

Head: Just let the head and neck flop forward as far as they will go; and then backwards – holding it for a few seconds in each position.

Shoulders: Push your shoulders up as high as you can into your neck; notice any tight areas; then release the muscles. Repeat.

Face: Open your *mouth* as wide as you can; really stretch it; then just relax it. Repeat the exercise. Now, screw your *face* up into a ball as tight as you can; then just let it relax. Repeat. Raise your *forehead* as high as you can; and then let it go. Smile the widest *smile* you can with the lips together, pushing the *cheeks* upwards; then let them go. Repeat. Screw the *eyes* up as tightly as you can; then let go. Repeat. Tense the *scalp*, and then let go. Repeat. People are often surprised at the tension they are holding in their scalp, and by the relief they feel when they let it go.

Concentrate your thought into the solar plexus – the area in between the ribcage and diaphragm, breathe deeply several times, letting whatever thoughts come flow through your mind, even if they are very emotionally painful; just let them flow and then let them go. This exercise can be done anywhere at any time, once you have got the hang of it.

Use plenty of essential oil diffused around the room in which you are sitting. Choose oils from the relaxing and tension-relieving lists. You can combine them with other oils that may be pertinent to your mood or emotions.

VISUALIZATION

As a technique, until very recently, visualization might have been considered a bit weird, not to say bizarre. All that has changed. Not only has medical research shown that mind and body *are* one integrated whole, visualization techniques have been shown to work. It is well known that visualization is very much a part of the eastern philosophies but less well known that the Greeks used it and that it was part of the western medical tradition until the mid 1600s, when the supposed mind-body dichotomy came into fashion. The first research into visualization was done by Edmund Jacobson in the 1920s who showed that a person's leg muscles would twitch involuntarily when he was visualizing himself running.

In visualization, the person imagines a scene or scenario they wish to occur happening. Most commonly, the technique is used to have an influence on the course of disease and the scene imagined is of the diseased cells being in some way or other destroyed or banished. The same principle applies to conditions of the mind, even love. For example, one might imagine oneself full of confidence striding up to the boss and asking for a rise and, crucially, he or she saying 'yes'; or one might imagine the perfect partner – in full detail physically, mentally and spiritually – coming into your life. This kind of imagining has to be repeated over and over again, reinforcing the reality you want to create.

It is not easy to visualize anything without practice – the practice of actually *seeing*, rather than passively looking. Start out by looking at a two-dimensional picture for two or three minutes and then trying to remember all the details. It needs time, but keep on practising until you have really noticed all the details in the picture and can remember them, and as you remember them, see them in your mind's eye. Then do the same exercise with a three-dimensional object, repeating once a day, until you can remember all the details of that object clearly and, as you remember, again, see it in your mind's eye. Eventually progress to a living image – the garden for example, and try to train your eye really to see what is going on there. Now progress to the image on which you want to work. Is it you being a fabulous success on the opening night of the dramatic society's latest show, or you working contentedly behind your desk and efficiently processing the papers from the in-tray to the out-tray? Whatever it is that you want to visualize and make happen doesn't matter, so long as you are consistent, and persevere.

Visualization is very often incorporated into meditation and relaxation techniques, and is also an integral part of autogenic training. Use essential oils during visualization that are specific to the reason for the visualization. If your image involves your being confident, use a confidence-boosting oil, and so on. Refer to the charts for mind, moods and emotions. Depending on whether you are utilizing a stimulating or relaxing image, choose from the essential oils below.

STIMULATING ESSENTIAL OILS FOR VISUALIZATION

Rosemary, Ginger, Black Pepper, Thyme

RELAXING ESSENTIAL OILS FOR VISUALIZATION

Lavender, Neroli, Chamomile Roman, Clary Sage

Chapter 10

THE HEALING PROFESSIONS AND ESSENTIAL OILS

PROFESSIONALS IN BOTH THE ALLOPATHIC AND COMPLEMENTARY fields can benefit from using essential oils, which can be used in conjunction with any form of healing. This book is concerned with the mind and emotions but, as we know, the mind has a powerful impact on the workings of the body. Attending to the mind, perhaps by using essential oils, can greatly benefit the well-being of the entire person, also in conditions that seem superficially to be quite unrelated to mental processes, while for those professionals that deal exclusively with the mind, such as psychotherapists, essential oils provide a marvellous tool for helping to release hidden problems and anxieties.

DOCTORS

Over the past five years there has been a complete shift in the attitude of the British Medical Association and doctors in general, away from ignorance and intolerance of complementary therapies and towards understanding. So much so, in fact, that doctors can now legally refer patients to complementary therapists, including aromatherapists. Also, some GP practices now employ aromatherapists as part of the team. All over the world there are courses introducing doctors to the fundamentals of complementary therapies, so they can better understand what benefits they have to offer. And of course, health authorities are now employing aromatherapists within the National Health Service. Ironically perhaps, this new attitude has partly been driven by financial considerations. If a practice can help a patient by complementary means and their overall budget is less, in today's new reorganized money-conscious system, that is all for the good; especially for the patient.

Because prescriptions now cost the patient so much money, and because doctors are being pressurized to bring their drug-budgets down, the logic of using essential oils – which are cheaper, non-addictive, effective and harmless – suddenly makes sense to people who, just a few years ago, wouldn't have considered this option. Also, a profound shift has occurred in the public's mind towards complementary therapies because millions of people now have tried them and found that they work. The proof is in the pudding. The word travels, of course, and attitudes change. Meanwhile, the media make the public very aware of the dangers that can come with certain allopathic medications, some of which take years to become apparent. Patients now appreciate a doctor who says, 'Look Mrs Smith, I can give you a prescription for sleeping tablets if you like but why don't you try having lavender baths instead? If that doesn't work, we can then try the pills.' It shows an openness of mind. Of course I wouldn't suggest that doctors give up their armoury of drugs, I don't know anybody who would, but if essential oils can do as well if not better, why not try them before resorting to stronger medication? There is no longer any reason *not* to.

We haven't reached the point where essential oils are sold at the doctor's surgery (and I look forward to that day) but there's no reason why doctors' surgeries shouldn't diffuse essential oils in the waiting room – they would certainly make the room more pleasant. Choose essential oils that could allay anxiety or, in times of 'flu epidemic, those with antibacterial or microbial action. As we all know, especially those of us who have attended baby clinics, waiting to see the doctor and having to sit next to someone who is coughing out germs, can actually *make* you ill! Essential oils can do away with this problem, which keeps many people away from the surgery when they should in fact be making a visit.

HOSPITALS

'I hate the smell of hospitals' is a thing you often hear. The aroma of institutional cleaning fluids reminds people of why they were in hospital or had to visit a hospital – because they or someone they loved was suffering. This association turns a moderately unpleasant aroma into a feared one. Hospitals are places where people are sick – literally, where they spill blood or where urine and faeces are expelled behind curtains in public wards. In crowded accident and emergency waiting rooms people have to wait for hours, sometimes next to people who didn't have time to wash before coming in, or those who are there because they simply have no home to go to. For many reasons then, hospitals need an aromatic uplift more than most places.

The waiting areas in hospitals should be diffused with aromas that are acceptable to a wide range of people. The citrus, floral and woody essential oils are among the best choices. The most frequently used essential oil, lavender, has an aroma that is not universally liked, although it is usually accepted as moderately pleasant and, of course, it's loved by some people. The ideal is to create a pleasant atmosphere which induces calm, using essential oils which are not too expensive. One also needs to give the impression of freshness and cleanliness, and use something which is refreshing – to take the edge out of the long wait. I would suggest lemon, pine, geranium, eucalyptus lemon (*E citriodora*) and, in mixes, lavender. The citrus essential oils tend to evaporate fairly quickly but they are cheap and have a calming effect, and they are acceptable to almost everyone. All the above can be used on their own or blend the following oils in these proportions:

| Lemon | 5 parts to | | Lemon | 5 parts to | | Lemon | 5 parts to |
| Pine | 1 part | | Geranium | 1 part | | Lavender | 1 part |

| Eucalyptus Citriodora | 5 parts to | | Eucalyptus Citriodora | 5 parts to |
| Pine | 1 part | | Geranium | 1 part |

For the partners' waiting room on the maternity ward, the lemon and geranium blend should be used because it is the most anxiety-relieving.

Obviously, in a public place such as a hospital one would not use a diffuser that involved the use of bare flame – candles – to heat the essential oil; and electric sockets may not be installed in convenient places, or the diffuser may not be fitted with the correct fuse and runs the risk of blowing the whole electrical system – so the electrical type of diffuser may be impossible to use. There is now, however, a small, portable diffuser on the market which uses neither candles nor electricity but which is very effective in small areas – please see the supplier list in Appendix III, where I also list companies which supply commercial diffusing units for larger areas.

The antiviral, antibacterial and antifungal properties of essential oils have been discussed in my two previous books, *The Fragrant Pharmacy* and *Fragrant Sensuality*; these are very important aspects of essential oil use and their benefits within the hospital environment are obvious. Indeed, it is something of a sick joke that if you don't have an infection when you go into hospital, you'll have one by the time you come out! There is a tremendous potential, then, for essential oils being diffused in hospital atmospheres, especially perhaps in operating theatres and intensive care units.

These anti-infection qualities of essential oils can be used, however, by individuals who are obliged to stay in hospital. In my experience there's never been a complaint from other clients and, indeed, they and the nurses are very interested in the whole subject. People like the idea that they – simply by being in the same vicinity – are receiving a certain amount of protection themselves and I've been requested on many an occasion to bring in a bottle of this or that essential oil for other patients. As a general rule, if you're in a large ward with many people try to stick to the citrus, floral and woody aromas which are the most generally acceptable.

HOSPICES

A marvellous woman, Elisabeth Kübler-Ross, encouraged the development of the hospice movement in the 1960s and since then it's gone from strength to strength, country to country, so that now there are hospices all over the world – usually supported by donations and in great part run by volunteers. They all deserve all the help they can get.

Hospices care for the dying, aiming to make the clients' last months as pleasant and pain-free as possible. Essential oils are about uplifting the spirit and allaying stress and anxiety, and obviously have a role here and can truly help a person pass over in peace and even happiness.

It would be nice to think that each hospice had a variety of essential oils available from which each client could choose an essential oil or make a blend of oils to be used in their room, or relatives might ask if there is a particular aroma they'd like brought in. In the more public areas it would be best, again, to choose the citrus or floral essential oils – something light, rather than heavy. I would suggest the following oils used singly or in combinations: lemon, eucalyptus citriodora, grapefruit, mandarin, geranium, petitgrain, coriander and lavender. Here are three blends which are light, refreshing, and acceptable to most people:

Coriander	1	Lemon	1	Coriander	1
Petitgrain	1	Geranium	1	Mandarin	2
Eucalyptus Citriodora	1	Grapefruit	1	Geranium	1

The odour should be only just perceptible, not very noticeable. The aim is not to perfume the area so much as impart a subtle pleasant fragrance. This helps to make the atmosphere of the whole building happy, relaxed, pleasant, fresh and lively. All this helps the friends and relatives visiting the building, who are often more distressed than the clients themselves. Indeed, I have often heard hospice clients say of relatives, 'I wish they'd relax, they're trying to put such a brave face on things they're really not themselves.' By imparting a sense of relaxation into the building with essential oils it helps everyone – clients, visitors and staff alike.

Also, if an aroma becomes associated with the patient in their last days it can act as a reminder of them in future times. I remember one woman telling me that her mother chose to have neroli diffused in her room during her last weeks here on earth and the daughter was so grateful there was something which so easily evoked the memory of her mother. She could pick up her bottle of neroli whenever she was feeling sad, sniff deeply, and the memory of her mother would all come flooding back – not her dying, but her living, happy days. It became their final link, their special way of communicating.

NURSES

It is among the nursing professions that there has been the greatest growing interest in aromatherapy over recent years. You can see why. Working in the front line, with clients, they can see that essential oils do what they say they can do. They're interested to delve further. And who can blame them when it is they who have to wipe Mrs Jackson's tears when she cries in pain. The trouble is, many are not getting good and long enough training. Unless they are professionally registered aromatherapists they are not insured by the hospital to carry out any work other than nursing.

Registered tutors of aromatherapy have to have been in practice for five years, at least, and have had several years experience as an assistant tutor. But nurses are often advised to go to a weekend workshop, which is often taught by someone who has little more than a weekend workshop training themselves. One weekend workshop is fine for self-help and home use which is what they are intended for, but to work in conjunction with the medical profession, you should be a clinical aromatherapist, and that takes training. Most 'aromatherapists' work to prevent disorders. Nurses on the other hand, are dealing with people who are already ill, often quite seriously. Another difference is that registered aromatherapists are literally hands-on, and nurses are, within the hospital environment, rather hands-off – traditionally, the doctors hand out the therapy. Nurses are certainly right to think essential oils could quite easily do away with many of the problems they see in hospitals every day, but aromatherapy is more than the application of essential oils, and to use essential oils correctly and safely, nurses may have to revise their thinking on how healing actually works.

In fact, it is very encouraging that nurses should be so excited by the possibilities in aromatherapy. It is not their fault that training is not standardized. There can't be anything wrong with more people learning more ways to care for other human beings. Of course it's fine to use a diffuser in the ward, if the other staff agree. There are more and more courses designed especially for nurses who, when properly trained, could effectively treat clients with aromatherapy.

DENTISTS

Some dentists are using essential oils to overcome the 'Oh no, I've got to go to the dentist' factor. They can see the fear and anxiety written all over the faces seen each morning in the waiting room. It can't be a great start to the day! In some clinics, a gentle diffusion of essential oils has proved of great value in calming patients before treatment. Good essential oils to use in this situation might be lavender, lemon, geranium, clary sage, juniper and grapefruit.

CHIROPRACTORS AND OSTEOPATHS

Although it appears that chiropractors and osteopaths deal only with the physical body, particularly the bones and nerves, they also deal with the stresses their clients undergo during the course of their day, not to mention life. They can *feel* them, in the form of rigid, tightly contracted muscles in their hands which make treatment more difficult. It is much easier and more effective to treat someone who is not so tense.

Using relaxing essential oils gently diffused in the treatment room may help the client and therapist alike. Even if the client isn't feeling particularly stressed, just anticipating the potential clunks and clicks when the bones are going to be manipulated is enough to make some people tense up, particularly as these people are in pain anyway. Essential oils can also be used in manipulative massage in whatever lotion or cream the practitioner usually uses, and this will help ease tense muscles further.

CARERS

Anyone who is at home caring for an elderly or sick relative knows the strain of wanting to have their own life while feeling obliged not to leave the relative alone. Carers need a lot of emotional support, but it doesn't always come easily. Who cares for the carer? – Carers National Association.[1] Using essential oils doesn't take away the jobs but they can help by making both carer and cared for calm and emotionally steady, which can lighten the workload tremendously. Use the charts for specific problems (pages 311–19), and gently diffuse the oils to help create a nice, gentle, pleasant atmosphere. The following oils are all helpful: grapefruit, juniper, geranium, lavender, mandarin, bergamot, chamomile roman, clary sage and sandalwood.

The carer can also try one of these bath blends after a heavy day. Blend the essential oils together in the following proportions, then use five drops in a bath. The synergistic blends below are enough for four baths each:

CARER'S CALMING BATH BLEND		CARER'S STIMULATING BATH BLEND	
Ormenis Flower	*2 drops*	*Cypress*	*2 drops*
Mandarin	*15 drops*	*Grapefruit*	*15 drops*
Geranium	*3 drops*	*Rosemary*	*3 drops*

HEALERS

Healers come into contact with all kinds of problems and they are continuously giving out healing energy to others. Diffused in the treatment room, the following essential oils protect the healing energies and can also help the healing process: rose otto, chamomile roman, neroli, frankincense, sandalwood, geranium, jasmine, bergamot, spikenard, myrrh, petitgrain.

COUNSELLING

Counselling is for everyone, including healthy people who find themselves unable to cope with life's problems or a particular situation. It might take time to find the right service, and the person within that service that suits you – compatibility is of prime importance. But it's worth the trouble, so keep looking. The Citizens Advice Bureau can help, as can the Westminster Pastoral Foundation 2 who can supply a list of counselling services and centres. Find out what the various qualifications mean – some people might have had a few months' training, while others have had years. It might seem odd to go to a stranger with your problems but it's often much easier and less embarrassing to talk them over with someone who is not involved. It's also easier to be honest about a situation to a stranger than to family and friends, who probably have their own interest in the matter.

All sorts of people go to counselling. You may need to discuss how your job is negatively affecting you, or proving difficult to do, or bereavement, debt or divorce. You may just have heard you have a terminal illness, or that someone close to you is suffering. You may feel unable to cope with life's ups and downs, or be depressed, stressed and tense, or perhaps have suffered a loss of confidence, or feel helpless or frustrated. These are the things counselling is there to help with – problems both large and (apparently) small. There is also specialist counselling, for people who have suffered trauma called 'post-traumatic stress syndrome', caused by incidents such as train crashes, air or boat disasters, or trauma caused by various

Chamomile

types of abuse. Some aromatherapists are now also training as counsellors to help them in their practice.

Counsellors can use essential oils in the same way as psychotherapists – gently diffusing essential oils in the waiting room or consulting room to help clients feel more at ease and more able to talk freely and confidently. Appropriate oils would be bergamot, geranium, lemon, lavender, clary sage, ormenis flower, cypress, sandalwood and grapefruit. However, rather than using the same essential oil(s) all the time, choose oils from the charts that seem appropriate for particular clients. You might also suggest that clients use the oils diffused at home, or in the bath.

PSYCHOTHERAPISTS

The basis of psychotherapy is talking, which is perhaps the way our ancestors dealt with the stresses and strains of life. These days, however, our family and friends are quite likely to live on the other side of the country, if not the world, and the telephone system is kept busy with people sharing their problems. Psychotherapists, however, are trained to help you express your feelings, problems and experiences and they deal with problems that may have been too deeply hidden to be dealt with by a chat with a friend. To a psychotherapist, you can reveal very personal experiences and they'll help you identify what is worrying you, and help you understand your behaviour. They'll give you advice, encouragement and privacy.

The idea with psychotherapy is that you can discuss your problems and look at things from a different angle, to gain a better understanding of why the problems started in the first place, thus enabling negative patterns of behaviour to be broken. Psychotherapists do not prescribe drug treatment or electrical shock therapy. They talk over any kind of problem including emotional problems, anxiety, stress, tension, depression, obsession, compulsions, insomnia, fears, educational or work problems, aggression, disruptive behaviour, phobias such as agoraphobia or claustrophobia, and sexual problems, among other things. There's no point in being reticent – they've probably heard it all before!

Many psychotherapists have been trained in special techniques, which can be carried out within the context of individual or group sessions. They'll organize the time you spend with them rather than 'simply' allowing the conversation to ramble on, and this may be a better option for some. Included among these specialist techniques are psycho-drama, regression therapy, behavioural therapy, hypnotherapy, Gestalt therapy, autogenic training, relaxation techniques and transactional analysis, amongst others. It's important to pick a qualified practitioner as in Britain anyone can call themselves a 'psychotherapist'. Your doctor may be able to refer you to someone or write to the Psychological Society.[3]

Psychotherapists can use essential oils gently diffused in the waiting room or consulting room to help clients feel more relaxed, and able to talk freely and confidently, and suggested oils for this are mentioned in the previous section, *Counselling*. But by using Chart 11.2 on pages 311–19 and the personality profiles given in Chapter 14 on pages 394–412, the psychotherapist will be able to pick out an essential oil that is best suited for his or her particular clients. These can be used in a diffuser in the consulting room. Aromatherapy courses are also available for psychotherapists and will give them a more comprehensive idea of the possibilities. The psychotherapist might also suggest that the client uses essential oils diffused at home, or in the bath. Clients undergoing psychotherapy could choose their own oils to be used in conjunction with the sessions, but do inform your therapist if you are using them at home or would like to use them during sessions.

Psychodrama

Psychodrama was invented by Jacob Moreno, a contemporary of Freud, who was inspired by an actress into the idea that acting out emotional problems in the form of a play or drama can help solve them. It usually takes place within the context of group therapy, everyone acting together under the guidance of a qualified professional. It might involve shouting and screaming, punching cushions or knocking foam bricks over, which might sound a bit dramatic – but that's what it's about! It helps people to discover and express and release feelings they would not otherwise be able to do.

Regression Therapy

Some psychotherapists use regression therapy to release persistent stresses and problems that do not respond to treatment. One of the best regressionists is Dr Roger Woolger,[4] a Jungian psychologist who uses simple techniques that allow the mind to regress to past lives. This process allows people to release not only mental problems, but also physical ones, as the mind-body connection re-enacts situations that troubled them in the past. This technique should only be undergone in the hands of a fully qualified practitioner as it can be very traumatic and distressing as situations are relived and re-experienced.

Dr Woolger says that he doesn't even know if his sessions show evidence of past lives as there are no scientific methods of analysis to establish that; however, the information people come up with during these sessions is often quite alien to their present-life experience and strongly suggests that they may in fact be past lives. The aim of regression therapy is to examine these past lives, which may contain what Woolger describes as 'unfinished business'. He encourages clients to recognize the conditions, problems and disorders that have arisen as a consequence of this unfinished business, and leave it behind, so the personality can advance forward in life.

Chapter Eleven

POSITIVE AND NEGATIVE MOOD AROMATHERAPY CHARTS

CHART 11.1
EMOTIONAL HEALING – POSITIVE STATES

The essential oils in italics are those used in classical aromatherapy, the others have been adopted for these uses in more modern times.

Alertness

Basil, bergamot, black pepper, cardamon, cinnamon, coriander, eucalyptus citriodora, *grapefruit*, juniper, lime, *peppermint*, petitgrain, pine, *rosemary*, thyme linalol

Assertiveness

Basil, cedarwood, cypress, fennel sweet, frankincense, ginger, patchouli, *ylang ylang*, black pepper, jasmine, *ormenis flower, bergamot*, coriander, carnation, *tuberose*, pimento berry, lime, *cardamon*, cistus, *litsea cubeba*

Concentration

Intellectual – *Lemon, basil*, lemongrass, *litsea cubeba*, cardamon, bergamot, orange, cedarwood, *rosemary*, eucalyptus, peppermint, *frankincense*
Spiritual – *Frankincense*, neroli, *chamomile roman*, rose otto, narcissus, hyacinth

Confidence

Cedarwood, *cypress*,
linden blossom, *cardamon*,
fennel sweet, ginger, bergamot,
grapefruit, jasmine, pine, rosemary, orange, coriander,
tuberose

Contentment

Rose otto, cypress, *lavender*,
neroli, *bergamot*, orange,
sandalwood, patchouli, clove,
ylang ylang, chamomile roman

Creativity

Bergamot, cistus, lemon, *frankincense*, geranium, *neroli*, rose,
jasmine, bay, clove, *carnation*,
mimosa, litsea cubeba, sandalwood, cypress, *juniper*

Focus

Thyme linalol, *lemon*, fennel,
bergamot, *basil*, basil linalol,
cedarwood, *cypress*, juniper,
lemongrass, *litsea cubeba*,
ginger, cinnamon, clove,
ylang ylang, linden blossom,
nutmeg, *rosemary*

Happiness

Orange, rose, jasmine, coriander, ginger, clove, cinnamon,
benzoin, carnation, *geranium,
pimento berry*

Joy

Sandalwood, frankincense,
lemon, rose otto, petitgrain,
orange, ylang ylang, *neroli*,
chamomile roman, *bergamot,*
linden blossom, *mimosa*

Peace

**Everyone has essential oils
that they can personally
attune to; these are guidelines only.**

Chamomile roman, neroli,
juniper, frankincense, rose otto,
melissa, angelica seed, spikenard, yarrow, jasmine, carnation

Performance

Bay, bergamot, cistus, eucalyptus citriodora, *frankincense,
lemon*, lavender, *grapefruit,
helichrysum*, rose maroc,
jasmine, geranium, tuberose,
ormenis flower, *cypress*

Positivity

**All essential oils used in aro-
matherapy have a positive
nature, and positive benefits
upon the human organism.
The following essential oils
are only a guideline**.

Basil, lemon, cedarwood,
grapefruit, pine, vetiver,
patchouli, juniper, myrrh,
cypress, cardamon, petitgrain,
geranium, frankincense, rosemary, pimento berry, bay

Restfulness

Lavender, geranium,
rose maroc, clary sage,
linden blossom, *neroli*,
marjoram, petitgrain,
sandalwood, mimosa

Self-Awareness

Clary sage, ylang ylang,
cypress, geranium, pine,
sandalwood, *bay*,
ormenis flower, *jasmine*, clove,
pimento berry, mandarin,
coriander, angelica seed, *sage*,
cistus, *myrtle*

Self-Esteem

Hyacinth, sandalwood, vetiver,
ylang ylang, rose maroc,
jasmine, carnation, *bergamo*t,
geranium, ormenis flower,
cedarwood, tuberose

Self-Image

Orange, lavender, melissa,
neroli, chamomile roman,
ylang ylang, rose maroc, jasmine, sandalwood, cypress,
juniper, cedarwood, bay, pine,
black pepper, frankincense,
mandarin, nutmeg, myrtle

CHART 11.2
EMOTIONAL HEALING – PROBLEMS

**The essential oils in italics are
those used in classical aromatherapy, the others have been
adopted for these uses in more
modern times.**

Abuse

Emotional

Ormenis flower, *rose otto,
chamomile roman*, melissa,
neroli, mandarin, benzoin

Hurt inner child

Geranium, lavender, neroli,
melissa, mandarin, benzoin,
rose otto

Addiction

General

Vetiver, narcissus, *helichrysum*,
basil, frankincense, spikenard,
benzoin

Alcohol

Helichrysum, *juniper*, lemon,
bergamot, marjoram,
clary sage,
eucalyptus citriodora

Drugs

Vetiver, helichrysum, spikenard, *valerian*, ormenis flower, *nutmeg*, juniper, *bergamot*, basil, clary sage, geranium, hyacinth, narcissus, tuberose

Hypnotics

Narcissus, jonquil, rose maroc, *hyacinth*, carnation, jasmine, hops, *valerian*, tonka bean, vanilla, *tuberose*, spikenard

Other useful essential oils

Marjoram, bergamot, chamomile roman, juniper, patchouli, bay, *clary sage*, *nutmeg*, cistus

Aggression

General aggression

Geranium, frankincense, sandalwood, grapefruit, *cedarwood*, *vetiver*

Soothing effect in aggression

Neroli, *lavender*, *clary sage*, *chamomile roman*, benzoin, *marjoram*, coriander, litsea cubeba, *valerian*, *spikenard*, *rose maroc*, tuberose, mimosa, carnation

Aloneness

Neroli, chamomile roman,

rose otto, jasmine, melissa, frankincense, orange

Amnesia

Confusion

Cardamon, tuberose, ginger, *black pepper*, bergamot, geranium, *petitgrain*, *helichrysum*, grapefruit, basil

Shock-induced

Mandarin, ylang ylang, rose maroc, rose otto, neroli, melissa, peppermint, lavender

Fear-induced

Sandalwood, chamomile roman, cypress, vetiver, lemon, bergamot, orange, cedarwood, neroli, geranium

Anger

Calming down

Chamomile roman, chamomile german, tuberose, lavender, linden blossom, vetiver, bergamot, rose maroc, rose otto, petitgrain, patchouli

Coping with

Black pepper, chamomile roman, linden blossom, vetiver, ylang ylang, rose maroc, valerian, spikenard, myrtle, benzoin

Expressing unrealized anger

Tuberose, black pepper, ginger, ormenis flower, cedarwood, patchouli, clove

Anorexia

See Anxiety, Obsession, Self-esteem, Confidence

Anxiety

General

Bergamot, *lavender*, mandarin, sandalwood, patchouli, *chamomile roman*, vetiver, cedarwood, *neroli*, rose otto, basil, *melissa*, *geranium*, juniper, frankincense

Apprehensive anxiety

Bergamot, *lavender*, neroli, rose otto, melissa, geranium

Depressed anxiety

Bergamot, melissa, neroli, *rose otto*, *sandalwood*, vetiver, cedarwood

Restless anxiety

Vetiver, *cedarwood*, juniper, chamomile roman, frankincense

Tense anxiety

Sandalwood, *clary sage*, chamomile roman, patchouli

Apathy

Cardamon, lemon, *ginger*, *black pepper*, bergamot, orange, jasmine, rose otto, ormenis flower, basil, peppermint

Bereavement

Benzoin, *rose otto*, neroli, *linden blossom*, lavender, melissa, *chamomile roman*, patchouli, cypress, rose maroc, mandarin, vetiver

Breakdown

Emotional breakdown

Lavender, cypress, geranium, sandalwood, rose otto, mandarin, benzoin, neroli, chamomile roman

General

Lavender, clary sage, lemon, orange, *chamomile roman*, *geranium*, *neroli*, helichrysum

Bulimia

See Rage, Guilt, Self-esteem, Confidence

Burn-out

Emotional

Vetiver, bergamot, rose otto, neroli, linden blossom, *melissa*, patchouli, sandalwood, *hyacinth*, marjoram, lavender, benzoin, clary sage, helichrysum, lemon, frankincense, chamomile roman, petitgrain, ginger, jasmine

Confusion

Cardamon, ginger, *black pepper*, bergamot, geranium, petitgrain, helichrysum, grapefruit, *ormenis flower*, basil, rosemary, peppermint, cypress, juniper, pine, thyme linalol, lavender

Dejection

Bergamot, frankincense, grapefruit, mandarin, geranium, nutmeg, *mimosa*, linden blossom, orange, rose maroc, jasmine, petitgrain, neroli, ylang ylang

Delirium

Peppermint, *eucalyptus globulus, eucalyptus radiatia, lavender*, marjoram

Delirium Tremens

Lavender, petitgrain, lemon, chamomile roman, *marjoram, valerian*, geranium

Dementia

Basil, cardamon, ginger, black pepper, *rosemary, rose otto*

Memory-evoking

Basil, rosemary

Appetite stimulating

Lemon, black pepper, coriander, cardamon, clove, orange, lime, grapefruit, nutmeg, *cinnamon,* ginger

Gentle oil, for restlessness and tremors

Rose otto, neroli, *lavender, geranium*, chamomile roman, jasmine,

Depression

Mandarin, chamomile roman, lemon, bergamot, grapefruit, orange, jasmine, ylang ylang, rose otto, rose maroc, neroli, geranium, petitgrain, helichrysum, eucalyptus citriodora, sandalwood, clary sage, marjoram, lavender, frankincense

Weepy depression

Rose otto, neroli, patchouli, chamomile roman, sandalwood, geranium, ylang ylang, benzoin

Agitated or anxious depression

Melissa, cedarwood, lavender, chamomile roman, bergamot, marjoram, nutmeg, orange, ormenis flower, valerian, lemon

Lethargic depression

Grapefruit, cypress, rosemary, melissa, helichrysum, peppermint, clary sage, eucalyptus citriodora, eucalyptus piperita

Hysterical depression

Mandarin, chamomile roman, linden blossom, vetiver, bergamot, neroli, narcissus, lavender, marjoram, valerian, spikenard

Depressive-Manic

Chamomile roman, chamomile german, frankincense, geranium, *grapefruit*, mandarin, rose otto, *lavender*, lemon, *neroli*, patchouli, sandalwood

Doubt

Coriander, litsea cubeba, *frankincense*, benzoin, angelica seed, ylang ylang, basil

Emotional Violence

Frankincense, juniper, geranium, rose otto, neroli, *chamomile roman*, jasmine, *carnation*, hyacinth, *benzoin*, melissa, lavender

Emotional Exhaustion

Cypress, bergamot, marjoram, *rosemary, eucalyptus globulus, eucalyptus radiata*, frankincense, litsea cubeba, grapefruit, black pepper, cardamon, ginger, lemon, pine, chamomile roman

Facing Death

Rose otto, rose maroc, *jasmine*, linden blossom, *frankincense*, neroli, chamomile roman, geranium, narcissus, benzoin, bay, carnation, *sandalwood*, cedarwood, bergamot, *juniper*, hyacinth, tuberose

The choice of essential oils depends very much upon culture and personal preference, and may differ from those above.

Fatigue

Intellectual fatigue

Black pepper, ginger, *rosemary*, basil, cypress, grapefruit, peppermint, lemon

Mental fatigue

Lemon, petitgrain, *basil, peppermint,* eucalyptus piperita, rosemary, eucalyptus citriodora

Fear

General

Sandalwood, chamomile roman, cypress, *vetiver*, lemon, bergamot, orange, *cedarwood*, neroli, ormenis flower, basil, *frankincense*, clary sage, *lavender*, galbanham

Fear of failure

Fennel sweet, *coriander*,

ylang ylang, basil, frankincense

Fear of gossip

Cypress

Fear of madness

Fennel sweet, *cedarwood*,
ylang ylang, *frankincense*

Fear of feelings

Fennel sweet, frankincense,
sandalwood, *neroli*

Fear of change

Ylang ylang, frankincense,
lavender, *ormenis flower*

Fear of sexuality

Rose maroc, ylang ylang,
patchouli, vetiver, galbanham

Fear of love

Rose maroc, neroli, *carnation*,
hyacinth, *benzoin*

Fear of loving

Neroli, ylang ylang, carnation,
benzoin, *rose maroc*

Fear of being unloved

Rose otto

Fear of letting go

Cypress, rose maroc, frankincense, *galbanham*

Fits – Emotional

Lavender, marjoram, eucalyptus citriodora, *litsea cubeba*,
chamomile roman

Forgetfulness

Cypress, lemon, ginger, cistus,
black pepper, frankincense,
rosemary, peppermint, basil

Grief

Dissipating grief

Cypress, chamomile roman,
rose maroc, *rose otto, helichrysum*, ormenis flower, frankincense, *narcissus*, bergamot,
carnation, vanilla, nutmeg,
spikenard

Difficulty in expressing
grief

Hyacinth, neroli, rose maroc,
rose otto, melissa, *helichrysum,
benzoin*, mimosa, vetiver

Guilt

Linden blossom, vetiver, jasmine, pine, *rose otto*, juniper,
clary sage, ylang ylang, nutmeg

Hypochondria

Marjoram, rosemary, valerian,
hops, basil, peppermint,
thyme linalol, ormenis flower,
tea tree, manuka, oregano,
galbanham

Hysteria

Mandarin, *chamomile roman*, linden blossom, *vetiver*, bergamot, rosemary, neroli, peppermint, narcissus, *lavender*, marjoram, *valerian*, spikenard, hops

Insomnia

Lavender, mandarin, linden blossom, clary sage, marjoram, cistus, *valerian, hops*, vetiver, sandalwood, *chamomile roman*, lemon

Irritability

Cypress, chamomile roman, chamomile german, coriander, litsea cubeba, neroli, ylang ylang, melissa, narcissus, *lavender*

Loneliness

Bergamot, *helichrysum*, narcissus, chamomile roman, neroli, *benzoin*

Memory – Lack of

Ginger, *basil*, *lemon*, grapefruit, *rosemary*, thyme linalol, *cardamon*, black pepper, coriander, pimento berry

Misery

Narcissus, petitgrain, *benzoin*, orange, neroli, *rose maroc*, jasmine, clove, cinnamon, *ginger*, carnation, *pimento berry*

Moodiness

Geranium, eucalyptus citriodora, neroli, *lavender*, lemon, ylang ylang, ormenis flower, patchouli, chamomile maroc

Mood Swings

Geranium, cardamon, lavender, coriander, angelica seed, cypress, *cedarwood*, linden blossom, helichrysum

Nervous Exhaustion

Rosemary, petitgrain, *juniper*, neroli, *lavender*, orange, chamomile roman, marjoram, clary sage

Obsessional Behaviour

Sandalwood, *vetiver*, cedarwood, *narcissus*, clary sage, orange, lemon

Pain

Betula alba (birch), nutmeg, clove, rosemary, *lavender*, chamomile roman, *sage*, clary sage, *helichrysum*, peppermint, basil

Inflammation and pain

Lavender, *chamomile roman*

Tension and pain

Lavender, clary sage, vetiver, *marjoram*

Relaxing with pain

Lavender, neroli

Panic Attacks

Lavender, frankincense, *helichrysum*, *marjoram*

Passivity

Rose maroc, ylang ylang, cedarwood, pine, jasmine, *tuberose*, orange, *patchouli*, bay

Phobias

To calm and relax

Lavender, linden blossom, *clary sage*, neroli, ylang ylang, marjoram, ormenis flower, *chamomile roman*, sandalwood

Quarrelsomeness

Clary sage, lavender, lemon, *sandalwood, patchouli*, cistus, clove

Rage

Chamomile roman,

ylang ylang, ormenis flower, *vetiver*, clary sage, lavender, marjoram, *galbanham*

Regret

Rose maroc, rose otto, *pine*, cypress, mimosa, *hyacinth*

Rejection

Pine, cypress, sandalwood, *benzoin, chamomile roman*, neroli, rose otto, ylang ylang, hyacinth, tuberose, *carnation*

Repression

Hyacinth, *jasmine, frankincense*, ylang ylang, *cedarwood, pine*, patchouli, vetiver, juniper

Schizophrenia

Lavender, mandarin, geranium, chamomile roman, rose otto, lemon

Self-Blame

Rose otto, lemon, geranium, *chamomile roman, bergamot*, orange, ylang ylang, carnation, tuberose, benzoin, *melissa*, eucalyptus citriodora, ormenis flower

Sorrow

Cypress, hyacinth, melissa,

benzoin, frankincense, sandalwood, rose otto

Stress

*Bergamot, chamomile roman,
ormenis flower,* frankincense,
geranium, grapefruit, *lavender,*
lemon, mandarin, melissa,
neroli, marjoram, rose otto,
*sandalwood, vetiver,
clary sage, ylang ylang,* bay,
jasmine, hyacinth, benzoin,
eucalyptus citriodora,
litsea cubeba, tuberose, narcissus, linden blossom, nutmeg,
hops, *spikenard, valerian,*
yarrow, osmanthus

Tiredness – Mental

Clary sage, lavender, marjoram, rosemary, litsea cubeba,
grapefruit, peppermint

Trauma

Thyme linalol, *lavender,*
geranium, lemon, *marjoram,*
petitgrain, *chamomile roman,*
clary sage

Withdrawal

from life

Narcissus, orange

of emotions

Bergamot, rose otto, hyacinth,
chamomile roman, neroli, mandarin, geranium

for peace

Cypress, frankincense, cedarwood, juniper, rose otto,
chamomile roman, neroli, carnation, bergamot, geranium

**Any essential oil can be used if
you feel personally attuned to
it.**

Worthlessness

feelings of

Frankincense, sandalwood,
cedarwood, clove,
ormenis flower, neroli, *juniper,*
chamomile roman,
geranium

CHART 11.3 ESSENTIAL OILS USED FOR POSITIVE STATES

Angelica Seed

Peace, Self-awareness

Basil

Alertness, Assertiveness,
Positivity, Focus

Bay

Creativity, Performance,
Positivity, Self-awareness,
Self-image

Benzoin

Happiness, Contentment

Bergamot

Alertness, Assertiveness,
Concentration, Confidence,
Contentment, Creativity,
Focus, Joy, Performance,
Self-esteem

Black Pepper

Alertness, Assertiveness,
Self-image

Cardamon

Alertness, Assertiveness,
Concentration, Confidence,
Positivity

Carnation

Assertiveness, Creativity,
Happiness, Peace, Self-esteem

Cedarwood

Assertiveness, Concentration,
Confidence, Focus, Positivity,
Self-esteem, Self-image

Chamomile Roman

Concentration, Contentment,
Joy, Peace, Self-image

Cinnamon

Alertness, Focus, Happiness

Cistus (rockrose, labdanum)

Assertiveness, Creativity, Self-
awareness, Performance

Clary Sage

Restfulness, Self-awareness

Clove

Contentment, Creativity,
Focus, Happiness,
Self-awareness

Coriander

Alertness, Assertiveness,
Confidence, Happiness,
Self-awareness

Cypress

Assertiveness, Confidence,
Contentment, Creativity,
Focus, Performance, Positivity,
Self-awareness, Self-image

Eucalyptus (radiata/globulus)

Concentration, Alertness

Eucalyptus Citriodora (lemon)

Alertness, Performance

Fennel, Sweet

Assertiveness, Confidence, Focus

Frankincense

Assertiveness, Concentration, Creativity, Joy, Peace, Performance, Positivity, Self-image

Geranium

Creativity, Happiness, Performance, Positivity, Restfulness, Self-awareness, Self-esteem

Ginger

Assertiveness, Confidence, Focus, Happiness

Grapefruit

Alertness, Confidence, Performance, Positivity

Helichrysum (Immortelle or Italian everlasting)

Performance

Hyacinth

Concentration, Self-esteem

Jasmine

Assertiveness, Confidence, Creativity, Happiness, Peace, Performance, Self-awareness, Self-esteem, Self-image

Juniper Berry

Alertness, Creativity, Focus, Peace, Positivity, Self-image

Lavender

Contentment, Performance, Restfulness, Self-image

Lemon

Concentration, Creativity, Focus, Joy, Performance, Positivity

Lemongrass

Concentration, Focus

Lime

Alertness, Assertiveness

Linden Blossom

Confidence, Focus, Joy,
Restfulness

Litsea Cubeba

Assertiveness, Concentration,
Creativity, Focus

Mandarin

Self-awareness, Self-image

Marjoram

Restfulness

Melissa

Peace, Self-image

Mimosa

Creativity, Joy, Restfulness

Myrrh

Positivity

Myrtle

Self-awareness, Self-image

Narcissus

Concentration

Neroli (orange blossom)

Concentration, Contentment,
Creativity, Joy, Peace,
Restfulness, Self-image

Nutmeg

Focus, Self-image

Orange

Concentration, Confidence,
Contentment, Happiness, Joy,
Self-image

Ormenis Flower (chamomile maroc)

Assertiveness, Performance,
Self-awareness, Self-esteem

Patchouli

Assertiveness, Contentment,
Positivity

Peppermint

Alertness, Concentration

Petitgrain

Alertness, Joy, Positivity,
Restfulness

Pimento Berry

Assertiveness, Happiness,
Positivity, Self-awareness

Pine

Alertness, Confidence,
Positivity, Self-awareness,
Self-image

Rosemary

Alertness, Concentration, Confidence, Focus, Positivity

Rose Maroc

Performance, Restfulness, Self-esteem, Self-image

Rose Otto

Concentration, Contentment, Creativity, Happiness, Joy, Peace

Sage

Self-awareness

Sandalwood

Contentment, Creativity, Joy, Restfulness, Self-awareness, Self-esteem, Self-image

Spikenard

Peace

Thyme

Alertness

Thyme Linalol

Alertness, Focus

Tuberose

Assertiveness, Confidence, Performance, Self-esteem, Self-image

Vetiver

Positivity, Self-esteem

Yarrow

Peace

Ylang Ylang

Assertiveness, Contentment, Focus, Joy, Self-awareness, Self-esteem, Self-image

CHART 11.4
ESSENTIAL OILS USED FOR EMOTIONAL HEALING

Angelica Seed

Doubt, Mood swings

Basil

Addiction – general, Addiction – drugs, Anxiety – general, Apathy, Confusion, Dementia

– memory loss, Doubt, Fatigue
– intellectual, Fatigue – mental,
Fear of failure, Fear – general,
Forgetfulness, Hypochondria,
Memory – lack of, Pain,
Rejection

Bay

Addiction, Facing death, Stress

Benzoin

Addiction, Aggression – soothing, Anger – coping with,
Bereavement, Breakdown,
Burnt-out, Doubt, Emotional
violence, Facing death, Fear of
love, Fear of loving, Grief –
expressing, Loneliness, Misery,
Self-blame, Stress

Bergamot

Addiction, Addiction – alcohol,
Addiction – drugs, Amnesia –
confusion, Amnesia – fear
induced, Anger – calming,
Anxiety – general, Anxiety –
apprehensive, Anxiety –
depressed, Apathy, Burn-out,
Confusion, Dejection,
Depression, Depression – agitated or anxious, Depression –
hysterical, Exhaustion, Facing
death, Fear – general, Grief –
dissipating, Hysteria,
Loneliness, Self-blame, Stress,
Withdrawal from life,
Withdrawal – for peace

Betula Alba (birch)

Pain

Black Pepper

Amnesia – confusion, Anger –
coping, Anger – expressing
unrealized, Apathy, Confusion,
Dementia – memory, Dementia
– appetite stimulant,
Exhaustion, Fatigue – intellectual, Forgetfulness, Memory –
lack of

Cardamon

Amnesia – confusion, Apathy,
Confusion, Dementia –
memory, Dementia – appetite
stimulant, Memory – lack of,
Mood swings

Carnation

Addictions, Aggression –
soothing, Bereavement,
Emotional violence, Facing
death, Fear of love, Fear of
loving, Grief – dissipating,
Misery, Rejection, Self-blame,
Withdrawal – for peace

Cedarwood

Aggression – general, Amnesia
– fear induced, Anger –
expressing unrealized, Anxiety
– general, Anxiety – restless,
Anxiety – depressed,
Depression, Depression –
agitated or anxious, Facing
death, Fear – general, Fear of
madness, Mood swings,

Obsessions, Passivity,
Repression, Trauma,
Withdrawal – for peace,
Worthlessness – feelings of

Chamomile German

Anger – calming, Depression –
manic, Irritability

Chamomile Roman

Abuse, Addiction, Aggression
– soothing, Aloneness,
Amnesia – fear induced, Anger
– calming, Anger – coping
with, Anxiety – general,
Anxiety – tense, Anxiety –
restless, Bereavement,
Breakdown – general,
Breakdown – emotional, Burn-
out, Delirium tremens,
Dementia – restlessness and
tremors, Depression,
Depression – weepiness,
Depression – hysterical,
Depression – manic, Emotional
violence, Emotional exhaus-
tion, Facing death, Fear – gen-
eral, Fits – emotional, Grief –
dissipating, Hysteria, Insomnia,
Irritability, Loneliness,
Nervous exhaustion, Pain, Pain
– inflammatory, Phobias, Rage,
Rejection, Self-blame, Schizo-
phrenia, Stress, Trauma,
Withdrawal – of emotions,
Withdrawal – for peace,
Worthlessness – feelings of

Cinnamon

Dementia, Exhaustion –

nervous, Misery

Cistus (rock rose)

Addictions, Forgetfulness,
Insomnia, Quarrelsomeness

Clary Sage

Addictions, Addiction –
alcohol, Addiction – drugs,
Aggression – soothing, Anxiety
– tense, Breakdown – general,
Burn-out, Depression, Fear –
general, Guilt, Insomnia,
Nervous exhaustion,
Obsession, Pain, Pain – with
tension, Phobias, Quarrelsomeness, Rage, Stress, Tiredness –
mental, Trauma

Clove

Anger – expressing unrealized,
Dementia – appetite stimulant,
Misery, Pain, Quarrelsomeness,
Worthlessness – feelings of

Coriander

Aggression – soothing, Doubt,
Dementia – appetite stimulant,
Fear of failure, Irritability,
Memory – lack of, Mood
swings

Cypress

Amnesia – fear induced,
Breakdown – emotional,
Breakdown – general,
Confusion, Depression –
lethargic, Exhaustion, Fatigue

– intellectual, Fear – general, Fear of gossip, Fear of letting go, Forgetfulness, Grief – dissipating, Irritability, Mood swings, Regrets, Rejection, Withdrawal from life

Eucalyptus radiata/globulus

Delirium, Exhaustion

Eucalyptus citriodora (lemon)

Addiction – alcohol, Depression, Fatigue – mental, Fits – emotional, Moodiness, Self-blame, Stress

Fennel, Sweet

Fear of failure, Fear of madness, Fear of feelings

Frankincense

Addiction – general, Aggression – general, Aloneness, Anxiety – general, Anxiety – restless, Burn-out, Dejection, Depression, Depression – manic, Doubt, Emotional violence, Exhaustion – emotional, Facing death, Fear – general, Fear of failure, Fear of madness, Fear of feelings, Fear of change, Fear of letting go, Forgetfulness, Grief – dissipating, Panic attacks, Repression, Stress, Withdrawal – for peace, Worthlessness – feelings of

Galbanham

Fear – general, Fear of sexuality, Fear of letting go, Hypochondria, Rage

Geranium

Abuse – the inner child, Addiction – drugs, Aggression – general, Amnesia – confusion, Amnesia – fear induced, Anxiety – general, Anxiety – apprehensive, Breakdown – general, Breakdown – emotional, Confusion, Dejection, Delirium tremens, Dementia – restlessness and tremors, Depression, Depression – weepy, Depression – manic, Emotional violence, Facing death, Moodiness, Mood swings, Self-blame, Schizophrenia, Stress, Trauma, Withdrawal of emotions, Withdrawal – for peace, Worthlessness – feelings of

Ginger

Amnesia – confusion, Anger – expressing unrealized, Apathy, Confusion, Dementia, Burn-out, Exhaustion, Fatigue – intellectual, Forgetfulness, Memory, Misery

Grapefruit

Aggression – general, Amnesia, Confusion, Dejection, Dementia – stimulating appetite, Depression,

Depression – manic, Exhaustion, Fatigue – intellectual, Fear – general, Memory – lack of, Tiredness – mental, Withdrawal – for peace

Helichrysum (Immortelle or Italian everlasting)

Addiction – general, Addiction – alcohol, Addiction – drugs, Amnesia – confusion, Breakdown – general, Burnout, Confusion, Depression – general, Anxiety – dissipating, Grief – expressing, Loneliness, Mood swings, Pain, Panic attacks

Hops

Addictions, Hysteria, Hypochondria, Insomnia

Hyacinth

Addictions, Addiction – drugs, Apathy, Burn-out, Emotional violence, Facing death, Fear of love, Grief – expressing, Regrets, Rejection, Repression, Stress, Tiredness – mental, Withdrawal of emotions

Jasmine

Addictions, Aloneness, Apathy, Burn-out, Dejection, Dementia – restlessness and tremors, Depression, Emotional violence, Facing death, Guilt, Misery, Passivity, Repression, Stress

Juniper

Addictions, Addiction – alcohol, Addiction – drugs, Anxiety – tense, Anxiety – restless, Confusion, Emotional violence, Exhaustion – nervous, Facing death, Guilt, Repression, Withdrawal – for peace, Worthlessness – feelings of

Lavender

Abuse – the inner child, Aggression – soothing, Amnesia – shock induced, Anger – calming, Anxiety – general, Anxiety – apprehension, Bereavement, Breakdown – general, Breakdown – emotional, Burn-out, Confusion, Delirium, Delirium tremens, Dementia – restlessness and tremors, Depression – agitated or anxious, Depression – hysterical, Depression – manic, Emotional violence, Exhaustion – nervous, Facing death, Fear – general, Fear of change, Fits – emotional, Hysteria, Insomnia, Irritability, Moodiness, Mood swings, Pain, Pain – with inflammation, Pain – relaxing, Panic attacks, Phobias, Quarrelsomeness, Rage, Schizophrenia, Stress, Tiredness – mental, Trauma

Lemon

Addiction – alcohol, Amnesia
– fear induced, Apathy,
Breakdown – general, Burn-
out, Delirium tremens,
Dementia – appetite,
Depression, Depression –
manic, Exhaustion, Fatigue –
intellectual, Fatigue – mental,
Fear – general, Forgetfulness,
Insomnia, Memory – lack of,
Moodiness, Obsession,
Quarrelsomeness, Self-blame,
Schizophrenia, Stress, Trauma

Lime

Dementia – appetite

Linden Blossom

Anger – calming, Anger – coping, Bereavement, Burn-out,
Dejection, Dementia – restlessness, Depression – hysterical,
Exhaustion – emotional, Facing
death, Guilt, Hysteria,
Insomnia, Irritability, Mood
swings, Phobias, Stress

Litsea Cubeba

Aggression, Doubt,
Exhaustion, Fits – emotional,
Irritability, Stress, Tiredness –
mental

Mandarin

Abuse – emotional, Abuse –
the inner child, Amnesia –

shock induced, Anxiety –
general, Bereavement,
Breakdown – emotional,
Dejection, Depression –
general, Depression – manic,
Hysteria, Insomnia,
Schizophrenia, Stress

Manuka

Hypochondria

Marjoram

Addiction, Addiction – alcohol,
Aggression – soothing, Burn-
out, Delirium, Delirium
tremens, Depression – agitated
or anxious, Depression – hysterical, Exhaustion, Fits – emotional, Hypochondria, Hysteria,
Insomnia, Pain, Panic attacks,
Phobias, Rage, Stress,
Tiredness – mental, Trauma

Melissa

Abuse – emotional, Abuse –
the inner child, Aloneness,
Amnesia – shock induced,
Anxiety – general, Anxiety –
apprehensive, Anxiety –
depressed, Bereavement, Burn-
out, Emotional violence,
Depression – agitated or anxious, Grief – expressing,
Irritability, Self-blame, Stress,
Withdrawal of emotions

Mimosa

Aggression – soothing,

Dejection, Grief – expressing

Myrtle

Anger – coping with

Narcissus

Addiction – hypnotic, Addiction – drugs, Depression – hysterical, Emotional exhaustion, Facing death, Grief – dissipating, Hysteria, Irritability, Loneliness, Misery, Obsession, Stress, Withdrawal from life

Neroli

Abuse – emotional, Abuse – the inner child, Aggression – soothing, Aloneness, Amnesia – shock induced, Amnesia – fear induced, Anxiety – general, Anxiety – apprehensive, Anxiety – depressed, Bereavement, Breakdown – general, Breakdown – emotional, Burn-out, Dejection, Dementia – restlessness, Depression, Depression – weepy, Depression – manic, Emotional violence, Exhaustion – nervous, Facing death, Fear – general, Fear of feelings, Fear of love, Fear of loving, Grief – expressing, Hysteria, Irritability, Loneliness, Moodiness, Misery, Pain – relaxing, Phobias, Rejection, Stress, Withdrawal – of emotions, Withdrawal for peace, Worthlessness – feelings of

Nutmeg

Addictions, Addiction – drugs, Dejection, Dementia – appetite stimulant, Depression, Depression – agitated or anxious, Grief – dissipating, Guilt, Pain, Stress, Tiredness – mental

Orange

Amnesia – fear induced, Apathy, Breakdown, Dejection, Dementia – appetite, Depression, Fear – general, Misery, Nervous exhaustion, Obsession, Passivity, Self-blame, Withdrawal – from life

Oregano

Hypochondria

Ormenis Flower (Chamomile Maroc)

Abuse – emotional, Addiction – drugs, Anger – expressing unrealized, Apathy, Confusion, Depression – agitated or anxious, Fear – general, Fear of change, Grief – dissipating, Hypochondria, Moodiness, Phobias, Rage, Self-blame, Stress, Worthlessness – feelings of

Patchouli

Addictions, Anger – calming, Anger – expressing unrealized, Anxiety – general, Anxiety –

tense, Bereavement, Burn-out, Depression – weepy, Depression – manic, Fear of sexuality, Moodiness, Passivity, Quarrelsomeness, Repression

Peppermint

Amnesia – shock induced, Apathy, Confusion, Delirium, Fatigue – intellectual, Forgetfulness, Hypochondria, Hysteria, Pain, Tiredness – mental

Petitgrain

Amnesia – confusion, Anger – calming, Burn-out, Confusion, Dejection, Delirium tremens, Depression, Exhaustion – nervous, Fatigue – mental, Misery, Trauma

Pimento Berry

Memory – lack of, Misery

Pine

Confusion, Exhaustion, Guilt, Passivity, Regrets, Rejection, Repression

Rosemary

Confusion, Depression – lethargic, Dementia, Exhaustion, Exhaustion – nervous, Fatigue – intellectual, Forgetfulness, Hysteria,

Hypochondria, Memory – lack of, Pain, Tiredness – mental

Rose Maroc

Addiction, Aggression – soothing, Amnesia – shock induced, Anger – calming, Anger – coping with, Apathy, Bereavement, Dejection, Fear of loving, Depression, Facing death, Fear of sexuality, Fear of love, Fear of letting go, Grief – dissipating, Grief – expressing, Misery, Passivity, Regrets, Self-blame, Stress, Withdrawal – of emotions

Rose Otto (Bulgar)

Abuse – emotional, Aloneness, Amnesia – shock induced, Anger – to calm, Anxiety – general, Anxiety – apprehensive, Anxiety – depressed, Apathy, Bereavement, Breakdown – emotional, Burn-out, Dementia, Depression, Depression – weepy, Depression – manic, Emotional violence, Facing death, Fear of being unloved, Grief – dissipating, Grief – expressing, Guilt, Regrets, Rejection, Self-blame, Schizophrenia, Stress, Tiredness – mental, Withdrawal – of emotions, Withdrawal – for peace

Sandalwood

Aggression, Amnesia – fear induced, Anxiety – general,

Anxiety – tense, Anxiety –
depressed, Breakdown – emotional, Burn-out, Depression,
Depression – weepy,
Depression – manic, Facing
death, Fear – general, Fear of
failing, Insomnia, Obsession,
Phobias, Quarrelsomeness,
Rejection, Stress, Worthlessness
– feelings of

Sage

Pain

Spikenard

Addiction – general, Addiction
– hypnotic, Addiction – drugs,
Aggression – soothing, Anger
– coping with, Depression –
hysterical, Grief – dissipating,
Hysteria, Stress

Tea Tree

Hypochondria

Thyme Linalol

Confusion, Hypochondria,
Memory – lack of, Trauma

Tuberose

Addiction, Addiction – drugs,
Aggression – soothing,
Amnesia – confusion, Anger –
calming, Anger – unrealized,
Confusion, Facing death,

Passivity, Rejection, Self-
blame, Stress

Valerian

Addiction, Addiction – drugs,
Aggression, Anger – coping
with, Depression – agitated,
Depression – anxious,
Depression – hysterical,
Delirium tremens,
Hypochondria, Hysteria,
Insomnia, Stress

Vanilla

Grief – dissipating

Vetiver

Addiction, Addiction – drugs,
Aggression – general, Amnesia
– fear induced, Anger – calming, Anger – coping with,
Anxiety – general, Anxiety –
restlessness, Anxiety –
depressed, Burn-out,
Depression – hysterical,
Fatigue – mental, Fear – general, Fear of sexuality, Grief –
expressing, Guilt, Hysteria,
Insomnia, Obsession, Pain –
tension, Rage, Repression,
Stress

Yarrow

Grief – dissipating, Stress

Ylang Ylang

Amnesia – shock induced,
Anger – coping, Depression,
Depression – weepy,
Dejection, Doubt, Fear of fail-
ure, Fear of madness, Fear of
change, Fear of sexuality, Fear
of love, Guilt, Irritability,
Moodiness, Passivity, Rage,
Rejection, Repression, Self-
blame, Stress

Part Three

AROMA-GENERA: HUMAN CHARACTERISTICS AND PERSONALITIES OF ESSENTIAL OILS

'The whole earth is a thurible heaped with incense, afire with the divine, yet not consumed. This is the most spiritual of earth's joys – too subtle for analysis, mysteriously connected with light and with whiteness, for white flowers are the sweetest – yet it penetrates the physical being to its depths. Here is a symbol of the material value of spiritual things. If we washed our souls in these healing perfumes as often as we washed our hands, our lives would be infinitely more wholesome.'

MARY WEBB
The Joy of Perfume

Chapter Twelve

WHAT IS PERSONALITY?

INTRODUCTION

PHYSICALLY, HUMAN BEINGS ARE MUCH THE SAME. WE ALL HAVE a skeleton, with muscles, respiratory system, cardiac and circulatory system, digestive organs, and so on which, if put under the microscope, would look very similar. Where we differ profoundly from one another is in our brain functions – our thoughts, emotions and behaviour. In other words, our personality. Just think about your family and friends for a moment – no two people are the same in terms of their ideas, attitudes, dreams, temperament and so on. Where does this difference come from?

Personality is not etched for ever into us, like a fingerprint. It changes both depending on who we are with at any given point in time, and at different times in our lives. I can think of a little six-year-old girl, for example, who is perfectly behaved and creatively occupies herself when she is with her friend, Celeste, but who behaves like an obstreperous teenager when she is with her friend, Mandy, and who is an out-and-out brat when she plays with Miranda, or a bossy tyrant when she is with the passive Susan, and who bursts into tears at the slightest thing when she plays with her next-door neighbour, Peter.

If she just had one person to play with all the time these differences would not be so apparent, and perhaps her mother would think that, indeed, her personality was etched into her like a fingerprint. As it is, we can see that her personality changes in relation to those people she is with. Personality also changes depending on life's experiences and so we hear people say 'his whole personality changed after he got that job', and so forth. People *do* change, quite dramatically sometimes – either because of an outside influence, new job or love for example, or because of an internal one – such as finding a spiritual home.

Psychologists have found that babies of seven to eight weeks display differences in terms of their activity levels, attention span, intensity of reaction, changeability of mood and degree of persistence and, when these babies were followed up later, these same differences could be observed despite the social and emotional environment in which the children grew up. Clearly we are born with a unique personality but exactly how much of our adult personality is due to genetic or environmental factors is the question that has fascinated researchers. In the search to get to the root of personality, identical twins have been under a great deal of scrutiny, especially those who were bought up in different homes. Take the case of the American 'Jim twins' who were adopted at birth by different families and didn't meet each other until they were thirty-nine years of age. By then, both Jims had worked as part-time sheriffs, both drove Chevrolets, both regularly holidayed in St Petersburg, Florida, both had married women called Linda, and divorced, both had remarried women called Betty, both had dogs called 'Toy', and both had sons called James – in one case it was James Alan and in the other, James Allen.

A review of forty studies into twins found that identical twins (with the same genes because they grew from a fertilized ovum which separated into two) reared apart from each other were more similar in their personality traits than fraternal twins (with different genes because they grew from two ova, which were fertilized by two sperm). On this basis, it could be said that *nature* has more impact on an individual than *nurture*, and we are also reminded that individuals inherit their sympathetic nervous system, which regulates blood pressure and heartbeat, from their parents, and can influence the way a person responds to circumstances, making it similar to that of their parents. But it is not that simple. Other research clearly shows that *nurture* has a powerful impact on an individual.

Any parent knows that if they have a fit of anger one day their child is liable to have a fit of anger the next. We can observe our children doing and saying what we do. It is thought that the personality traits most likely to be reactive to parental influence are bad temper, aggression, anxiety, timidity, impetuosity and altruism. Anxiety, depression, phobias, compulsions and obsessions are also very likely to have their roots in the high level of emotional drama in their childhood home life. And simply by growing up around our parents we could adopt their political leanings and religious beliefs, and may even go into the same professions as they.

Another important influence on our personality is whether we were the first-born child. Research shows that first-borns are more likely to be achievement oriented, conservative and reserved and it is thought this is because they made themselves more acceptable to their parents as a way of overcoming the displacement they felt with the arrival of siblings. But parents are often more protective of the first child, believing all manner of harm will come to them whereas with subsequent children the parents have learned that the child will survive. Also, older children take on responsibility for their younger siblings and even have to protect them – either from other children or from the parents. First-borns are also given more responsibility by their parents in that they have to do jobs around the home to help out while the younger ones are just not capable.

Younger siblings, on the other hand, are never asked to help their older brothers and sisters get dressed or washed and I don't know any younger siblings who have sat for hours and helped the first-born with their reading, unless the first-born had learning difficulties. Younger siblings tend to be given more freedom because the parents aren't as worried as they were with the first; they have less responsibility and have not needed to develop skills in protecting others. All this can make them a little 'wild', a fact usually attributed to their being rebellious because they feel they are not as loved as the older child, or to their hating their older sibling. I find this theory rather dubious because in my experience younger siblings are as likely to idolize their older siblings as to hate them.

Finding the roots of personality is not easy. Children from similar environments have very different personalities and may, in fact, have a similar personality to a child who grew up in a totally different environment. Also, two children from very strict homes may develop in different ways – one may become cautious and correct and the other may rebel and go completely the other way. The old *nature versus nurture* debate seems to have come to the conclusion that it is 50 per cent due to inborn factors, and 50 per cent to environmental ones.

Personality, then, comes from many areas. There is a certain genetic factor, and being male or female has a powerful influence, both in terms of hormones and socially expected behaviour (probably the latter being more influential). Our parents influence us, as do siblings and our age relative to them, the environment we grow up in is important (whether that is in Somalia, Sarajevo or Surrey), as are the people available for us to play or work with. Are we then just a mish-mash of influences, clay in the hands of circumstance? The answer to this is no. We are born individuals, as research also shows, and in a sense, it is our adult prerogative to recover our individuality and shake off those influences we no longer desire.

It is easy to feel like a piece of flotsam adrift on the sea of life, sent here and there by the tides of time. Powerful eddies are created by other people imposing their ideals and behaviour patterns on to us, and they are forces which are difficult to fight, especially when they are our nearest and dearest. We go around and around, wondering where we are, and where we will end up. And powerful, dangerous tides are created by life circumstances such as illness, unemployment and bad relationships. Meanwhile strong forces within us created by abuse, violence and fear project us on to shores we do not really want to be on.

Yet in our mind's eye we probably all have an image of the

ideal place where we would like to end up, the perfect person we would like to be. Among the qualifications we might aim for are thoughtfulness and sensitivity towards others, integrity, tolerance, trust and openness, professional creativity, and a concern for justice, peace and freedom in the world. Psychologists agree that conformity is not necessarily good for us and being true to ourselves is. We need to develop control over our lives, deep personal relationships, time for reflection, the imagination to overcome problems and a zest for living. Then, we might be happy!

But who are 'we'? The answer is ever elusive. Dr Roger Woolger, a Jungian psychologist writes about regression therapy: 'Each other life that comes to us, however brief or fragmentary, is a piece of another self. The personality is not single, it is multiple – not in the psychiatric sense of multiple personality, but in that there are many levels to the self like many skins to an onion. We peel off these selves as we look into our past lives or as we look into our own dreams'[1]

Multiple Personality Disorder (MPD) is the other aspect of complexity, and extremely interesting from a mind over matter point of view because it proves, if nothing else does, that there is still much to learn. People with MPD (known as 'multiples') switch from one personality to another and have been shown to have different brainwave patterns depending on which personality they are 'in' at any given time. They can even have different physical disorders, present or not present, depending on the personality they are expressing. There are many scientifically recorded incidences of this, with people having and then 'disappearing' symptoms when the well personality takes over. Not only can allergic reactions, scars, burn marks, swollen insect stings and cysts disappear almost immediately, even the eye colour can change! A multiple with diabetes can lose all the symptoms when in a non-diabetic personality, and it has even been reported that a person with cancer can 'disappear' the tumour when 'in' the personality that doesn't have the cancer.[2]

Although MPD is an extreme, we are all to some extent 'multiple personalities'. The little six-year-old girl mentioned earlier is a different personality depending on whether she plays with Celeste, Mandy or Peter. And we know that we ourselves can have different personalities depending on who we are with. We would not, for example, behave in the same way we do at the rugby club ball as we do when we're asking the bank manager for a business loan (unless your rugby club is *extremely* sedate!). We are, in a sense, multi-faceted like a diamond, throwing out different reflections and colours in response to the light coming from outside. This phenomenon is well recognized in psychology, which considers Jung's theory of a total 'Self' comprising many sub- or secondary personalities to be one of his most enduring contributions to the study of the human mind. The beauty of the human mind is that we have this complexity, fluidity and potential which need not merely be reactive but can be controlled to a certain extent. Let's just hope it's controlled to your advantage when you go for a personality test!

PERSONALITY TESTS

Without doubt, personality is important. It is how you portray yourself to the outside world. It is what you will be judged on when people first meet you, both socially and professionally. When you apply for a job you are very likely to have to fill in a lengthy form of questions designed to show the potential employer what your innermost feelings are on a diverse range of subjects such as money – getting it and spending it – exercise, party-going, pets, companionship, hobbies, family, dreams, desires and so forth. By the time you've filled one of these forms out you may know more about yourself than you did before, and your potential employer will know as much as you! What all this invasive busybody 'personality testing' is about, so we are told, is to identify management potential and see how you would fit into a team. However, it may also identify for your potential employer whether you'll toe the company line and not sway the corporate boat by standing up for the workers when a tricky decision has to be made regarding redundancies. 'Personality testing' is about making sure you are, in no way, shape or form, a threat to the company and its profits. No longer are exam passes and other achievements, even hobbies and experience, enough.

Personality testing is carried out in the form of long questionnaires and, also, is assessed through graphology. These methods are employed by companies and other employing organizations, career counsellors and clinical psychologists. Whether they have any true value is a matter open to question, and in a hundred years' time they may laugh at us all, but in the meantime our personality is not our own – it's in the personnel department's files! For that reason, if no other, perhaps it's worth spending a little time considering what our personality is, and whether or not we want to change it.

PERSONALITY IN PERFUMERY

It takes years to design a perfume, and millions of pounds to market it. And who knows if anyone will buy it? Perfume houses, then, have had a tremendous interest in trying to establish personality types, so they can more effectively create perfumes that people want, and market them efficiently. In market research people will be asked whether a perfume reminds them of a glamorous, cultivated lady, a successful career woman or a fresh and sensitive young girl, so the perfume houses can have a clearer idea of people's perceptions of the 'character' of any particular perfume, so they can market them accordingly. As part of the drive to know the market, the fragrance house H&R (Haarmann & Reimer) in conjunction with the Research Institute for Applied Esthetics of Freiburg, Germany, have adapted the Luscher colour test to identify personality types which, in turn, can be linked to particular fragrances. According to their system, there are seven groups of female fragrance buyer, classified as A–G: extroverted, introverted, emotionally ambivalent, emotionally ambivalent with extroverted mood trend, emotionally ambivalent with introverted mood trend, emotionally stable with extroverted mood trend and emotionally stable with introverted mood trend. Each of these personality groups is further defined. For example, the Group D personality is described as '. . . lively, cheerful and vivacious, yet easily injured. This group reacts spontaneously to its environment . . .', and so on, and is designated with the 'fragrance need' floral, floral-fruity. Group A '. . . quickly impart life to a boring group . . .'; Group B '. . . would rather stay home than go to a boring party'; Group C 'enjoy dreaming about things that cannot possibly ever come true . . .', and so on. These are of course just glimpses of the much fuller descriptions given to the personality types which are interesting because they are the links between colour preference and fragrance need, as far as this system of classification is concerned.

Classifications are, of course, variable and dependent upon the requirements of particular groups. The fragrance industry needs to be able to tie in its product, which has a particular fragrance, with the marketing approach they need to take to achieve maximum returns on their considerable investment. The Luscher colour test is itself used extensively by educational and behavioural psychologists to ascertain personality traits so people can be encouraged to perform better in life, while 'colour imagers' have another attitude to colour – choosing clothes to suit the skin tone and hair colour of a particular woman (and 'colour therapists' use colour light-filters projected on to their patients for healing, while mental colour therapists use colour projected from their minds to heal – which might sound strange until one considers the fact that all life is vibration – which colour is too). The fragrance industry recognizes very well that people choose different perfumes for different activities, to complement the moods they may be in at any particular time.

CHARACTEROLOGY AND TYPOLOGY

Most of us know our astrological birth sign, and many of us will know whether we are an 'earth', 'fire', 'air' or 'water' sign. This is a form of typography, a classification system, which is also about character, characterology. We talk about someone being 'too earthy' or 'too fiery', 'an air-head' or 'wet', and when we do this we're continuing a tradition that stretches back in time, for as long as we can see. Classifying people's characters in various ways has been done throughout time and throughout the world. The Sufis have the nine characters of the enneagram, the Chinese have yin/yang and the five elements of water, fire, wood, metal and earth, the Indians have Ayurvedic medicine which recognizes the three personality and energy types vata, pitta and kapha, while the Greeks had the four 'humours', a concept that was continued in western medicine until the seventeenth century and beyond. The father of psychology, C. G. Jung, also adapted these four humours of air, fire, water and earth into the concept of the four aspects of a human being: thinking (air), intuition (fire), feeling (water), and sensation (earth).

We might talk about someone being in good or bad 'humour', by which we mean their mood, but this word comes from 'humoral', which once described a person's basic physical or mental qualities or disposition. The man who most influenced the course of western medicine – the ancient Greek, Galen – used the categories of *sanguine* (fire) – optimistic and happy; *melancholic* (earth) – depressed and anxious; *choleric* (air) – irritable and impulsive; and *phlegmatic* (water) – listless and not easily moved. The different combinations of the four humours in any one individual constituted their 'complexions' or 'temperaments' – their physical and mental qualities – and the ideal was to have an equal proportion of all four. Balance, in other words. Although the words sanguine, phlegmatic and so on are still used in the English language, they have lost the psycho-physical significance they had in ancient Greece. The choleric person, for example, was not only irritable and short-tempered but yellow-faced, lean, hairy, proud, ambitious, revengeful and shrewd. These characterizations were the basis for diagnosis for over 1,500 years in the western tradition, and a person who was innovative and a 'born' leader would be described as a fire personality, someone who used their five senses in a practical way would be an 'earth' personality, someone who was sensitive and feeling would be a 'water' personality, while the thinkers and philosophers were the 'air' type, and medications or treatments would be given taking the personality into account.

Diagnosing people by a combination of physical and mental

attributes is still today not in the slightest bit unusual.
Homeopaths do it every day. Dr Ronald Livingston, for
example, describes the patient who would most benefit from
the homeopathic remedy natrum muriaticum: 'withdrawn,
moody, taciturn, seclusive, sullen and silent when questioned;
and attention and sympathy make him resentful and un-
gracious to the point of tears'.[3] Likewise, a practitioner of
Ayurvedic medicine will diagnose you in terms of the three
energy forces or *doshas* – *vata, pitta* and *kapha*, which he or
she will aim to bring into harmony with ayurvedic medicines,
diet, massage, meditation, yoga or essential oils. Vata dosha
types are described as enthusiastic and lovers of new experiences but when out of balance they become anxious,
exhausted and depressed. Pitta dosha types have a fiery
temperament and are ambitious, perhaps overbearing and
demanding, but will suffer stress, tension and anxiety when
out of balance. Kapha dosha types are calm, strong and steady
but when imbalanced become insecure, lethargic and lazy. A
person might have two dominant personality types and the
skill of the practitioner depends on their being able to identify
these and bring them into harmony with one another.

Balance is all in the 4,000 year-old Chinese Taoist system,
not only between yin and yang, but between each of the five
elements which are expressions of their interaction – water,
fire, wood, metal and earth – and which are expressed within
an individual in terms of their psychological disposition, as
well as their physical body. Macrobiotics, a nutritional system
developed in the 1880s by a Japanese doctor called Sagen
Ishizuka, aims to balance the yin/yang qualities which exist
within us all by the means of foods, which are designated
either yin or yang. People who are more yin than yang are said
to be relaxed, peaceful, calm, sociable and creative; while
those who are more yang than yin are said to be energetic, alert
and precise. Too much yin brings lethargy, loss of concentration and depression, while too much yang causes irritability
and tension. If you went to any person practising a therapy
relating to yin/yang energies, your personality would be
assessed to help diagnose where the imbalances are.

Achieving balance is also the aim of the Polynesian

Kahunas, medicine men and women of the Huna faith. The whole basis of this system of medicine is the belief that man is a spiritual/intellectual/emotional being and that these three aspects have to be in harmony if disease is not to occur. Indeed, the mind is believed to be the source of all ill health even that arising from accidents – because your mind told you to be in the wrong place at the wrong time! The condition of the mind, then, is a crucial aspect of diagnosis while massage and chanting are aspects of the healing process.

When Dr Edward Bach devised his Bach flower remedies in the 1930s, he intended psychological and emotional characteristics to be part of the diagnosis, so that a remedy would be chosen depending on the feelings of a person at any given time, and depending on the life-circumstances at the time. Whether chosen by a therapist or by oneself, as well as considering any illness, other things such as relationships or work should be taken into consideration. Sweet chestnut will be recommended for utter dejection, bleak outlook and despair, for example, while red chestnut is more appropriate for someone who is obsessed by care and concern with others. Honeysuckle is for people who are homesick, nostalgic or living in the past, and water violet is for those who are proud, reserved and aloof. Dr Bach believed that each person's personality and nature could be matched with a 'type remedy', which might be taken for a long period of time whereas other remedies could be used on a short-term basis to deal with passing problems.

C. G. Jung was very impressed with the old Greek and medieval idea of the four humours and adapted them into his psychoanalytic theory. The four elements were expanded into eight as follows: *Air* (thinking); *air-fire* (intuitive thinking); *Fire* (intuition); *water-fire* (intuitive feeling); *Water* (feeling); *water-earth* (sensory feeling); *Earth* (sensation); and *air-earth* (empirical thinking). Jung thought that one of these functions was the predominant, and that the functions to either side were auxiliary while the function furthest way from the predominant function (if one sees these classifications as a circle) was subconscious and difficult to express. This view has been critized, however, because a person can be, for example, both feeling (water) and thinking (air) – as a concert pianist, for example.

Another system of personality classification exists in the enneagram – a word which combines ennea, meaning nine, and gram, meaning diagram. This system was made popular by the spiritual teacher George Ivanovich Gurdjieff in the early twentieth century although the enneagram can be traced back in time to the secret brotherhoods of the Sufis in the tenth and eleventh centuries and may go back very much further than that. The ancient Egyptians were very seriously into the number nine believing, for example, that Atum of Heliopolis, as it says in the Pyramid Texts, 'came forth from between the thighs of the divine Nine'. Whatever, according to the ennead there are nine personalities: the reformer, the helper, the status seeker, the artist, the peacemaker, the thinker, the loyalist, the generalist and the leader. These are of course further defined so, for example, the thinker is not only perceptive and analytic, but paranoid. As with all systems of characterology and typology, each personality type has the potential to be positive or negative.

Webster's dictionary lists 17,953 different descriptions of personality traits, which shows the immense complexity that there is in the human character. Trying to classify these traits into distinct personality types has been, as we have seen, an aspect of human endeavour, and it continues to be so. These days we tend to talk in terms of psychology, so people are defined in the literature as hysterical, obsessional, schizoid, paranoid, depressive, cyclothymic, anxious or narcissistic. These all sound very negative but in fact it is, as usual, all about potential. So, for example, we are told that the anxious personality can be very competent and decisive.

All the systems of characterology and typology stress that no character is 'better' than another and that balance is what it's about. Fire, for example, is enlivening and warming but it can, if taken to extreme, destroy. Water can be a refreshing stream or a tidal wave that pushes asunder all in its path. It is great to be a thinking 'air' personality but a tornado can rearrange things that were previously well placed. Earth is a good foundation but an earth slide destroys all in its wake. Balance and connection with our universal self is, as ever, the ultimate human goal.

Chapter Thirteen

AROMA-GENERA: HUMAN PERSONALITIES OF ESSENTIAL OILS

INTRODUCTION

WE PLACE PEOPLE INTO TYPES ALL THE TIME. WE SAY 'SHE is a born worrier', 'he won't stand for any nonsense', 'she's always apologizing', and so on. Phrases like this are short but they conjure up a whole personality which is a composite of all the other people we've known who are 'born worriers', for example. Likewise, when we say 'she spends money like water', our mind quickly scans our past experience and comes up with all the other people we've known to spend money like water, giving a category into which we shall slip this latest entry – 'Oh, another one of those, *that* type'.

In a sense this is unfair because we are all individuals and there is no one 'type' of person. The person spending money, for example, may be spending it on other people, or on themselves, and some may be spending money they actually have, while others are spending somebody else's money, or the credit card company's money! Already, this makes five sub-types. But in fact there are millions of sub-types and it would be impossible for our minds to keep all the information we have about them if we didn't file them away under some form of 'type' classification. Classification helps to keep our mind tidy, even though it may sometimes be unfair and even in-accurate. Personality classification is a trade-off between accuracy and mental overload.

Professional therapists similarly use personality classifica-tions to help us choose, from the wide range of options, the right combinations of oils for a particular person. It will not be to one personality type we refer, but to several layered one upon the other. These factors should be taken into consider-ation in addition to the therapeutic value of possible essential oils in relation to the physical or emotional problem(s) the client presents with. Some of us do this because we have been trained to do so, while others do it subconsciously based on their practical experience, or intuitively. Utilizing this 'harmony with' relationship between particular people and particular oils opens up a whole new vista of potential in terms of physical result, but also in terms of emotional and spiritual upliftment.

For the practitioner, as a practical aid, personality profile assessment takes no more time than the initial consultation, which should also include questions relating to personality traits such as 'are you a person who rushes everywhere, or do you take things easy?', 'do you express your anger, or bottle it up?'. Questions such as this provide answers which can be as illuminating as knowing where the physical pain is.

This is a book about mind, mood and emotion – aroma-psychology – and therefore in this context the personalities of the essential oils are extremely important and the interesting thing is, when you get a harmony between a particular person and a particular oil, the physical problem can clear up more quickly. Not only that, people who are using this system have seen some almost miraculous recoveries simply from choosing the essential oils *only* on the basis of their personality typology, not taking the therapeutic values into account at all. The results are beneficial on all levels, body, mind and spirit. This is true whether the problem being treated is a physical or an emotional one.

During workshops I have given both here and abroad I've noticed a growing awareness of the need to be more easily able to formulate the perfect blend for each individual's psyche. What I am presenting here is an introduction to the subject of

Aroma-Genera, which will be covered in more detail in a forthcoming publication.

The subject of personality types in relation to essential oils was introduced to me many years ago when I was an apprentice of clinical herbal medicine in Switzerland, and working in Germany, Italy and other European countries. Phytotherapy, as it is known in mainland Europe, uses herbs, essential oils and naturopathy as an integrated system. It was, and still is, a normal part of diagnosis and treatment to consider the emotional and mental characteristics of individual patients. So, one might say of an insomniac for example, 'they're angry all the time, we shall use this tea', or 'this person changes direction too quickly, we shall use that tea', and so on. Both patients present with insomnia but the diagnosis and treatment will depend on whether valerian tea is used or chamomile. In classical phytotherapy it is taken for granted that a person's mental state will affect their physical body and that, conversely, a treatment using herbs or essential oils could affect the mind. Aromatherapy also incorporates these ideas – it is only a question of degree, and consciousness.

The personality profiles presented in the following chapter have been collected by myself over many years of practical application, through which I have learnt to be acutely aware of personality traits. However, it has become clear to me that there is a system to the use of essential oils *vis-à-vis* personality, whether or not in conjunction with the treatment of physical ailments, and it is this system that I present in this chapter, under the new name, Aroma-Genera, which means the different types of personalities, here classified for the first time as *Florals, Fruities, Herbies, Leafies, Resinies, Rooties, Seedies, Spicies* and *Woodies*. These are of course variations on the personality groupings classically accepted in modern-day psychology. Many hundreds of people have been through my workshops where these classifications have been elucidated. The feedback I have since received from these people has been most enthusiastic and I have been asked countless times to provide the material in book form. People's emotional state is expressed through their 'personality' and, conversely, personality is a key in the treatment of the emotional state.

AROMA-GENERA

The human being is all about potential. We all have good days and bad days, the question is, how many good or bad days do we have in any given week or year. The aim of Aroma-Genera is to maximize the potential so that we more often operate on the positive end of the spectrum of possibility. The nine groupings which follow are arranged as *Abundant Self, Generally,* and *Impoverished Self,* reflecting this potential fluidity. The aim is to become more often abundant, that is positive, and less often impoverished, or negative.

To choose one's Aroma-Genera group requires honesty. Read each group carefully and see which most closely reflects your own personality traits. This may be done with a friend or family member, someone who knows you very well but, although other people will know your patterns of behaviour, they may not know your innermost thoughts. It is then, ultimately, up to each individual to ascertain into which group or groups they fall.

I often find in workshops that, at first, people will choose the Aroma-Genera class which fits not the person they are, but the person they *wish* they were. This is, in a sense, 'jumping the gun' because while personality can certainly be encouraged in more positive directions, as we shall see later, the starting point is to establish where one actually is right now.

From a practitioner's point of view, one of the most fabulous aspects of aromatherapy is the potential of the blending process. Throughout this book I have referred to synergistic blends – mixtures of several essential oils – and these are the mainstay of our work because blending brings into play the old truism that something can be 'more than the sum of the parts'. This same dynamic comes into play with Aroma-Genera. Very few people display the characteristics of one group alone – they are complexes of two, three, or even more groupings. You may then find yourself saying 'I'm a bit of a herbie but also a bit of a leafie'; this is fine, and to be expected, and choosing oils and blending them may be based on two, rather than just one, grouping.

One of the challenges of aromatherapy, at least as perceived by the general public, is that there is so much choice. People stand in front of a row of essential oils in the shop and ask themselves 'which one is for me?' Aroma-Genera helps' us answer this question. There *are* oils which are better suited to a particular individual and the success of the aromatherapist and lay person alike depends upon being able to make good choices. My aim here is to introduce the possibilities inherent in the confusing diversity of options available, and I present the information with confidence because experience has shown me that it works. When people find the oils that best suit them they can progress in leaps and bounds and become the person they truly wish they were. Another advantage in the system is that it provides a certain amount of lateral thinking and people find themselves considering essential oils they would never previously have thought of using. And, as we shall see, some of the most unusual combinations have a profound impact, not only on the body but on the whole person – mind, body and spirit.

THE MAGNIFICENT NINE

Working with the products of nature on a daily basis I have over the years been constantly amazed by the beautiful, and effective, aromas that can be made when combining particular essential oils. However, sometimes life can be stunningly beautiful in its simplicity. This was the thought that ran through my mind when I discovered the aromas that could be made when blending only those oils that belong to a particular Aroma-Genera. For example, if you take one drop of every floral essential oil and mix them all together, the effect can be simply divine. A depth of effect is reached which goes well beyond the physical and into the etheric, so that a kind of electrical shudder or wave of energy reaches throughout the whole body. And this extraordinary effect is achieved simply by smelling this combination from the bottle of mixed drops. Something very interesting is happening here, and it happens when you make mixes using exclusively essential oils from each of the other eight Aroma-Genera groups as well.

What we're talking about here is an effect which is felt on

the non-physical level, as well as the physical. To take a sniff from a bottle and have a shudder run through, not exactly the body, but the space taken up by the body and beyond, that can be felt like a wave, is something everybody who has experienced this finds staggering. It is humbling as one realizes that nature has its own simple system, which is expressed in sheer beneficial beauty.

Clearly I have a large collection of essential oils and can make mixes using a large number of *just* floral essential oils or absolutes, or *just* seedie essential oils, or *just* woodie essential oils and so on. But anyone with a fair collection can do the same. Even three essential oils taken from a particular Aroma-Genera group can give some idea of the potential of this mixing, but the more oils one can use, the better. If you do not have more than one essential oil from a particular group, ask your friends to let you have three drops from their bottles of essential oils that you don't have in your collection. Swop drops with each other, and see how deep and rich the Aroma-Genera mixes can be. As you're only asking for three drops of each, even your meanest friends will let you have some of their jasmine, or neroli, vanilla or carnation, which are among the most expensive and precious oils and absolutes.

What is so interesting about this experiment is that you will find yourself mixing oils which, normally, one would never put together, simply because you'd think the aromas would be incompatible. In fact, when blended together the oils from each Aroma-Genera group can blend together fabulously. Indeed, the reason I have called this sub-section *The Magnificent Nine* is because people's reaction to the Aroma-Genera mixes is most usually 'Oh, that is magnificent!' – and this is from people who are used to the fabulous aesthetic potential of essential oils. It is not simply that the aroma is splendid, but that the effect is immediately felt as a 'rush'. Somehow, an extraordinary balance seems to be created when blending in this fashion, a balance that has a deep and powerful effect on the whole person.

I suggest to people that they take nine bottles and label them 'floral', 'fruitie' and so on and put in them just three drops of each essential oil you have that falls into that group. Add to the mixes as and when additional essential oils are made available to you, and observe how the aroma gathers depth as more essential oils are added. When you have these nine bottles, which should contain a minimum of three essential oils of that group, they act as an additional means of choosing a person's Aroma-Genera type, working on the principle that people are attracted to the aromas that will ultimately do them most good, however emotional that journey may be.

WHEN IS A FRUITIE A FRUITIE?

As you can see from the chart at the end of this section, some essential oils fall into two groups. For example, lavender is both a floral and a herb, whereas clove is a fruit and a spice. The reason that an oil can fall into two groups is that two parts of a particular plant may be used in the distillation process – for example, lavender oil is extracted from the flowers, but sometimes also from the rest of the plant and is generally known as a herb in aromatherapy. Clove, on the other hand, is distilled from the buds – which is the fruit of the plant, but it is and has been known to be for centuries a 'spice'. Clearly, people around the world have different definitions of what is, or is not, a spice, depending upon whether their culture uses the material as a condiment in traditional cooking. Resins and roots are exceptions as they are usually only distilled from the part of the plant which defines their category, the resin or the root. The fruities also tend to be categorized under one heading although, for example, cardamon and pimento berry are also classified as spices. Do not let these overlaps bother you – they don't bother nature which, although simply beautiful, is also beautifully complex!

MOVING ON

It is not the purpose of Aroma-Genera to have everyone neatly classified under one group. Indeed, it is possible that the most highly evolved persons carry the abundant self-characteristics of all groups! So, for example, the ideal person might have the enthusiasm of a floral, the good nature of a fruitie, the practical caring skills of a herbie, the vision of a leafie, the wisdom of a resinie, the peace-making qualities of a rootie, the spirituality of a seedie, the joy of a spicie and the courage of a woodie. However, none of us are this perfect! All we can do is aim to be as positive as we can, given the real life circumstances with which we have to deal.

Only you truly know where your weak points are. You might think you need to get out more and meet people and get more stimulus, or you may feel that you need to be more in touch with your spiritual self. Only you may know how depressed you can get, or how isolated you can feel. The aim of Aroma-Genera is not only to help you identify these weak areas, but help you adjust your personality so the negatives have less influence and impact on you. We want to replace the negative with the positive, and with the essential oils you can, literally, do that. You can add a drop of joyfulness, or a drop of spirituality, in the form of essential oils which deliver those qualities. Nature *adds* positivity – and it comes in no form more concentrated than in essential oils.

The fact is that people do change for the better. It is not a question of becoming 'better' as far as other people are concerned, but 'better' as far as *you* are concerned, and that is judged in terms of happiness as well as in terms of good health. These are the natural states, in which we feel most at ease. Aroma-Genera helps us attain this ease, this fulfilment, but it cannot be done overnight. Aim first to identify your group(s), and aim to become the abundant self of those groups, gradually adding a bit of this, a bit of that, making yourself a fully rounded individual. This will not be the aim of everyone. Many people will be perfectly happy, and rightly so, being their abundant self within the context of one group. That may be their destiny, and they may have great things to achieve in that Aroma-Genera group. We are all individuals with individual hopes, expectations and desires. It is not for us to dictate what makes a person 'perfect', but for each individual to establish that for themselves. And, we have the measure – a happy, smiling face!

The following groupings are examples of essential oils and absolutes which fall into the nine Aroma-Genera groups. Following these are the nine Aroma-Genera human personality groups.

Florals are defined as those essential oils (and absolutes) which are extracted from the flowers or petals of plants or trees. For example:

FLORALS

Boronia, Cananga, Carnation, Cassia, Chamomile German, Chamomile Roman, Champaca, Genet, Helichrysum, Hyacinth, Jasmine, Lavender, Lemon Flower, Linden Blossom, Marigold, Melilotus, Mimosa, Narcissus, Neroli, Ormenis Flower, Osmanthus, Rose Maroc, Rose Otto, Tagetes, Tuberose, Ylang Ylang

Fruities are defined as those essential oils which are extracted from the fruit of a plant or tree. For example:

FRUITIES

Bergamot, Black Pepper, Cardamon, Clove, Cubebs, Grapefruit, Hops, Juniper, Lemon, Lime, Litsea Cubeba (May Chang), Mandarin, Orange, Pimento Berry, Schinus Molle, Tangerine, Tonka Bean, Vanilla, Mace

Herbies are defined as those essential oils which are extracted from plants generally thought of as herbs. For example:

HERBIES

Melissa, Basil, Calamintha, Clary Sage, Geranium, Hyssop, Lovage, Marjoram, Peppermint, Spearmint, Oregano, Rosemary, Sage, Thyme Red, Thyme Linalol, Thyme Lemon, Yarrow

Leafies are defined as essential oils which are extracted from leaves of trees or plants. For example:

LEAFIES

*Bay, Birch, Buchu, Cajeput, Cinnamon, Cistus, Cypress,
Eucalyptus, Eucalyptus Citriodora, Eucalyptus Piperita,
Eucalyptus Radiata, Fir, Myrtle, Niaouli, Patchouli,
Petitgrain, Pine, Ravensara, Tea Tree, Violet Leaf*

Resinies are defined as essential oils which are extracted
from the resin or balsam which exudes from trees or shrubs.
For example:

RESINIES

*Benzoin, Canadian Balsam, Copaiba Balsam, Peru Balsam,
Tolu Balsam, Borneol, Elemi, Frankincense, Galbanham,
Myrrh, Opopanax, Styrax Levant*

Rooties are defined as essential oils extracted from the roots
of plants. For example:

ROOTIES

*Angelica, Galangal, Ginger, Orris, Snakeroot, Spikenard,
Turmeric, Valerian, Vetiver*

Seedies are defined as essential oils extracted from the seeds
of plants. For example:

SEEDIES

*Ambrette Seed, Angelica Seed, Anise (Star), Aniseed, Caraway,
Carrot Seed, Coriander, Cumin, Dill, Fennel (Sweet), Nutmeg,
Parsley Seed*

Spicies are defined as essential oils extracted from various
parts of plants or trees commonly known as 'spices'. For
example:

SPICIES

*Anise, Aniseed, Black Pepper, Caraway, Cinnamon, Clove,
Coriander, Cubebs, Cumin, Galangal, Ginger, Mace, Nutmeg,
Pimento Berry, Turmeric*

Woodies are defined as essential oils extracted from twigs, wood, chippings or shavings from trees. For example:

WOODIES

Amyris, Cabreuva, Cade, Camphor White, Cascarilla Bark, Cedarwood, Cinnamon, Guaiacwood, Linaloe, Pine, Rosewood, Sandalwood, Spruce

Ylang Ylang

THE NINE PERSONALITY GROUPS

Florals

Aspirations: to have status and be admired, to be impressive and stand out from the crowd.

Florals' Abundant Self can be:

Attractive; enterprising; artistic; well-liked; energetic; dynamic; confident; loving; genuine; flexible; seeking self-improvement; ambitious; enthusiastic; passionate; sensuous; desirable; high ideals; striving for perfection and excellence; inner-directed aesthetic nature.

The floral type make the best of themselves physically, are good fun and well-liked. Their lives are filled with enthusiasm, energy and enterprise – dynamism in other words. They are totally confident and ambitious, not in a nasty way but positive to achieve something in this world and aim to have fun while doing it! Love blossoms from them when in the abundant state and they are passionate, sensuous and very, very desirable. Self-improvement is their aim, which is part of the striving for perfection. The floral type loves perfumes and anything that makes them feel good. Being extremely tactile, they'll choose to wear the best suit they can afford, preferably in the lightest, most flowing wool or silk material that moves sensuously with them. If they wear jeans, they'll have a designer label, or the pair that has the most style credibility at any given time. The house will always be full of flowers and plants, scents, candles and music. Florals have a very aesthetic nature.

Although they can appear very superficial, florals are very sensitive, soft-hearted individuals, who can pick up on the most subtle mood changes in others and will try their hardest to uplift spirits if they are down. Florals bring a lot of happiness and joy into this grey world and will help other people in any practical way they can – in terms of adding beauty to life. Although very caring, trusting and naive in many situations, florals are often the object of jealousy, much misunderstood.

Florals generally are:

Flirtatious; romantic; sexual; full of fantasies; seductive; caring; vulnerable; sensitive; concerned with appearance; image and status conscious; pretentious; competitive; conceited; friendly; successful; exhibitionist; self-promoting; self-important; calculating; unrealistic dreamers.

From an early age, about one minute old, the floral personality starts to utilize its powers of flirtation – on daddy if it's a girl, and mummy if it's a boy. This will develop later into great powers of seduction – made possible by the fact that they are very sexual. Full of fantasies, the young floral girl will have her head full of princes on white chargers and she will have her wedding planned, down to the choice of dress and bouquet of flowers. Florals worry about other people and are very inquisitive, especially when discussing other people's romantic liaisons. They never feel guilt – it is simply not in them or if it is they just blank it out, particularly when it concerns them!

Florals are very much concerned with their appearance, are narcissistic, image and status conscious, and can be totally pretentious. Competition is part of their nature, especially when it comes to love and romance so you find in a group of teenagers, a floral goes forward and starts talking to the group of the opposite sex, wanting to get there first and monopolize the most attractive. Florals will use their sexuality for everything. Floral women have no feelings of being inferior to men and will employ every trick in the book to get what they want from them, if necessary, including short skirts and very high heels. They are not exploited, but exploiting. 'Go for it' could be their catch phrase, to which you could add 'and never mind how'! Self-assurance marks florals out, and they get this confidence in themselves because they feel desirable. They are charming and popular and will appear to be very nice people, even though in their minds they may be thinking what an awful dress you're wearing. Florals are very artistic, lovers of dance, art, music, all the good things in life. Generally, florals are very successful, or have attached themselves to someone who is very successful. They feel very self-important and will self-promote without any compunction. Florals are calculating, exhibitionist, unrealistic dreamers.

Reward is the word that is etched into the mind of the floral type. If they don't have the reward of someone's admiration, life is not worth living. If they don't have a lover who can provide this reward of admiration, they're desperate, half-people, people-in-waiting. They believe themselves to be outstanding and they need to be shown to be that – the winner who gets all the acclaim and admiration. Their image is extremely important to them, it gives them credibility so packaging themselves is a number one priority – so they can get the rewards they cannot live without: love, money, success.

Florals' Impoverished Self can be:

Insensitive; exploitative; difficulty in loving and sharing; shallow values; manipulative; underhanded; devious; disloyal; envious; power-crazed; vindictive; liars; saboteurs.

The floral type can be insensitive and exploitative and have very shallow values. They can become manipulative, power-crazed liars, even vicious, malevolent and underhand. Impoverished florals can be deceptive and misleading if that suits their purpose. Driven by their need to have the greatest status, florals can be disloyal and betray, and driven by a jealousy of other people's success they will sabotage that person's plans to gain the advantage. This can even extend to interfering with other people's lives and relationships because this gives florals a sense of triumph, power. When impoverished, the ability to truly love goes, although sex can still be employed as a tool to get what they want. They feel no compunction in marrying for money and then taking on lovers. They can have a problem with intimacy and commitment (because there is always someone better over the hill), and can be phony.

The floral type cannot help comparing their lives with other people's and are very serious social climbers – opportunistic, calculating and pragmatic. They have grandiose ideas about themselves, imagining themselves living in huge detached houses with a big drive (if they don't have it already), impressing people with the huge diamond ring on their hands. Florals will self-pityingly cry for hours if they think that will achieve them something but they'll be wearing waterproof mascara and looking over their hanky to make sure they are getting the desired reaction. When people don't take florals' advice they can become arrogant and contemptuous. Their exhibitionist nature can lead them into exhibitionist behaviour, sometimes bordering on the decadent.

Orange

Fruities

Aspirations: to feel harmony within themselves, have security, respect and approval.

Fruities' Abundant Self can be:

Appealing; lovable; engaging; faithful; loyal; trustworthy; reliable; dependable; dedicated; co-operative; companionable; bright; joyful; emotionally balanced; independent; self-aware; enthusiastic; nice to be with; passionate; sensuous; inspirational; empathetic; benevolent.

If you are an employer looking for the perfect employee, the fruitie is for you. This personality is hard working, friendly, committed, supportive and encouraging, *plus* they take responsibility (both for the task in hand and for themselves) but do not have great ambition and will not be after your job. This personality loves seeing projects coming to fruition and will enthusiastically put all their energies into something, saying 'let's make this work'. And they can make it happen because they are great organizers. Put an advert in the paper for one now!

Fruities are self-aware, emotionally balanced and are usually very nice, happy people. They are liked by almost everyone because of their engaging positivity and friendliness. In fact, fruities are a sheer delight to be around because they're bright, joyful and playful, and have an altogether benevolent character. This makes them appealing, endearing and lovable. In addition (their good qualities are many), fruities have empathy with others, and are inspirational. Fruities are faithful and dependable to their friends, as well as to their bosses, and are sensuous and passionate with their lovers.

Fruities generally are:

Compliant; dutiful; conventional; organizers; respectful; submissive; jovial; willing to please; supportive; assertive; self-confident; realistic; loving; artistic; emotionally secure; endearing; responsive; commited; dislike authority; can be rebellious.

You can't define a fruitie as introvert or extrovert because they swing between the two in equal proportion. These are the kind of people who keep their friendships from primary school right through life, even to the grave. Although they have many acquaintances, they have few they would call true, deep friends but to all they offer jovial companionship. Fruities are supremely self-confident which can make them very familiar with other people, not in an unpleasant way but just as an aspect of their warmth, which is rooted in their loving nature. Fruities have a great need to *belong*, and will make sure that relationships with friends and family are good. This is easy for them to achieve because they are very willing to please, even compliant and dutiful when the rest of us have run! Their respectful nature can turn into a submissive one, although generally fruities are assertive. Bonding is extremely important to fruities and if their trust is broken, they will be devastated. Fruities can be taken advantage of and when this occurs they become anxious and depressed, quite unlike their usual selves.

Fruities need to express themselves and are very creative in their relationships. They have a very independent nature, great faith in themselves, and tremendous courage. Although fruities are conventional, they do have a rebellious streak and can react against authority if they believe it is behaving unjustly.

Fruities' Impoverished Self can be:

Contradictory; indecisive; hesitant; cautious; defensive; insecure; clingy; anxious; unreasonable; feelings of inferiority; self-sacrificing; illogical; self-abasing; impatient; over-sensitive; disheartened; stagnant; devious; spiteful; sarcastic; immature; masochistic; aggressive.

It is very sad to see a fruitie impoverished, which can happen if they are taken advantage of, becoming world-weary and depressed. They can become tired and faded, defensive and indecisive. The fresh, child-like quality that was once so appealing now becomes immaturity and a tendency to cling to other people, full of inferiority complexes, untypically insecure. Self-criticism takes over, along with self-sacrifice and servility and, in bad cases, masochistic actions. Disheartened with life and people, the fruitie stagnates and stays at home, becoming more and more impatient, touchy and over sensitive, and aggressive if people try to help. To protect themselves from prying people, devious methods are subconsciously employed to avoid being used and hurt again. A sharp tongue and spitefulness are sure signs of their impoverishment.

Clary Sage

Herbies

Aspirations: to love and be loved unconditionally, to be appreciated and needed.

Herbies' Abundant Self can be:

Loving; empathetic; charitable; compassionate; unselfish; big-hearted; humanitarian; bounteous; generous; welcoming; caring; supportive; helpful; giving; encouraging.

Herbies are the salt of the earth. They will fix your fence, make sure the old folk down the road are secure when there's been a snowstorm and collect food parcels for charitable organizations. Not only do they do any little job you ask them to do, they'll see where they can help and do it before you ask. In fact, they are always looking for things to do for people. So, for example, if a herbie is in the garden and sees a plant that would look nice crawling up your fence, they'll take a cutting and give it to you. Herbies are nice, solid, dependable people. If your father is a herbie and you have a crisis on, he'll take it over for you, sort it out so you can get on with your life. Herbies never overcharge on a job, they're steady, reliable and constant. Herbies want to give service, whether that is in the form of ironing your shirts, taking out the rubbish, baking you a cake, anything. They are always helpful, giving and generous. Thoughtfulness is their middle name, they plan ahead to help people, doing whatever they can or whatever they think people might need. If you've ever wondered who buys birthday books, it's the herbies. They never forget a birthday. Herbies are interested in other people and consider it a privilege to be allowed into their lives.

Herbies generally are:

Friendly; congenial; sympathetic; neighbourly; welcoming; well-intentioned; emotional; demonstrative; motherly/fatherly attitudes; self-sacrificing; complacent; enthusiastic; smothering; gushing; nosey; down-to-earth.

This group is sympathetic and have good intentions. They are the stay-at-homes, which is where they really want to be. Herbie females can be made to feel inferior by those feminists who think all women need to be fulfilled in some area outside the home. Herbies *need to be* at home and are happiest there –

preferably with a friend sitting on the sofa having a cup of tea and telling them all the latest drama in their lives. Although male herbies will go down the pub with the lads, they secretly wish they were in their shed at the bottom of the garden – which is not an escape to them, but an extension of their home where they can do 'man' things. Herbies feel themselves to have been given the saintly role, and they are very charitable and humble and worry about everyone and everything. They're very demonstrative, give a lot of attention and flattery, and can be over-enthusiastic. They love to talk about love, and some herbies hug a lot, putting their arms around you and so on.

Herbies can be extremely nosey. They'll exasperatingly ask question after question, never-endingly. The reason they do this is that they are living vicariously through other people. Although they are happy, herbies' own lives are not usually very exciting so they enjoy listening to other people's exciting experiences. If you've climbed a mountain and tell a herbie about it, they have climbed the mountain too. This is where they get their excitement, and without something to get nosey about they can get miserable. Gossip is as important as food to them, it feeds their imagination. This is the way they balance out their stay-at-home lives. This is usually OK for women, who invariably have their pulse on what's going on, but men can get left out so the herbie male will badger his wife until she gives him the latest neighbourhood gossip, while the herbie female will badger her male partner to get the office gossip!

Herbies have great empathy and feeling for others. They are caring and sincere, warm-hearted, and encouraging – they genuinely want people to succeed. They will appreciate you if you appreciate them. They see the good in others – which can backfire on them sometimes and they get hurt. But they often disparage themselves, thinking they should be doing more with their lives. They can also feel undeserving. Herbies do their best for other people, often at the expense of themselves, and often they do too much. This is the type that keeps every-thing and everyone together – that is their role in life, and they know it.

A typical herbie is Paula. The mother of five children, Paula keeps a chart of the children's many activities, which she organizes with military precision, ferrying them all to their various classes and activities. She also manages to find time to make clothes, cakes, jams and chutneys. Her husband doesn't have to lift a finger and wouldn't even dream of changing a toilet roll. When the demands of a family are not enough, Paula also has her elderly mother to organize and care about, the garden to tend, and the meals she cooks for the homeless to deliver. Non-herbies often wonder how it is physically possible to organize so many people and activities but it is possible because herbies usually engage in few activities for their personal satisfaction and have very little social life.

Herbies' Impoverished Self can be:

Resentful; anguished; exploitative; manipulative; domineering; demanding; self-serving; slovenly; guilt-inflicting; sympathy-seeking; hypochondriac; psychosomatic illness; martyrdom.

Herbies can resent the fact that they seem to do everything for other people and don't usually realize that this is a drive within them. They may feel resentful, but they still can't help themselves taking on everyone's little jobs. The herbie type can become very smothering. They don't like the children to leave home and will not understand why they do this unless it's for a good reason, like getting married or getting a job in another town. 'Why are you leaving?', they ask, 'I do everything for you, your washing, cooking . . .' They pretend not to understand the natural desire to break free. When the children leave home, a whole source of information and vicarious living leaves too so herbies can feel a void in their lives, which they usually fill with long telephone conversations after which, vicariously refreshed with new input, they can enjoy an evening watching soap operas and eating the cake they have just made. They may say to themselves, 'I'll get a little part-time job to occupy myself,' although they don't really want to because they're much happier pottering around the house.

One of herbies' failings is to get too intimate – too nosey until the person gets so exasperated they cut off all contact. This causes withdrawal symptoms in the herbie, who feels they are entitled to the information. This is when the herbie can become very intrusive and turn nasty – 'how dare you not tell me everything'. They hover around, wanting to meddle in everything and find out all they can about your business.

When they're impoverished, herbies want a *lot* of thanks – to be overthanked. Indeed, all the favours have to be repaid. They can also get very possessive and jealous of the people they have helped over the years. Although, in fact, many of the jobs they have done for people were less for those people than for themselves – because they needed something to occupy themselves, just as they need to be involved in other people's lives. In a negative frame, they can exaggerate their usefulness to other people so, for example, if you ask them to go and buy you a pint of milk they will do this but tell other people they had to buy you a week's groceries because you had nothing in the house.

Herbies will complain that they've never done anything for themselves, always for other people, and that nobody appreciates them. Guilt will be inflicted on all those concerned, and will be used as a form of manipulation. Hypochondria and psychosomatic illnesses will develop.

Leafies

Aspirations: to connect with the environment, understand the global perspective and gain wisdom.

Leafies' Abundant Self can be:

Visionary; knowledgeable; creative; wise; ingenious; perceptive; innovative; intuitive; focused; insightful; cooperative; observant; attentive; understanding; involved; inspirational; enlivening; rejuvenating; contributive.

The leafies are the wise visionaries who know where we have come from and where we're in danger of going. These

Cypress

people's minds are always alert, they take in everything in an instant, shake it down into its component parts and store it away for future reference. Knowledge is their sustenance and they'll spend hours in libraries, getting more of it. They want to understand the world, the universe and everything, and often do. Einstein was probably a leafie, as many brilliant geniuses are. Lateral thinking is a standard procedure for this type of person, as is looking at things holistically. Because they are innovative thinkers, often inventors, they're quite likely to have several original theories kicking around at the same time. The intellectual leeches of this world hang around leafies, hoping to pick up clues, often grasping them and presenting them to others as their own.

The leafie is not only extremely curious and knowledgeable, but also perceptive, intuitive, focused, insightful and inspired. Hard work and concentration doesn't frighten leafies and they'll research a subject thoroughly, from top to bottom, so they have all the details to consider. Although they can become very specialized in their particular field, they never lose sight of the whole. These are profoundly creative people, intellectually, and they have an ingenious, original approach. No research lab should be without one.

Leafies generally are:

Cerebral; thoughtful; logical; solitary; introspective; idealistic; imaginative; extremist; revolutionary; detached; complicated; non-conformist; invigorating; refreshing; stimulating; vulnerable; melancholic.

Leafies are pacifists and can't abide aggression in any form. If an intellectual rival starts shouting or being rude, leafies wince as if receiving actual blows to the head. Although often categorized as intellectuals, leafies are complicated individuals interested in subjects well outside their usual fields of enquiry, which may have nothing to do with academic pursuits. They are genuinely interested in what people have to say because, with their lateral thinking, they can see relevance to their own interests in many diverse subjects. These are the networkers, who can link facts from ten specialist areas and see a new law of nature.

Because leafies spend so much time thinking, they can forget to experience life and when they do, it can all come as a bit of a shock to the system. They can react to the new input in bizarre ways, trying to incorporate the different levels of experience into one whole. Personally, leafies are thoughtful, introspective, detached and solitary. Politically, they are idealistic and sometimes extremist. If you were to meet a leafie at a party you'd say to yourself, 'Here is an eccentric and non-conformist,' and you'd listen in wonder as he or she expounded on everything under the sun, often coming up with some very original ideas. Esoteric knowledge is, for leafies, just like any other knowledge – there to be researched and understood.

However, leafies can suffer intellectual delusions, almost as if reality were not important. They are also very vulnerable to criticism and can feel threatened by the slightest word.

Melancholia can settle over this personality very easily and they can retreat into solitude and refuse to answer the phone.

Leafies' Impoverished Self can be:

Compulsive; obsessive; paranoid; cynical; scornful; hostile; hypersensitive; easily intimidated; mean; vulnerable; fool-hardy; critical; confused; defeatist; suppressed; prone to insanity.

Although leafies are brilliant they can be wrong sometimes but when they're impoverished, they refuse to accept it. They'll take great umbrage if people disagree with them. Intellectually, they can reduce a subject so much it doesn't reflect the whole reality, and may make inaccurate conclusions because they can ignore facts which don't fit into their theory. This foolhardiness is not the only danger – they can also become stale.

On a more personal level, the impoverished leafie can become compulsive, ill-humoured, scornful, and defeatist. Recluses are often impoverished leafies, who already have a leaning towards secretiveness and isolation. Mental instability is also a danger at this time, starting with melancholy, confusion and suspicion, even paranoia, and going on to delusions and obsessions. Impoverished leafies can become out-of-touch, not to say out out-to-lunch!

Resinies

Aspirations: to have position and purpose.

Resinies' Abundant Self can be:

Liberal; charitable; merciful; wise; non-judgemental; reasonable; realistic; balanced; conscientious; moralistic; ethical; objective; fair-minded; truthful; spiritual; sagacious; sympathetic; principled; honest; kind; caring; benevolent.

Frankincense

Morality, truth and justice are the forces that drive this personality, often into professions which can utilize in a practical way these overriding concerns. Right and wrong are the signposts that direct their lives, and purity of thought is their ideal state of mind. Ethical considerations are behind their every move; spirituality is their goal. If all judges were resinies we would have no doubts about the legal system because justice would most certainly prevail. Realism and tolerance temper their advice, which is given honestly and with genuine care. Although they have such high expectations of themselves, resinies have a basic human charity and 'sympatico' which allows them to relate to others with a non-threatening, kindly air. These people command respect because their high principles are obvious for all to see, it directs their every move and can be heard in their every word.

Resinies generally are:

Perfectionists; efficient; orderly; strong-willed; knowledgeable; balanced; persistent; persuasive; campaigners; workaholics; self-controlled; high-minded; utopian; precise; difficult; responsible; emotionally withdrawn; religious fanatics.

What the resinie is aiming for is a spiritually perfect life so, if they believe in reincarnation, they will not have to return to this earth again, or if they believe in heaven and hell, will be going in the right direction. Resinies are very helpful to people, allowing them to offload their spiritual concerns on to them. Resinie's heart is in the right place – each and every day. They know very well their responsibility to the planet and to the human race, even if they don't realize they have a right for a little sustenance and fun too. That may, in fact, be the point of it all! Resinies need to become less the bombastic pulpit-basher and more the laughing, joking Tibetan monk.

Driven as they are by high ideals, the resinie works constantly like a beaver trying personally to stop the tide of wrong-doing and disharmony in the world. They don't much like parties unless they think there might be someone there who can contribute to their latest altruistic or campaigning project and who, faced with resinies' persuasive arguments and persistence, will usually be persuaded to contribute. Their strong wills carry resinies forward, like explorers across the huge frozen wastes of Antarctica, plodding step by small painful step towards their goal. Hardship doesn't bother them, they take it all in their stride, falling back on their organization and efficiency, which will see them through to the end. Often, people find them difficult because they can be one-dimensional and, frankly, not much fun.

Resinies are not concerned with sensual beauty, preferring spiritual beauty. It's not that they don't *like* sensual beauty or beautiful things, but these things are incidental in their life. Because resinies find it difficult to relax and enjoy themselves, a drop or two of a floral essential oil does them a great deal of good, providing balance. Although generally warm and caring, resinies can also sometimes be emotionally withdrawn, while repressing their sexuality can be resinies' way of denying their human state. Promiscuity holds no interest whatsoever for them.

Resinies' Impoverished Self can be:

Critical; indignant; angry; unbalanced; abrasive; arrogant; proud; intolerant; menacing; obstinate; dogmatic; unprincipled; judgemental; discouraged; depressed; rash; deprived.

If resinies make a moral mistake they are desolate and find it difficult to forgive themselves. If they are critical, they are most critical of themselves. The constant drive for perfection takes a terrible toll on resinies because they become disappointed with people, themselves and life in general. They can break like a twig under the foot of reality. When they're impoverished, resinies can become self-righteous, dogmatic, abrasive, intolerant, and very, very angry.

If things do not progress forward in a positive manner, and people are a disappointment, discouragement sets in, often leading to nervousness and depression. Resinies feel it is them against the negative forces, so when they're impoverished, there is a strong sense of being threatened. Battle weary, they reproach themselves for their lack of success. Perfectionists as they are, especially in regard to themselves, if they've made a mistake resinies are overcome with shame, guilt and self-reproach, which is difficult to shake off until they realize that they, too, are human.

Rooties

Aspirations: peacemaker; to have union with everything and traditional values.

Rooties' Abundant Self can be:

Peaceful; responsive; open-minded; helpful; hopeful; patient; strong-minded; supportive, encouraging; loyal; assured; content; composed; tranquil; unpretentious; kind; caring; good-natured; observant; giving; thoughtful; unselfish; humble; solid; reliable; loyal.

Ginger

The rooties are very good-natured, easy-going, laid back and serene. They accept life as it is. The whole world might be in a panic but rootie can dismiss it all, not too bothered. Stability is a definite characteristic of this personality as they can accept everything with equanimity, perhaps because they trust themselves and others. Some people might dismiss them as naive because they are simple souls, unpretentious and gentle, but they also have a capacity to be profound. This is the peacemaker – ever kind and supportive, always making people feel comfortable. If you've had a row or been made miserable, these are the people to visit because their healing influence will make you feel better simply from being around them. Partly, this reassuring quality is made possible by the fact that they are caring and deeply receptive. Rooties are generally very nice people, always willing to help anyone with their plans, giving encouragement and offering genuine optimism. Rooties are assured in an unpretentious sort of way, composed, solid, and rather more strong-minded than one might at first expect.

Rooties are the ultimate mediators because they are fundamentally harmonizers and healers. Because they are complete in themselves, they can establish profound relationships with all kinds of people, which instils an air of trust when disputes come to be settled. People will take rooties' advice, realizing that peace is their ultimate goal, and because they are impressed by their great dignity. Among their many good qualities are humility, a capacity to give, great powers of observation, reliability and loyalty.

Rooties generally are:

Easygoing; passive; good listener; down-to-earth; dedicated; tries to please; puts others first; original; dislikes change; modest; pacifier; controlled; conventional; traditionalist; environmentalist; satisfied.

It's easy to pass the rootie by unnoticed. They don't have the flamboyance of a floral or the obvious drive of a woodie. Some people might call them a plodder, although they do have original ideas, but they are not sparkling in an obvious sense and so are often misunderstood as dull. However, rooties have many very good qualities without which the world would be a less gracious place. They are modest and dedicated and genuinely aim to please. Composed and controlled, they'll step in as the most effective peacemaker.

Rooties could be called conventional traditionalists because they dislike change almost as much as they dislike arguments and disruptions. They'll turn a blind eye to any problem and leave things to sort themselves out. Rooties only see what they want to see and ignore the rest. If the wife or husband is having an affair, a rootie will 'blank' it out and if their child is being bullied at school, they'll say, 'Oh yes dear, you'll sort it out dear' – or, in other words, don't bring dispute into the house. This stubborn denial of problems, the walking away from conflict, is a form of unresponsiveness and it gets them into serious relationship problems, ironically perhaps. They must decide whether they are really satisfied with their lives, or merely resigned to them.

Rooties' ideal life would be to live in the country in a nice cottage, leading a quiet conventional life. Ecology is one of their main concerns. Of all the personality types, rooties are grounded firmly in this earth, which gives them great stability.

Rooties' Impoverished Self can be:

Neglectful; suppressed; obstinate; disorganized; confused; muddled; easily upset; inertia; slackness; absent-mindedness; disinterested; moody; uncaring; downhearted; sad; low-spirited; sneaky; apathetic; depressed; emotionally weak.

Rooties have to watch out that they do not become too submissive, the doormat type – especially if they are female and are linked to a woodie partner. This tendency stems from their adherence to sexually stereotyped roles, an aspect of their basic conventionality. They can take on too much and, if there's a crisis, collapse into an apathetic heap. Obstinacy is a way they handle conflict, which is of course an anathema to them. The impoverished rootie can be neglectful, disorganized, low-spirited, easily upset and depressed. Inertia overtakes them and they become emotionally very weak and unstable. If they have been suppressing their opinions (probably in the name of peace), they can become caustic, moody and sneaky. You can tell whether a rootie is in an impoverished state because they become unfocused and start going on and on and on endlessly – moaning, muddled and confused. Disinterest overtakes them as they retreat into themselves. Feeling lost is a classic symptom of an impoverished rootie who needs, at all times, to be grounded.

Seedies

Aspiration: to create beauty and understanding in themselves and others.

Seedies' Abundant Self can be:

Creative; inspirational; intuitive; knowledgeable; full of life; energetic; mindful; observant; considerate; self-aware; honest; emotionally balanced; harmonious; non-judgemental; sensorial; sensitive; honest; forthright; virtuous; genuine; joyful.

The seedie personality strives to be spiritually rich. Their powers of intuition are so finely tuned they can pick up other people's feelings as if they were radios picking up waves from all the radio transmitters. This intuition is also apparent when it comes to themselves, they know what is and what isn't right for them, and are very much in touch with their feelings. Seedie personalities are sensitive, self-aware, considerate and insightful.

Seedies have a remarkable ability to go through the same experience over and over again, going to the corner shop for example, seeing it and feeling it as a completely new experience each time. It is as if everything is new and exciting, and they notice something new on each trip, marvelling at it all. These powers of observation contribute to their considerable creativity, which is occasionally nothing short of inspirational. Not only are they observant – the information goes into their minds and stays there, stored away for future use. Seedies are totally alive – aware, sensitive, mindful and energetic.

Beauty is like spring water to the seedie; it is what uplifts them and makes their lives rich. Romance too is vital to their well-being. Seedies have an uncanny ability to avoid bad situations by just sliding away and, if anyone could do it, the seedie could hitch-hike around the world without coming against any trouble because their intuition would sense danger around corners. Another extraordinary capacity is to change like a chameleon, and seedies are constantly re-inventing themselves, changing their job or appearance in a flash. One endearing quality is that they don't take themselves too seriously, and another is that they are true to themselves and those around them. Seedies are honest, forthright, virtuous, funny and joyful. A few are also geniuses.

Seedies generally are:

Imaginative; creative; artistic; self-assured; introverted; expressive; caring; giving; spiritual; over-sensitive; deeply feeling; fragile; misunderstood; uncertain; insightful; intuitive; self-sacrificing; amiable; tolerant; even-tempered; self-indulgent; dreamer; harmonized.

Seedies are delicate souls, overly sensitive sometimes and deeply feeling. This can give them a fragile quality and, indeed, they can be hurt. Florals and seedies make a disastrous combination in a relationship, but a woodie personality can stabilize a seedie and bring them down from their dreaming world of beauty and wonders. Generally, they are emotionally balanced with inner harmony, well able to deal with their own feelings but, in certain circumstances, they will withdraw, become shy, and not go outside the front door if they can help it. Indeed, seedies are perfectly happy on their own and can go weeks without seeing anybody, getting on with whatever they are doing, enjoying the chance to grow in their own space, taking time to explore activities which enhance their state of consciousness.

Crowds make seedies feel self-conscious, perhaps because they are so sensitive to everyone's feelings they imagine people can see through them too. They can be very hurt by people, lovers in particular, and are often manipulated, used, or taken advantage of by less evolved souls. Seedies perhaps give too much of themselves, part of their self-sacrificing, over-tolerant nature. Respect of others is seedies' starting point in relation-

Angelica

ships, and they will be discreet to a remarkable degree, yet, if you find yourself in conversation with a stranger who suddenly tells you something profoundly revealing and honest about themselves, it's probably a seedie.

Seedies are quite easy to recognize because they are highly individualistic and stand out in a crowd. They are sensual, gentle and rather too generous for their own good. If they are criticized, they'll swallow it bravely, possibly because they do have self-doubts, but can be hypersensitive, vulnerable and easily hurt. They are often misunderstood.

Seedies' Impoverished Self can be:

Self-pitying; melancholy; disillusioned; disrespectful; disdainful; hopeless; self-destructive; emotionally cold; apprehensive; suspicious; aloof; contemptuous; can feel an outsider; lost to reality; emotionally burnt-out.

When seedies become emotionally overwhelmed or mentally exhausted, depression can set in. The negativity is often turned inwards so they become insecure with feelings of worthlessness, and have no hope for themselves. The self-indulgent streak which is usually harmless enough becomes, when they are impoverished, an addictive personality – perhaps turning to drink or drugs. Emotional burn-out causes seedies to become suspicious, undemonstrative and emotionally cold. Self-pity, melancholy and disillusionment become the order of the day and a seedie feels like an outsider, an observer of life, unwilling to join in. Even the creativity goes, and despite occasional flurries of activity it proves to be unproductive, like the writer who types page after page but is dissatisfied with them all and throws them all in the bin, or the painter who paints over canvases, never getting it right.

Spicies

Aspirations: to have it all – the hedonistic lifestyle.

Spicies' Abundant Self can be:

Joyous; zealous; animated; exhilarating; appreciative; fascinating; charming; magnanimous; vivacious; sparkling; congenial; warm-hearted; debonair; gracious; loving; seductive; self-assured; practical; dynamic; multi-faceted.

The spicie personality is joyous, exhilarating and animated. When Londoners were huddled in the tunnels of the underground system during the Second World War, it would have been a spicie who started the singing, 'It's a long way to Tipperary, it's a long way to go . . .', and so everyone's spirits would have been lifted. Spicies love life and at their best are sparkling, happy, warm-hearted, spontaneous and entertaining. As the ultimate sensation-seekers, they can be very seductive personalities. Spicies can be very intelligent people, multi-faceted and multi-talented, and are also extremely productive and practical – a combination which can lead to a brilliant career. They are often entrepreneurs but in any case dynamic, go-getting achievers. Spicies are dynamic and self-

Nutmeg

assured with a zealous appreciation of life. Their energy and intelligence can make them fascinating people, and at their best they are charming and loving.

Extrovert; entrepreneurial; connoisseur; materialistic; sophisticated; exhibitionist; pleasure-seeker; entertaining; achiever; dynamic; sensationalist; passionate; emotional; power-seeking; status-seeking; perfectionist; attentive; controlling; arrogant; over-confident; wilful.

Spicies generally are:

You can recognize spicies from their over-the-top reactions to everything. If you were looking at Niagara Falls the spicie would be saying 'it's *fabulous*, just *fabulous*' in a very loud voice. Nobody reacts as strongly as they do, to everything. If you do something for them, their gratitude and appreciation gushes forth in a torrent. Spicies are extremely excitable and definitely extroverts. They get excited about everything, especially about those things that relate to them. Indeed, they can spend so much time thinking and talking about themselves, they can forget that other people have far greater problems or stories they'd like to tell if only they could get a word in edgeways.

I can think of one, a brilliant linguist for whom the authorities had to make special dispensation so she could go to Cambridge University at age sixteen. One friend went on holiday with her and said she spent so long getting herself made up and dressed (a major preoccupation of spicies) by the time they reached the beach it was too hot and they had to go in again! Exasperating was the word mentioned. Nevertheless, these two remained friends and over the years have had tremendous fun going to zillions of parties and clubs in the spicie's gold Rolls-Royce.

Spicies have got to have money, which doesn't interest them from a power point of view, only a spending one, and they can shop till they drop. Their wardrobes will be full of clothes they never wear and their cupboards are full of special gourmet treats they simply couldn't resist buying. If they don't have money they'll go mad with the credit cards or find some way to pretend they have masses of dosh, like borrowing a friend's most expensive clothes. Spicies are deeply materialistic and will, if necessary, attach themselves to someone who can indulge them. Also, if they have the money themselves, they'll have toyboys or floozies to enjoy life with. Spicies do not know how to deny themselves, for them life is there to enjoy.

Spicies are the pleasure-seekers of this world, often connoisseurs of art, antiques and all the beautiful things in life. They are worldly, sophisticated people (or wish to be), and, often, their aim in life is to be a socialite. They can be great trendsetters and, sometimes, shockingly exhibitionistic. Generally, spicies are selfish, but fun.

Spicies' Impoverished Self can be:

Superficial; insensitive; boorish; discourteous; impolite; ill-mannered; impulsive; debauched; compulsive; mean; shabby; loathsome; greedy; self-centred; jealous; demanding; resentful; hysterical; panicky; depressed.

I remember once meeting a Brazilian diplomat who was the classic impoverished spicie. Having had full opportunity over the years to indulge himself in life's pleasures, he sat there totally jaded. Nothing would excite him, even the two young girls brought in for the purpose. He sat there in his silk Givenchy shirt and very expensive suit with a large Scotch in his hand, a tray of caviar on the table in front and two nubile floozies on either side, and he looked totally miserable! The debauchee was at the end of the road, with no pleasure left to explore, no new exciting purchase to be made, burnt-out and bored.

Spicies can become impoverished both by such burn-out and by frustration of their dreams. At their worst, spicies are superficial, impatient, insensitive, boorish, crude, demanding, resentful, self-destructive, mean and impolite. I say 'impolite', but that's being polite because impoverished spicies can actually be extremely rude and ill-mannered, abusive and insulting. They think of everyone as a servant and become very demanding, as if the whole world were designed to feed their need for pleasure. If they want to drive at a hundred miles an hour through a built-up area, they will, and they'll peep their horn as if to say 'get out of my way, I'm much more important than you'. This loathsome behaviour can be made worse by their greedy, addictive nature.

To the impoverished spicie, people are there to be used and their needs are completely irrelevant. They might buy you a new outfit, but it'll be one *they* like to see you in, not the one you want. As lovers, they can be jealous and overpowering, and tetchy from morning to night. If the typical impoverished spicie cannot find in their wardrobe the pair of shoes that will *exactly* match their outfit, they'll throw a tantrum, scream, shout, throw things around and generally behave like a very spoilt little child. They'll do this regardless of whether they have an audience or are alone. Hysteria, panic attacks and depression are common. The greatest fear of an impoverished spicie is to be bored and without a credit card.

Woodies

Aspirations: to be in control and have an impact on the world through self-determination.

Woodies' Abundant Self can be:

Steadfast; loyal; wise; courageous; eminent; magnanimous; inspiring; supportive; defender; authoritative; protective; ethical; honest; trustworthy; principled; honourable; strong-minded; decisive; confident; powerful; gallant; champion of causes; visionary; warm-hearted; energetic; expansive; compassionate.

Woodies are very strong, independent people, bold and forthright. They know what they want and they go for it, striving for their place in the world. Woodies are ruled by intellectual culture, civil rights, civil justice and wisdom, which they pursue with intelligence, dynamism and assertion. Because they are very quick thinkers, woodies often talk very fast, backed up by their considerable education.

'Action Man' was probably a woodie: bold, powerful, independent, ever able to take the initiative and get a task done. This strong, silent type are real nature lovers and will work tirelessly for the environment, perhaps as a Greenpeace hero, perhaps on the committee to stop road development in their area. Although aggressively ambitious, woodies have a nice disposition, being compassionate at heart, faithful to friends and ideas, honourable in their dealings and, if a man, gallant with old ladies!

Woodies will do anything they can for a cause in which they believe, once they've established the validity of it. 'Tell me again,' they'll say, questioning your motives about a project, 'tell me again' and 'again' and, when they know you are genuine and right-minded, will climb mountains for you, fight the dragons or do whatever it takes to establish rightness in the world. Having great courage and fortitude, and an endless

Sandalwood

capacity for hard work, woodies achieve a great deal in their life, both professionally and in terms of social ideals. Woodies are often turned to for help because people recognize that they are ethical, trustworthy and wise.

When in balance, woodies are intuitive, perceptive, warm-hearted people who will not nag you into the ground about any mistakes you may have made. They seem to be a bit above all that, steadfastly carrying on with their own plans, motivated by an inner moralism and driven by boundless confidence and persistence.

Woodies generally are:

Forceful; intellectual; individualistic; self-reliant; assertive; moral; self-confident; motivated; influential; controlling; content; perceptive; solid; unmovable; enterprising; persistent; earnest; conventional; faithful; steadfast.

Woodies are not puritanical at all so although they may run a youth club, for example, they won't chastise the youngsters for any wrongdoing. They are unhappy in tightly controlled religious groups and, being natural leaders, may start their own less puritanical and more tolerant breakaway group. Other people can find woodies rather daunting and powerful (because they know what they want), and may feel insecure in their presence but woodies are very fair-minded people and do not treat people unjustly. Although their children may tend to steer clear of their powerful woodie parents, they also know that woodie will give them space to grow and, if they have a problem, a woodie will swing into action and sort it out for them. Grandchildren love woodies and are not fearful of them in the same way because they appreciate knowing the parameters of expected behaviour, plus this personality has a tremendous amount of patience, especially as they grow older, and are also very caring and generous.

Woodie personalities must be in touch with nature. If they live in town, they belong to a golf club – not for the social aspects, nor for the game itself, but for the joy of walking on grass and looking at the nature around them.

Although woodies do like power, and miss it terribly when they retire, for example, they abhor injustice and can genuinely try to see other people's point of view. Their protective nature makes them good union leaders or managers, resistance fighters or politicians, even doctors, reporters and lawyers. Their principled, strong-minded, decisive nature makes them ideal for high positions of power, in business or politics, to which they can bring an element of vision and inspiration which could truly change the balance sheet – or the world!

Woodies' Impoverished self can be:

Domineering; dictatorial; hostile; threatening; unscrupulous; ruthless; moody; argumentative; expressionless; suffocating; unyielding; harsh; vengeful; egotistical; tyrannical; severe; mean.

The impoverished woodie can easily become a dictatorial tyrant, wilful, hostile, ruthless and moody. This is the type of personality we'd all hate to have as a boss. A woodie can become expressionless, under which one senses unexpressed aggression – which can be highly intimidating, an aspect of their power when in an impoverished state.

An elderly city businessman I met once fell into this category. He was dictatorial in all the ways mentioned above but what really sticks in my mind is the meanness of his attitude not only towards certain members of his family but towards his daffodils. On his kitchen wall he kept a chart recording the performance of the daffodils in his large garden. Each daffodil bulb was followed each year to make sure it was regenerating at maximum potential – i.e. increasing the number of flowers – and if it wasn't, it was simply replaced no matter how beautiful. Now, that's ruthless!

CHART 13.1 ESSENTIAL OIL GROUPS

These are just some of the essential oils which could be included in the following nine groups.

Extraction Methods: Steam distilled: SD; Other: O

ESSENTIAL OIL	LATIN NAME	CHARACTER	OTHER GROUP	EX-TRACTION

Florals: This section contains the most absolutes – essential oils that cannot be extracted by steam distillation.

Boronia	*Boronia megastigma*	Floral		O
Cananga	*Cananga odorata*	Floral		SD
Carnation	*Dianthus caryophyllus*	Floral		O
Cassie	*Acacia farnesiana*	Floral		O
Chamomile German	*Matricaria recutica*	Floral	Herbie	SD

Chamomile Roman	*Anthemis nobilis*	Floral	Herbie	SD
Champaca	*Michelia champaca*	Floral		O
Genet	*Spartium junceum*	Floral		O
Helichrysum (Immortelle/				
Italian everlasting)	*Helichrysum angusti folium*	Floral		SD
Hyacinth	*Hyacinthus orientalis*	Floral		O
Jasmine	*Jasminum officinale*	Floral		O
Lavender	*Lavandula angustifolia*	Floral	Herbie	SD
Lemon Blossom	*Citrus limonum*	Floral		SD
Linden Blossom	*Tilia vulgaris*	Floral		O
Marigold	*Calendula officinalis*	Floral		O
Melilotus	*Melilotus officinalis*	Floral		O
Mimosa	*Acacia dealbata*	Floral		O
Narcissus	*Narcissus poeticus*	Floral		O
Neroli	*Citrus aurantium*	Floral		SD
Ormenis Flower	*Ormenis multicaulis*	Floral	Herbie	SD
Osmanthus	*Osmanthus fragrans*	Floral		O
Rose Maroc	*Rosa centifolia*	Floral		O
Rose Otto	*Rosa damascena*	Floral		SD
Tagetes	*Tagetes minuta*	Floral		SD
Tuberose	*Polianthes tuberosa*	Floral		O
Ylang Ylang	*Cananga odorata*	Floral		SD

Fruities:
Fruities: Although some of the following are not generally thought of as 'fruits', they are included here because they are in fact extracted from the fruit.

Bergamot	*Citrus bergamia*	Fruitie		O
Cardamon	*Elettaria cardamomum*	Fruitie	Spicie	SD
Clove	*Eugenia caryophyllata*	Fruitie	Spicie	SD
Cubeb	*Piper cubeba*	Fruitie	Spicie	SD
Grapefruit	*Citrus paradisi*	Fruitie		O
Hops	*Humulus lupulus*	Fruitie	Herbie/Floral	SD
Juniper	*Juniperus communis*	Fruitie	Woodie	SD
Lemon	*Citrus limonum*	Fruitie		O
Lime	*Citrus aurantifolia*	Fruitie		O

				Cubeba
Litsea Cubeba				
(May Chang)	*Litsea cubeba*	Fruitie		SD
Mandarin	*Citrus reticulata*	Fruitie		O
Orange	*Citrus sinensis*	Fruitie		O
Pepper, Black	*Piper nigrum*	Fruitie	Spicie	SD
Pimento Berry	*Pimenta dioica*	Fruitie	Spicie	SD
Schinus Molle	*Schinus molle*	Fruitie		SD
Tangerine	*Citrus nobilis*	Fruitie		O
Tonka Bean	*Dipteryx odorata*	Fruitie	Seedie	O
Vanilla	*Vanilla planifolia*	Fruitie		O

Herbies: The majority of herbie essential oils are distilled from the flowering tops or whole plant and are categorized accordingly.

Basil	*Ocimum basilicum*	Herbie	Leafie	SD
Calamint	*Calamintha officinalis*	Herbie	Leafie	SD
Chamomile German	*Matricaria recutica*	Herbie	Floral	SD
Chamomile Roman	*Anthemis nobilis*	Herbie	Floral	SD
Clary Sage	*Salvia sclarea*	Herbie	Floral	SD
Geranium	*Pelargonium graveolens*	Herbie	Leafie	SD
Hyssop	*Hyssopus officinalis*	Herbie	Leafie	SD
Lavender	*Lavandula angustifolia*	Herbie	Floral	SD
Lovage, Leaf	*Levisticum officinale*	Herbie	Leafie	SD
Marjoram	*Origanum marjorana*	Herbie	Leafie	SD
Melissa	*Melissa officinalis*	Herbie	Leafie	SD
Oregano	*Origanum vulgare*	Herbie	Leafie	SD
Ormenis Flower				
(Chamomile Maroc)	*Ormenis multicaulis*	Herbie	Floral	SD
Peppermint	*Mentha piperita*	Herbie	Leafie	SD
Rosemary	*Rosmarinus officinalis*	Herbie	Leafie	SD
Sage	*Salvia officinalis*	Herbie	Leafie	SD
Spearmint	*Mentha spicata*	Herbie	Leafie	SD
Thyme Lemon	*Thymus citriodorus*	Herbie	Leafie	SD
Thyme Linalol	*Thymus vulgaris chem. linalol*	Herbie	Leafie	SD
Thyme Red	*Thymus vulgaris*	Herbie	Leafie	SD
Yarrow	*Achillea millefolium*	Herbie	Floral	SD

Leafies: The extraction of leafies sometimes includes the twigs and stems.

Bay	*Laurus nobilis*	Leafie		SD
Birch, White	*Betula alba*	Leafie	Woodie	SD
Buchu	*Agothosma betulina*	Leafie		SD
Cajeput	*Melaleuca cajeputi*	Leafie	Woodie	SD
Cinnamon	*Cinnamomum zeylanicum*	Leafie	Spicie	SD
Cistus (Rock Rose)	*Cistus ladaniferus*	Leafie		SD
Cypress	*Cupressus sempervirens*	Leafie	Woodie	SD
Eucalyptus	*Eucalyptus globulus*	Leafie	Woodie	SD
Eucalyptus Lemon	*Eucalyptus citriodora*	Leafie	Woodie	SD
Eucalyptus Piperita	*Eucalyptus dives/ piperita*	Leafie	Woodie	SD
Eucalyptus Radiata	*Eucalyptus radiata*	Leafie	Woodie	SD
Fir	*Abies alba*	Leafie	Woodie	SD
Myrtle	*Myrtus communis*	Leafie		SD
Niaouli	*Melaleuca viridiflora*	Leafie	Woodie	SD
Patchouli	*Pogostemon cablin*	Leafie		SD
Petitgrain	*Citrus aurantium*	Leafie	Woodie	SD
Ravensara	*Ravensara aromatica*	Leafie	Woodie	SD
Spruce (Black)	*Picea mariana*	Leafie	Woodie	SD
Spruce (White)	*Picea glauca*	Leafie	Woodie	SD
Tea Tree	*Melaleuca alternifolia*	Leafie	Woodie	SD
Violet Leaf	*Viola odorata*	Leafie		O

Resinies:

Benzoin	*Styrax benzoin*	Resinie	SD
Borneol	*Dryobalanops aromatica*	Resinie	SD
Canadian Balsam	*Abies balsamea*	Resinie	SD
Copaiba Balsam	*Copaifera officinalis*	Resinie	SD
Elemi	*Carnarium luzonicum*	Resinie	SD
Frankincense	*Boswellia carteri*	Resinie	SD
Galbanham	*Ferula galbaniflua*	Resinie	SD
Myrrh	*Commiphora myrrha*	Resinie	SD

Opopanax	*Commiphora erythraea*	Resinie		SD
Peru Balsam	*Myroxylon balsamum*	Resinie		SD
Styrax Levant	*Liquidambar orientalis*	Resinie		SD
Tolu Balsam	*Myroxylon balsamum*	Resinie		SD

Rooties:

Angelica	*Angelica archangelica*	Rootie		SD
Galangal	*Alpinia officinarum*	Rootie		SD
Ginger	*Zingiber officinale*	Rootie		SD
Orris	*Iris pallida*	Rootie		SD
Snakeroot	*Asarum canadense*	Rootie		SD
Spikenard	*Nardostachys jatamansi*	Rootie		SD
Turmeric	*Curcuma longa*	Rootie		SD
Valerian	*Valeriana officinalis*	Rootie		SD
Vetiver	*Vetiveria zizanoides*	Rootie		SD

Seedies:

Ambrette Seed	*Hibiscus abelmoschus*	Seedie		SD
Angelica Seed	*Angelica archangelica*	Seedie		SD
Anise (Star)	*Illicium verum*	Seedie	Spicie	SD
Aniseed	*Pimpinella anisum*	Seedie	Spicie	SD
Caraway	*Carum carvi*	Seedie	Spicie	SD
Carrot Seed	*Daucus carota*	Seedie		SD
Coriander	*Coriandrum sativum*	Seedie	Spicie	SD
Cumin	*Cuminum cyminum*	Seedie	Spicie	SD
Dill	*Anethum graveolens*	Seedie		SD
Fennel (Sweet)	*Foeniculum vulgare*	Seedie		SD
Nutmeg	*Myristica fragrans*	Seedie	Spicie	SD
Parsley Seed	*Petroselinum sativum*	Seedie		SD

Spicies: Because the spice oils are mostly taken from seeds and fruits these oils are also categorized under those groups.

Anise (Star)	*Illicium verum*	Spicie	Seedie	SD
Aniseed	*Pimpinella anisum*	Spicie	Seedie	SD

Black Pepper	*Piper nigrum*	Spicie	Fruitie	SD
Caraway	*Carum carvi*	Spicie	Seedie	SD
Cardamon	*Elettaria cardamomum*	Spicie	Fruitie	SD
Cinnamon	*Cinnamomum zeylanicum*	Spicie	Leafie	SD
Clove	*Eugenia aromatica*	Spicie	Fruitie	SD
Coriander	*Coriandrum sativum*	Spicie	Seedie	SD
Cubeb	*Piper cubeba*	Spicie	Fruitie	SD
Cumin	*Cuminum cyminum*	Spicie	Seedie	SD
Galangal	*Alpinia officinarum*	Spicie	Rootie	SD
Ginger	*Zingiber officinale*	Spicie	Rootie	SD
Mace	*Myristica fragrans*	Spicie	Fruitie	SD
Nutmeg	*Myristica fragrans*	Spicie	Seedie	SD
Pimento Berry	*Pimenta dioica*	Spicie	Fruitie	SD

Woodies:

Amyris	*Amyris balsamifera*	Woodie		SD
Cabreuva	*Myrocarpus fastigiatus*	Woodie		SD
Cade	*Juniperus oxycedrus*	Woodie		SD
Camphor White	*Cinnamomum camphora*	Woodie		SD
Cascarilla Bark	*Croton eluteria*	Woodie		SD
Cedarwood	*Cedrus atlantica*	Woodie		SD
Cedarwood	*Juniperus virginiana*	Woodie		SD
Guaiacwood	*Bulnesia sarmienti*	Woodie		SD
Linaloe	*Bursera glabrifolia*	Woodie		SD
Pine	*Pinus sylvestris*	Woodie	Leafie	SD
Rosewood	*Aniba rosaeodora*	Woodie		SD
Sandalwood	*Santalum album*	Woodie		SD
Spruce (Black)	*Picea mariana*	Woodie	Leafie	SD
Spruce (White)	*Picea glauca*	Woodie	Leafie	SD

Chapter Fourteen

INDIVIDUAL PERSONALITY TYPES

IN THIS CHAPTER WE SHALL BE LOOKING AT THE INDIVIDUAL personalities of essential oils, that is to say, the human characteristics that each oil displays. People who use oils invariably begin to talk about them as if they were people. Someone might talk about *needing* geranium, as one might need a dear friend or partner, to offer comfort and solace after a hard day in the concrete jungle. Or another person might talk about frankincense as a source of spiritual upliftment – as if they gave the same kind of stimulation and peace as a discussion with a spiritual mentor. Aromatherapists and general users alike seem to come to the same conclusions about oils, the most common generalizations being that lavender is like the mother, mandarin is 'the child within', cypress is strength, while ylang ylang is the gentle seductress.

Associations such as these have grown and expanded in my mind over the years so that I now have a rather complex image of the personalities of each essential oil, and I've come to know which particular oils could be best suited to each particular person at any given time. Experience has taught me that a certain psyche-matching takes place – the personalities of particular oils match particular personality-types of people. Look at it another way – certain essential oils do *not* match certain people. There doesn't seem to be an affinity.

Of course it is very difficult to explain why such a harmony or disharmony should happen. It is simply one of those things which therapists experience on a daily basis. But it is not a haphazard phenomenon because a certain pattern emerges. Certain *types* of people have a certain relationship with particular oils, either for good or not for good – which in this case does not mean bad. 'Bad', or 'not good', in this context simply means that they do not induce the required beneficial effect as quickly as one might expect . . . and certainly as one might expect with the essential oils which *are* in harmony with the particular person.

I have included in this introduction oils which are readily available and/or are required study for those undergoing aromatherapy training. The full spectrum of potential extends much further, not only because many essential oils have not been included here, but because each essential oil has chemotypes. What this means is that slight variations on each oil arise because of the different growing conditions. For example, the lavender that is grown in the valleys is not the same, chemically or in terms of personality, as the lavender that is grown high in the mountains. Although the plants may *look* much the same, and are of the same botanical species, the components within them are determined to a degree by the growing conditions, including the type of soil, the other species of plants which are growing nearby, the amount of sun they receive, or rainfall and so on. All these factors contribute to the making of different chemotypes which, in professional aromatherapy, are taken into consideration when treating patients.

Just as a human has a personality and sub-personalities so do essential oils in the form of chemotypes. Therefore, when we view the spectrum, we have in essential oils a system that can incorporate personality, sub-personality and multi-personality, and with all the possible combinations of blends can cover all 17,953 states of the human emotional condition noted in Webster's dictionary.

CHOOSING YOUR PERSONALITY TYPE

When looking through the individual personality profiles bear in mind that very few people are 'classic' types. We may have a 'predominant' personality and many other personalities as well. So, for example, if you read Jasmine and find yourself saying, 'Yes, that sounds like me but there are some aspects of this character that don't fit', don't worry because you would not expect them all to match exactly – very few people have all the personality traits outlined under any particular essential oil. No two human beings are the same; we are composites of characters here described.

As you read through the personalities you may recognize people you know or see portions of a particular person's character or personality. We are multi-faceted beings and the reason essential oils have such potential is that we can dip into different personalities and create, mix or formulate an individual blend which includes and reflects the many facets of each individual person.

We all use essential oils each day – perfumes, toiletries, foods and drinks – and we're not about to give up these pleasures because the essential oil contained in our favourite soft drink, for example, doesn't happen to fit our own personality type. There are many ways to use essential oils, and by Aroma-Genera or individual essential oil personality choice, we simply have another dimension to enjoy. With the personality profiles, you may find that there are oils you hadn't really thought of before as having an affinity with you, and now you may be encouraged to use that oil for the first time.

Think of essential oils as drops of positivity, whose purpose is to bring us into harmony with the whole. They are more than fabulous fragrances. They bring well-being, both in terms of physical and emotional health. Use them with positive thought because all life is vibration and thought is vibration too. Essential oils are *positive additions* to life. They can help us move beyond the limitations imposed by circumstance and ego, and make connection with the greater whole, the spiritual dimension, our universal self.

AN INTRODUCTION TO ESSENTIAL OILS AND ABSOLUTES AND THEIR HUMAN PERSONALITIES

Although the personalities here outlined are extensions of the larger Aroma-Genera groups of florals, fruities, herbies, leafies, and so on, either section can be read and practised as a system in its own right. The essential oils chosen in this and the previous section can be used in all the usual ways.

BASIL
HERBIE
Ocimum basilicum

CHARACTER
Uplifting, Awakening, Clarifying, Stimulating

USE TO COUNTERACT THESE NEGATIVE ATTRIBUTES
Indecision, Mental fatigue, Mental exhaustion, Negativity, Lack of Direction, Fear, Burn-out, Confusion, Intellectual fatigue, Apathy, Bitterness, Resentment, Addiction, Conflict, Fear of intimacy, Shame, Doubts, Melancholy, Sadness

USE FOR THESE POSITIVE ATTRIBUTES
Positivity, Purposefulness, Concentration, Assertiveness, Decisiveness, Straightforwardness, Trust, Integrity, Enthusiasm, Clarity, Cheerfulness, Strength

BASIL PERSONALITY PROFILE

Basil personalities are often the entrepreneurs of the world and, male or female, are able to see what others may not even know exists. For them, opportunities abound. Ambition, flair, drive and enterprise get them where they want to be and, unless someone bars their way unjustly, they will get there without harming others, and by being honest. Basils have a wisdom far beyond their years plus a fair amount of luck – often missing ruin by the skin of their teeth, as a brilliant flash

of inspiration gets them out of difficult situations. It sometimes seems as if Basils have spiritual intervention in times of
crisis – an advantage not a lot of us have.

The Basil personality can be very direct and blunt, particularly if you don't always get their point. They may seem
patronizing but they mean no harm and may even feel they're
doing you a favour by being blunt. Power holds a great attraction for these personalities and they often become the bosses
in commercial organizations, although they can also be found
in jobs that involve aspects of law or espionage. They're often
the genies of life – the eccentric artists, the mad poets, the
sacrificed writers – and perhaps it is their deep wisdom that
allows them to glance into unknown realms. Basils will not
criticize or think badly of any action, believing that everything
has its place, and there is a reason for everything. Perhaps this
explains their basic optimism. Basils could be called the pro-
tectors of ideas, imagination and free will.

The sordid or seamier side of life often holds a fascination
for Basils, and they could be found indulging in pursuits which
the less adventurous would shudder at. It is by walking the
fence between what is expected and what is not that gets them
into trouble. If they lean too far, they can fall in it – even
though their intelligence tells them not to. It is not unusual for
Basils to go on to disaster, mental confusion and madness.

The Basil personality enjoys academic pursuits far more
than sporting ones, but although philosophy books may be on
the bedside table, so too will be those discussing Tantra, the
ancient Indian cult of ecstasy. Basils believe in the communication between mind, body and spirit and this will extend to
their lovemaking. To them, sex is synonymous with spirituality, while marriage is more of a mental commitment – which
they'll take very seriously. Generally, Basils are charming and
sexy lovers of life, full of *bonhomie*, despite their calm, sometimes sullen exterior.

Basils are drawn by the mysterious and can be very
spiritual, and this interest can take many forms. For example,
they may join a sect – possibly rising to become leader; or
become very involved with a world religion; they may search
through meditation; or explore other, much darker, sides.

Basils are certainly fascinated with the paranormal and will apply cool logic to all that is found, describing it with flair and imagination. This fascination can lead to a lifelong exploration of things unknown and can occasionally get them into some very hot water. Basils will also experiment with hallucinogenic mind-altering drugs as they search for the surreal, and spiritual communication.

The eccentric aunt, the intellectual, those who go crazy with passion – all could be Basil personalities, who will fight for the right to be who they are, but are wise enough to let go if they cannot win the battle. The Basil doesn't care because, if need be, there are far more interesting things to pursue.

Norma Gilbert, MIFA, Reg., MIRCST, MBSR, aromatherapist, cranial sacral therapist and tutor:

'Strong, powerful, discerning and cerebral, like a monarch basil requires to be treated with dignity and respect and in return will be most trustworthy. Warming and balmy in small quantities, it can bring about a sense of true balance and strength.'

BERGAMOT
FRUITIE
Citrus bergamia

CHARACTER
Joyous, Refreshing, Uplifting, Encouraging

USE TO COUNTERACT THESE NEGATIVE ATTRIBUTES
Depression, Anxiety, Helplessness, Apathy, Bitterness, Burn-out, Despondency, Emptiness, Exhaustion, Grief, Hopelessness, Sadness, Loneliness, Stress, Tension, Emotional imbalances

USE FOR THESE POSITIVE ATTRIBUTES
Concentration, Confidence, Balance, Strength, Joy, Motivation, Good cheer, Harmony, Completeness

BERGAMOT PERSONALITY PROFILE

The Bergamot personality is young, fresh, caring and considerate – everything a granny would expect from the younger generation. Being around Bergamot can be as joyful an experience as walking through a field of the sunflowers that inspired Van Gogh. Although Bergamot types are not necessarily young in years they will always be young at heart and have a joyful approach to life. While they acknowledge the bad or negative things in life they don't allow them to overcome all the beauty and happiness that can be found. Indeed, they view good and positive things as all-embracing.

This personality is caring, considerate and full of energy. They're often found in the caring professions or in any job that requires large amounts of energy, skill and enthusiasm. Being very positive, confident and outgoing, Bergamots are never afraid to put themselves in line for the best position. They often drift towards the media, in which they enjoy being upfront – maybe as a presenter or spokesperson, a role in which they can display a charismatic personality – a feature too of their personal life. The Bergamot personality is also very good with children as their energy level is very compatible, and they understand the thrill of new adventure. Fun, for a Bergamot, might be climbing up Mount Everest or rowing down white water in a canoe.

However, this is the outward personality. Inwardly, Bergamots may suffer depression and, just as many other personality types can, they can easily plummet quite quickly into the depths of despair when things get too much, even for them to bear. But Bergamot never really allows anyone to really see just how down they can get, or how sad they're feeling – it just isn't in their nature to do so. Because of this, people are inclined to think they haven't a care in the world. Nobody may suspect that behind the mask, a Bergamot may be inwardly crying with emotional pain. Only the empathy exhibited towards others who are feeling distressed may give them away.

This might be said of a Bergamot: 'You wouldn't think he (or she) would be able to understand how I feel. He is always so cheerful, but he understood, and I felt I could tell him everything. I always feel so much better after I have seen him.' Of course this person may be feeling better but poor old Bergamot would have shouldered the distress and, unless they're really on top of things at the time, it could compound the low feelings they already have.

Another phrase that is applied to someone with Bergamot in their personality profile is 'they'll be all right, they're tough, they can handle it and never let anything get them down'. If only people knew! Bergamot can certainly get down, but whenever you meet this personality it will be a tonic, and you'll feel all the better for it.

Vivienne Lunny, MD, MBBS, MDMA, MIFA Reg., MISPA, RQA, aromatherapist and tutor:

'Bergamot comes into the room smiling, bright, happy and in balance, at ease with the world and is discriminating, loves nature, is tactful, practical, highly imaginative, caring and productive. Bergamot can see both sides of any issue which enables him/her to rebalance feelings and emotions.'

BLACK PEPPER
FRUITIE/SPICIE
Piper nigrum

CHARACTER
Security, Comforting, Directional, Endurance

USE TO COUNTERACT THESE NEGATIVE ATTRIBUTES
Emotional blockages, Compulsions, Confusion, Disorientation, Fatigue, Begrudging, Indecision, Irrationality, Anger, Frustration, Emotional coldness, Apathy, Mental exhaustion

USE FOR THESE POSITIVE ATTRIBUTES
Comfort, Stamina, Endurance, Motivation, Changeability

BLACK PEPPER PERSONALITY PROFILE

Black Pepper is the older, sterner personality among the essential oils but having said that, it can also be the livelier, older type of personality. Black Pepper people often seem old for their age, whether they're the baby who seems to be thirty or the twelve-year-old who acts as if he were forty-two. This type of person will reprimand you for not having behaved correctly at a social gathering – particularly if you are a carefree Melissa type. Indeed, Black Peppers can be very upright and extremely self-righteous (providing it suits them) and, if allowed to be, dictatorial. On the other hand, they can be charming, trustworthy, kind and very loyal if they wish, and if they like you.

As parents, their children may not understand Black Pepper until they themselves are middle-aged, and although often stern and forbidding to their children, they can instil a sense of security, which can be comforting in that the children know exactly what to expect. Once understood, Black Pepper is very predictable.

In the workplace and at home Black Pepper can be very stimulating, encouraging everyone to succeed, and tend to take on responsibility for everyone in their family circle. However, these are more likely to be the financial responsibilities rather than the emotional ones, provided that their advice is being taken. If a male Black Pepper has a son, he'll have to compete with the son, and will have to be lord and master. If female, Black Pepper will be of the 'she who must be obeyed' type. They'll bale their family out of trouble not so much for their family's sake, but for their own reputation, and will have no qualms about cutting a son or daughter out of a will and leaving them penniless.

Black Pepper can be very flirtatious and may boast about their sexual conquests, but this is more to convince themselves that they can be passionate. In truth, they may have an inability to let themselves be free enough to release passion. Although Black Pepper is a hot, warming essential oil, the person personality Black Pepper is not warming in love. If they ever recognize true love it's likely to be discarded for a better social match. Black Pepper goes through life having a multitude of lovers, trying to find, once again, the true love they let go – but they'll never admit it of course.

This type will tolerate anyone for the sake of appearances or if they think the other person might be useful to them in some way – until they get out of earshot, but Black Peppers make loyal friends. They're unashamed show-offs and have to be better than anyone else at everything (even if they're not), and they love to show off their knowledge – whether or not it's got something to do with their chosen career, or hobby. They're not unknown to adopt a 'holier than thou' attitude. Where Black Peppers are welcome is when they help with financial problems, give advice on stocks and shares, or tax returns, procedures in law and so on. They'll know how to get the most out of the welfare state and how, in monetary terms, to exploit the system to their advantage.

Black Peppers can sometimes be exasperating in their lack of empathy towards other people, and their complete lack of lateral thinking. They will lament the number of homeless, for example, but wonder 'why do people put themselves in that situation?' Black Peppers will ignore the plight of the majority of the world, as they're only interested in themselves and their families. Yet they often have charismatic power that tricks people into thinking they are leaders of men – which they definitely are not, but frequently arrange to be! They just don't have the compassion or understanding needed and will become the dictators, if allowed. Also, having a fiery temperament, Black Peppers can often blow their tops with indignation and frustration, usually over the stupidity of others.

Black Peppers are found in all walks of life, to a degree, but prefer jobs that give power and money – which they love, or which involves linear thinking – a career in which they do not have to use their imagination or creativity too much. Black Peppers would excel at being lawyers, judges, solicitors, bankers, accountants, financial advisers, or at a life in the military services – army rather than navy or air force, prison services, traffic wardens and traffic police. They are often found in unsuitable jobs and will never be happy unless they are in charge. The family will take the brunt of Black Pepper's frustration and anger as they take it all out on the family when they get home. Negative Black Peppers will blame everyone else for their emotional state and can be irritable, cold, stunted emotionally, and very emotionally violent. Luckily, it is very rare to find a completely negative Black Pepper personality.

One such character was a retired insurance underwriter from Lloyd's of London, who'd made a packet from being in the know and being with the right syndicate. From an extremely modest background, he changed his accent, conveniently forgot his roots, fought and rose to become a most respected member of the community. When it became apparent that his wife no longer fitted the picture, he embarked on a series of affairs, to show off to his friends and colleagues that he was a hit with the ladies, while dragging out his divorce for seven years while he hid his assets so his wife would get the bare minimum. His son, who had been treated as a rival since birth, was dumped with the mother, while the flattering daughter was given all the attention – and money! But, to save family face, when the unloved son went wild, the cold Black Pepper father picked up the bill. All his children wanted was for him to say 'I love you', but for Black Peppers, even when they feel love, these are the hardest words to say.

CARDAMON
FRUITIE/SPICIE
Elettaria cardamomum

CHARACTER
Clarifying, Stimulating, Encouraging, Enthusiastic

USE TO COUNTERACT THESE NEGATIVE ATTRIBUTES
Mental stress, Apathy, Confusion, Inflexibility, Judgemental, Intolerance, Unreasonableness, Burn-out, Suspicion, Sluggishness, Self-pity, Bewilderment, Rigidity

USE FOR THESE POSITIVE ATTRIBUTES
Clarity, Concentration, Direction, Motivation, Straightforwardness, Enthusiasm, Confidence, Courage, Fortitude, Purpose

CARDAMON PERSONALITY PROFILE

Cardamon is a strong, forthright personality, full of fortitude, stimulating and straightforward. You know exactly where you are with them – what you see is what you get! There are no hidden motives to their actions and they're direct and encouraging. This personality type gets motivated by good ideas and instils inspiration in others. Their being so enthusiastic could tend to get wearying if Cardamon wasn't also very balancing and able to harmonize everything. This is really their strength – no matter what happens to them, how fraught people may get when they're pushed by Cardamon, in the end harmony will reign. This characteristic of the Cardamon personality makes them very good leaders. They will push and push but in the end others will appreciate the sense of it all. Also, Cardamons believe in fairness and justice, and that too always comes through.

Cardamon

Cardamons wear an air of detachment much of the time, as if nothing really worries them, but when they get steamed up they go for the jugular! You don't mess with a Cardamon! If you happen to be confused and in a bad situation, Cardamon will come to the rescue, but not on a white charger and bearing gifts. They are much too frugal for that. It couldn't be said that they're mean but they won't squander their hard-earned cash on anyone but themselves. If you go out for dinner together don't expect them to pick up the bill. If you don't offer to pay yourself they'll split the bill straight down the middle and if there's one penny left over, they'll suggest you toss for it. Being so financially careful has its advantages – for one thing, Cardamon never gets into any dodgy deals. And Cardamon does like to have a few pennies tucked away for impulse buys.

The Cardamon personality loves flattery, but they rarely get it, so when a floral comes along full of sweet words, Cardamon will fall for it all. They can be a passionate personality, which may come as a surprise, and they love romance. Indeed, they'll dream up all kinds of crazy, exciting things to do, which can seem quite out of character. Who would have thought such a heart beats in them?

Female Cardamons are perfectly comfortable with their masculine side, which makes them very interesting to men, who feel that women don't usually understand them. No Cardamon is dull and all lead interesting lives, making everything seem like an adventure. They will respect the wishes of other people, especially in a love relationship but, as parents, they can be very strict and expect their children to embrace their high morals. Partners are expected to be individuals, and are respected for it, but this isn't always the case with children – who Cardamons expect to be carbon copies of themselves, and enthusiastic and motivated about their schoolwork to boot. They have great difficulty understanding a teenager's need to slump on the sofa listening to loud music.

When a Cardamon gets negative it can be quite alarming. Mostly, they suffer mental stress which can make them apathetic, inflexible, judgemental or self-pitying. They become suspicious of everyone who tries to help and can become rigid in their outlook and bewildered when anyone with enough courage points it out to them. If the negativity is allowed to carry on for too long, Cardamons can completely lose interest in life, becoming losers, their sense of fair play and good judgement gone for ever.

However, a positive Cardamon is good in leadership roles, provided that they learn to delegate, and they make excellent teachers. They aren't overly creative but they have the stamina to carry ideas forward which, in the end, can make them achieve more than a more creative personality.

CARNATION
FLORAL
Dianthus caryophyllus

CHARACTER
Secretiveness, Stillness, Originality, Liberating

USE TO COUNTERACT THESE NEGATIVE ATTRIBUTES
Disregard, Neglect, Detachment, Cynicism, Disorientation, Doubt, Mental loneliness, Aloneness, Emotional domination, Emotional solitude, Neglect, Self-criticism

USE FOR THESE POSITIVE ATTRIBUTES
Self-worth, Communication, Radiating, Creativity, Independence, Tenderness, Nurturing, Encompassing, Cushioning, Openness, Releasing

CARNATION PERSONALITY PROFILE

The Carnation personality will fill your days with love and promise you the earth – and really mean it! Bright ideas and a powerful imagination fill the head of the Carnation personality, who will always have pictures of flowers, trees or angels in heaven around. They also love all the sensuous things of life such as perfume, silks, expensive gourmet snacks. Being the ultimate floral, if they wished, Carnations could become the classic temptress or Don Juan, but that role is not for them. If the Carnation is female, men will want to take care of her, and if the Carnation is male, women will want to mother him. Everyone can sense Carnation's child-like innocence and trust in people.

Carnations tend to be very gentle people who sometimes cannot quite get a grasp on life events, tending to dream just a little too much, particularly when things aren't going as well for them as they think they should. One characteristic which can cause sadness and depression is their getting too involved with other people's problems, which they take on board but which brings them down, particularly if they feel unable to help.

There is no way a Carnation would hurt a hair on any person's head, and they can be a great comfort to people suffering loss or hardship. With inner wisdom and knowledge, they may be a devotional kind of person, but there is a warmth to this personality which can invite closeness and is, sometimes, unfortunately misinterpreted as sexual advance or social climbing by other people with a more lowly nature.

History in all its forms holds a fascination for this personality and they're quite likely to search for their family's roots or read history books – more likely being interested in the Renaissance than the Tudor period. Carnations also enjoy art tremendously and although they may not take it up as a profession – because they don't have the confidence to promote their work – they'll paint for pleasure, or take up flower arrangement or interior design, anything in fact in which this natural artistic inclination can be expressed.

Carnations are found in all walks of life but they tend to drift towards those jobs which do not push them into the spotlight. Any job that hides them behind a desk to which the public come is ideal, such as working in an employment agency, or in a bank; anything that brings them into contact with the public but not in an extroverted way. Carnations tend to be delicate in stature, movements and mannerisms and their discipline and grace would make them good classical dancers.

Although Carnations don't seem to have much luck themselves, they never win lotteries for example, they do seem to have a magical effect on those around them. If you go to a casino, take a Carnation with you and have them stand next to you at the roulette wheel – luck might just then come your way!

Monogamy is the only kind of relationship Carnations want and understand. Infidelity would never even cross their minds. To them, a perfect, faithful marriage is the true joy of life, an essential aspect of being in love. Being monogamous, knowing the partners are for one another only, gives Carnation a special feeling, and repelling advances from outsiders gives Carnations a kick far more exciting than affairs or promiscuity. Carnations need love like a flower needs the sun and, if they don't have it, they'll kid themselves they do, or go looking for a partner. Carnations cannot go through life alone, and if one lover leaves, you can be sure there will be another coming around the corner fairly soon. Without love the Carnation is very down and depressed.

One of the most noticeable traits of Carnations is that they cannot communicate their own sorrows and despairs, which they often have. It seems as if they are always there for everyone else but that nobody is there for them. This is particularly tragic because Carnations find it difficult, at times, to love themselves. The delicate temperament of Carnation leaves them vulnerable to spiteful words and actions and they can bruise very easily and become extremely hurt and sad. As parents, Carnations are very soft and gentle and not very hot on discipline. Consequently, their children take advantage of them and get away with everything.

When they're in a negative frame of mind, Carnations can be self-destructive and depressed, and they cut themselves off from life. They can grieve for years over the death of a parent, for example, or over a love that has been lost. Delicate beings as they are, Carnations can nurse a bruised ego for years, or hide the abused or hurt inner child for a lifetime. It is not unusual, after an episode of being hurt, for a Carnation to go to bed, pull the covers over their head, and stay there for a week, not emerging even to answer the phone.

Carnations give too much of themselves away. They'll burn themselves out worrying about what they should be doing with their lives instead of simply doing what they enjoy. Partly, this is because they lack the courage of their convictions. When they're on form, however, Carnations are full of laughter, love and care. Indeed, the one thing Carnations always have is copious amounts of love to give to all living things.

Susan Worwood, MIFA Reg., aromatherapist and author:

'Carnation is a comforting, yet sensual personality which makes one feel euphoric, as if sitting in a sanctified place with a sense of inner calm, expectant of the pleasures life has yet to provide.'

CEDARWOOD
WOODIE
Cedrus atlantica

CHARACTER
Grounding, Strengthening, Dignified, Powerful

USE TO COUNTERACT THESE NEGATIVE ATTRIBUTES
Scattered thoughts, Thoughtlessness, Fixation on past, Anxiety, Obsessions, Mental strain, Irrationality, Emotional sensitivity, Touchiness, Gloomy thoughts, Worry, Fear, Too analytical, Paranoia, Selfishness

USE FOR THESE POSITIVE ATTRIBUTES
Focus, Concentration, Strength, Confidence, Balance, Stability, Comfort, Persistence, Fortitude, Nobility of spirit

CEDARWOOD PERSONALITY PROFILE

The majestic stature of the Cedarwood personality is easy to spot – they seem to glide through life as if they had a royal charter! They may appear haughty and just too grand to be approached about anything mundane, but this would be entirely wrong. Cedarwoods are towers of strength in almost all situations, seemingly in total harmony with the forces of nature, having an ancient air about them, as if they are the repositories of all the world's history. This isn't necessarily the case, even if they make you feel it is. Cedarwoods instil confidence and security in people less able to cope with life's stresses and strains, and can be a great comfort in times of trouble. This ability puts them in the role of family adviser – the person you phone to ask how to deal with your tax return, or ask how you should approach a financial dispute. You wouldn't ask them to advise you on your choice of friends, or new outfit (or how to get something you don't really deserve) – for that, you'd turn to a Bergamot personality. Cedarwoods appear to be knowledgeable on almost everything and will become hurt if a member of the family turns elsewhere for advice. This rarely happens . . . you wouldn't dare!

However, Cedarwoods are not infallible and are, indeed, frequently wrong because they can be quite dogmatic in their views. The older ones are the worst because they may not even be aware that the world has changed over the last fifty years. If you have this personality for a father or grandfather it can be quite difficult, especially if he holds the family to emotional and financial ransom. This personality excels in the scholarly professions, such as teaching, librarianship, antiques, architecture and history. They're also inclined towards the sciences and conventional religion although they often have a curiosity about the paranormal too – from a purely scientific point of view, of course!

Unless the Cedarwood is partnered to a balancing type such as a Fruitie, they will dictate the complete running of the household, and all who are in it. Children may not see the loving side of this personality (and may even believe them to be incapable of love), but if trouble strikes, the world had better watch out as Cedarwoods will defend their brood to the last. Although Cedarwood is essentially a masculine personality, it's often found in women.

Cedarwoods can become extremely obsessive. They must always have their right seat in their place of worship and their favourite chair at home – and woe betide the visitor who inadvertently sits in the wrong place, who will suffer scowls. Cedarwoods always fold their newspapers in the same way and like the cupboards to be organized in a certain fashion. Although their mannerisms lead you to think they would only be at home in a palace, this isn't so, they're perfectly content in the humblest of places – even though these characters believe themselves to be truly magnificent.

Cedarwoods of either sex often become confirmed bachelors. It's not that they can't love deeply and affectionately, but it just seems like so much bother! This isn't a passionate personality – not about sex anyway. Excitement is reserved for projects, particularly if archaeologists or historians, and Cedarwoods may sacrifice their lives to trying to find the Holy Grail or uncover a particular document, but would never sacrifice themselves to love or abandon themselves to a carefree life.

When negative, Cedarwoods can be hell on earth – demanding, arrogant, selfish, overly controlling and paranoid. They'll turn every little upset into an international plot against them and may retire to bed with a psychosomatic illness – terminal of course – refusing help from doctors and medicines, and any attempt to make them comfortable, and then say that nobody cares. Subconsciously they seek out partners who are very long suffering, but loyal.

When they're positive, however, the Cedarwood personality is kind, dignified and very understanding. They can make things seem very precious, even sacred, as they willingly impart their knowledge, often appearing honoured to be asked to do so.

CHAMOMILE GERMAN
HERBIE/FLORAL
Matricaria recutita

CHARACTER
Strong, Peaceful, Healing, Cooling

USE TO COUNTERACT THESE NEGATIVE ATTRIBUTES
Nervousness, Frayed nerves, Anger, Frustration, Emotional dramas, Emotional tension, Irritability, Temper, Tenseness, Over-sensitive, Moodiness, Stormy, Bitterness, Resentment, Indifference, Deep emotional baggage

USE FOR THESE POSITIVE ATTRIBUTES
Communicative, Relaxed, Understanding, Organized, Soothing, Empathy, Patience, Calm

CHAMOMILE GERMAN PERSONALITY PROFILE

This deep blue Chamomile is a bountiful type of person, very deep and emotionally strong. They're experts at all activities that require sacrifice and determination. Blues are the father that tucks you in at night, the teacher who helped you with a difficult project, telling you not to worry, and the police officer who helped you home when you were in distress – the type of person you remember as being kind and caring even though you were a stranger to them.

Chamomile Germans have emotional depth and the ability to draw out the best in other people, but seem to keep their own feelings to themselves, preferring to use metaphor to disguise how they feel. The Chamomile German type is liable to be very down-to-earth, quite up-front, and always appears to be solid in thought – not at all frivolous. However, they can dramatize things and are often drawn to jobs which involve a certain amount of drama or communication. They may be involved in religion, and feel they have the calling as a priest, for example, but whatever religion it is they are drawn to they'll strive to have a deep understanding of it. Philosophy, archaeological digs, ancient monuments and architecture may be enjoyed by this personality, who is also fascinated by the lives of ancient people and their rulers.

The blue Chamomiles are well suited to a profession in teaching or anything to do with books – publishing or writing, particularly non-fiction. Being great organizers, they'll organize everything if you let them – including what you have for lunch and who you should invite to your party. If their suggestions aren't taken up, the Blues can get upset, although this doesn't last too long and is soon forgotten. This is a very contented personality, and seems to take everything in its stride.

The negative side of the Chamomile German personality is dark moods and heaviness of heart. In arguments they become irritable as they try to get their point of view across, and confused, tense and easily frustrated, speaking loudly and impatiently – the complete opposite to their normal behaviour. When in negative mode they can get easily upset, which disarms people who are used to seeing Chamomile in charge of everything. Often adopting an air of indifference, it leads to break-ups of relationships because it can be difficult for the partner to understand what sparked off Chamomile's bad mood. But this type often lives in the past and some subconscious cue could have reminded them of a past mistake or bad experience. Or it could have been a build up of things, an explosion (the Blues need to express themselves, not bury it) which gets aimed at the thing or person nearest to them – usually the family or partner.

Of course a strong relationship will ride out the storm, as most of these episodes are short-lived, but while they last, Chamomiles have everyone running for cover, including the dog. The deep blue Chamomile Germans are good to have around in an emotional storm, or when grieving, as they provide a strong, solid shoulder to cry on if needed.

CHAMOMILE ROMAN
HERBIE/FLORAL
Anthemis nobilis

CHARACTER
Harmonizing, Peaceful, Soothing, Spiritual

USE TO COUNTERACT THESE NEGATIVE ATTRIBUTES
Nervousness, Irritability, Temper, Anger, Depression, Hysteria, Fear, Anxiety, Exhaustion, Worry, Stress, Tension, Grief, Emotional imbalance, Broken heart, Grumpiness, Moroseness, Discontent, Impatience, Short temper, Over-sensitivity, Melancholy, Spiritual disconnection

USE FOR THESE POSITIVE ATTRIBUTES
Stillness, Calm, Softness, Gentleness, Relaxed, Serene, Spiritually aware, Emotionally stable, Inner peace, Understanding, Co-operative

CHAMOMILE ROMAN PERSONALITY PROFILE

Chamomile Roman is like someone who has been blessed with sunshine and joy, a harmonious disposition and emotional life. They are serene and gentle, and can sometimes seem to be in a dreamlike state, as if communicating with unseen angels. Chamomiles often have a strange power over ordinary mortals, on whom they have a calming, almost sedative effect, and people will follow them anywhere, believing implicitly in everything they say.

When a Chamomile Roman commits, they really commit themselves – either to a project or person. Half measures are not for them. They are great company and people will always be eager to visit them, as they are relaxing to be with, and have lots of interests, are entertaining, amusing and charming. In fact they can charm the birds out of the trees . . . and probably understand the birds' conversations as well. Chamomile Romans do not possess an ego as such and can appear overly humble in certain situations, being embarrassed if lavish praise is heaped upon them, although they may be secretly pleased that someone appreciated their work. This is not false modesty, but just a surprise that anyone would consider they had done anything out of the ordinary.

The inner peace that Chamomile Romans appear to have can be misleading because inner conflicts can torment them – mainly on the issue of their living on earth, and not in heaven! They are liable to have changeable moods and emotions, particularly in relationships – and this can cause them (and other people) emotional stress. Chamomile Romans can also become allergic to people – cutting them off, putting notices on the door saying 'keep away', and being generally disagreeable so nobody wants to visit. However, this is necessary to enable them to refresh themselves. They pick up on other people's feelings, pain and distress, and sometimes need time alone to recollect themselves before facing the world again. Romans are not only allergic to people, they can also be allergic to emotional problems or stress – and develop bloating and other intestinal problems, for example. Romans can become very depressed, unable to see anyone's point of view, and get distressed beyond belief if an injustice is done to them.

A negative Chamomile Roman will tend to externalize everything and have what could be called verbal diarrhoea. They will tell you every little detail of their day, how hard done by they were, what their work colleagues did to them, and how unjust everyone and everything has been towards them. No details will be left out and it may go on a bit. This is just a Roman's way of discharging distasteful episodes in the day but it can be annoying to the partner because when Roman has finished talking they're emotionally exhausted and drained, and won't want to hear anything a partner might have to say about their day. Anyhow, they will shortly bloom again and will no longer wish to speak about any of it. In fact, to be asked to repeat the events just makes them throw up their hands in horror because, as far as they're concerned, it's now over and done with. This cathartic experience can leave others annoyed to say the least, and can often lead to misunderstandings.

Chamomile Romans are more feminine than their brothers, the deep blue Chamomile Germans, and some human beings carry the characteristics of both. But above all, Romans are in touch with their spiritual selves. When they're children this can take the form of seeing fairies or imaginary friends, and it can quite easily carry on into adulthood. Chamomile Roman profiles are gentle and delicate with a serenity many would like to achieve, but which hardly any other personalities do – except perhaps Neroli.

Teddy Fearnhamm, IScB France, MRQA, aromatherapist and tutor:

'Chamomile Roman has every quality attributed to caring – it presents a small waterfall of comfort. Think of it: a cascade of Chamomile Roman and you immediately feel loved.'

CINNAMON
LEAFIE/SPICIE
Cinnamomum zeylanicum

CHARACTER
Warming, Secular, Fair-minded

USE TO COUNTERACT THESE NEGATIVE ATTRIBUTES
Instability, Severity, Bleakness, Malice, Spitefulness, Coldness,
Fear, Nervous Exhaustion, Debility, Introversion, Superficiality

USE FOR THESE POSITIVE ATTRIBUTES
Invigorated, Steadfast, Benevolent, Strength, Practicality,
Energized, Realistic, Direct

CINNAMON PERSONALITY PROFILE

Cinnamon is the larger-than-life, affable type of person – practical, intelligent and with a strong personality. They can be very conservative in thought and nature, preferring the comfort of the establishment rather than the risk and discomfort of the unknown. This isn't to say they're unadventurous, far from it, as they do enjoy a bit of excitement now and again – provided that it doesn't interfere with their well-being.

They are usually large, gregarious types – if not in stature, then in largesse. Both males and females can be aggressive rather than assertive but neither have a sexist frame of mind – they believe everyone has an equal part to play, just so long as it doesn't interfere with their own plans. Although they may appear sexist to others, Cinnamons simply do not think in those terms. To them, people are people. If women want to play football, 'good on 'em'.

Cinnamons take their home life very seriously and will defend everyone in it – partner, children, brothers, sisters, parents and grandparents. They don't take kindly to anyone criticizing any member of their family and if the children are harmed, either physically or verbally, Cinnamon will instantly be on the warpath. And, indeed, may deal with anyone who seriously hurt their loved ones.

Male Cinnamons are often admired by their peers as someone who is in control and has everything running smoothly, even if this isn't always the case. Males are often thought, incorrectly, to be having exciting affairs, especially as Cinnamon never denies it, while the Cinnamon woman may very well be hiding a real secret! This personality is often described as strong, or as an 'all-round chap' (or chapette), and a good companion – if a little vain. Cinnamons enjoy being well-dressed and usually have an expensive car, or at least a respectable one, a nice home and all the material possessions the western world deems necessary for a comfortable life. The home will be full of all manner of electrical gadgetry (even if it's never used), and plenty of gardening equipment that looks good leaning against the garden fence. If something wears out, Cinnamons don't bother mending it, they prefer to go out and buy a new one.

Unlike the sacrificing Juniper who puts everyone else first in the queue, Cinnamons will first and foremost please themselves. They stand up for their rights and want what is their due – and usually get it. The taxman or VAT inspector will be fought with and if the hospital isn't treating grandma right, the nurses, doctors and administrators will certainly get to know about it. Cinnamons expect service and honesty from everyone they deal with, and they never lie or short-change themselves.

Although Cinnamons wouldn't become local vigilantes, they do like law and order, with everything in its place, and no disturbances. They consider themselves fair-minded and despise unlawfulness, lying or cheating. Direct and forceful, Cinnamons can be too opinionated for their own good sometimes, particularly if an ideal is at stake. Although they try to keep it hidden, they have a strong moralistic streak, which often seems out of character for these street-wise people. Illness seemingly does not affect this character, but Cinnamons are sometimes clumsy and can be accident prone.

Athletics or other sporting activities appeal to their competitive nature. If they're allowed to be, the Cinnamon personality can be manipulating and, because they like to be in charge, overly controlling. They don't use cunning in their manipulation of others, being far too open for that, but will use brute strength of character, so people often find it easier just to let them get on with it. It makes life more peaceful. If someone close does argue with Cinnamon, they'll sulk for weeks rather than give in – which is, of course, another way of getting control.

Negative Cinnamons become very superficial, hollow and conceited. They may start to buy the most ostentatious objects and can become unstable – bullying their partner and friends. Infidelity is an easy temptation for them, mentally if not always physically, but they'll blame their partner for it. If they get found out there will be heated arguments and Cinnamon will become very insecure. Verbal aggression is to be expected at this stage, and Cinnamons can slide into mental stagnation, becoming withdrawn and lacking in motivation. Negativity robs them of the incentive to do anything worthwhile, and despondency can set in. With a little encouragement and praise, however, Cinnamon can soon be back in the game.

Because of their need for material wealth, which Cinnamons believe is necessary for their happiness, they often find themselves in jobs which aren't really suitable for their character. They are better off (mentally, if not financially) in jobs such as probation officer, security, social worker and sports teacher. Although not really entrepreneurial, Cinnamons are happy being self-employed in service businesses that are steady and always in demand, such as plumbing, electronics, carpentry, building and decorating. Being very trustworthy, they instil confidence in their customers and do well financially.

As friends and lovers Cinnamons are steady, lively company and everyone always knows exactly where they are with them. In their positive mode, they hold few surprises, are warmhearted and generally good people to know. They're very approachable and will try to help someone out of trouble if they can, even though they won't consider it their responsibility to do so.

CLARY SAGE
HERBIE
Salvia sclarea

CHARACTER
Euphoric, Restoring, Harmonizing, Warming

USE TO COUNTERACT THESE NEGATIVE ATTRIBUTES
Nervousness, Stress, Tension, Changeability, Worried, Anxious,
Claustrophobic, Compulsive, Depression, Nightmares, Hostility,
Hyperactivity, Lethargy, Obsession, Panic, Mental strain, Fear,
Paranoia, Melancholy, Burn-out, Delusions, Emotional debility,
Absentmindedness, Weepiness, Guilt

USE FOR THESE POSITIVE ATTRIBUTES
Calm, Soothed, Confidence, Grounded, Regenerated, Inspired,
Tranquil, Revitalized, Uplifted, Balanced, Strength, Relaxed,
Restores equilibrium

CLARY SAGE PERSONALITY PROFILE

Clary sage's personality is not that of the wiser and more mature
common Sage personality, but is more gentle, melancholy and
thoughtful. Clary will not be rash in their words but will think
carefully before they speak, measuring the effect their voice is
having on others – making sure it is not offensive. Because
Clary sage has the ability to probe deeply into the psyche of
others, they are very aware of the effect they can have on other
people. Although they may appear pensive at times they are
also playful and don't dwell on things too long, even if they
give that impression. If gut feeling or intuition tells them
something is finished, they will move on.

The Clary sage personality has the ability to stir up many
long forgotten feelings in people, good or bad, and it can be
quite unnerving for some other types – such as the Tea Trees,
who do not hide their feelings about anything. Having said
that, Clarys are very warm and friendly and enjoy people

along with all their idiosyncrasies. Never judgemental, which is much in their favour, Clarys have the ability to be comforting in times of need, especially during periods of grief.

Clary sages manage the pressures of daily life well and can handle all kinds of situations. Having an intriguing, fascinating nature, people are drawn to them (although the Clary sage often cannot figure out why). They are extremely creative and contradictory – being the wise man one minute and the fool the next, and not giving it a second thought, and why not?

In work, Clarys will not rest until they're sure a job has been done correctly, using their psyche as well as their head, they intuitively know when a task is complete. Being so adaptable they can tackle almost any job and shine in creative occupations, such as art, composing, writing, designing, or being involved in advertising, journalism, photography, video or film.

For most of the time Clary sages are perfectly balanced between male and female characteristics. If a woman, she may have been called a tomboy when young and if a man, he may have been called a sissy. Both would have been puzzled by this, as they simply don't have this type of sexist attitude. In later life, they can be mistakenly thought to be falsely trying to be 'one of the boys' or 'one of the girls' but any sarcastic comment on this is met with an answer that will set the ears burning for a week!

Clary sages are very sexual people and enjoy sensuality in all its forms. When they fall in love it will be completely – with mind, body and spirit. Because of the balance between their male and female sides, a relationship with Clary sage can be a very harmonious experience. However, they are sometimes drawn to the more unconventional type of relationship, if only for the experience. They are deeply romantic and not at all frivolous about their relationships – but can have a lapse of morals where love is concerned. Undoubtedly there is a secret life somewhere, which nobody will suspect. This secret life can be mundane – like going train-spotting without telling anyone, or exotic – being a spy!

The female Clary sage will be very feminine, one of the most feminine of the herbie types, and have lots of aspirations,

dreams and hopes. She's probably waiting for a knight in shining armour to sweep her off her feet. The male Clary sage will
search for the princess with the long shining hair, and the fact
that none might exist for him does not dampen the dream.
Indeed, Clary sages will dream their dreams until the day they
die.

When in negative mode, both male and female Clary sages
can succumb to outside pressures instead of dealing with them
– and this may happen as a mid-life crisis. It can make them
hypersensitive and hesitant, and they'll start to find fault in
their otherwise exciting relationships, claiming they are dull
and uninspiring – being altogether temperamental. It is often
when negative moods affect them that Clary sages will choose
the wrong friends and lovers. Negativity cramps their style,
and creativity. Clary sages will become isolated in their feelings, may suffer emotional crises and, by choosing the wrong
partner, emotional abuse. They will suffer with nervous and
emotional burn-out, they'll become compulsive, lethargic and
nervous, and may be prone to addiction. The negative Clary
sage can suffer paranoia and fears, and become obsessive. The
shift from positive Clary sage to negative one can be very dramatic. This is very rare, however, because the Clary sage personality is more likely to be intelligent, confident and assured.
Generally, they are very courageous and nice people.

Shirley Price, MIFA Reg., MISPA, aromatherapy tutor and
author:

'Not everyone likes Clary's aroma, but she is one of those people
who "grows on you" – and the more you get to know her, the
more you like her and realize how dependable she is.

  'Among her many talents, she is perceptive, recognizing that we
like to stay young . . . Not least, she is a charmer – helping us to
succumb to the advances of our partner if we find them inconvenient or demanding when we are tired.'

CORIANDER
SEEDIE/SPICIE
Coriandrum sativum

CHARACTER
Enlivening, Motivating, Encouraging

USE TO COUNTERACT THESE NEGATIVE ATTRIBUTES
Emotional tiredness, Weariness, Irritability, Nervousness, Stress,
Nervous debility, Doubt, Fear of failure, Sulkiness,
Being unco-operative, Vulnerability

USE FOR THESE POSITIVE ATTRIBUTES
Creativity, Imagination, Good memory, Confidence, Motivation,
Optimism, Sincerity, Expressiveness, Enthusiasm

CORIANDER PERSONALITY PROFILE

Coriander is a light, sweet, frivolous type of personality – but
with hidden depth! They are sincere, imaginative, full of
optimism, and very warm and inviting. They're always surrounded by people asking favours and their opinions and,
being so accommodating, Corianders never turn anyone away.

Coriander

Corianders enjoy expressing themselves and are masters of body language in getting their point across – throwing their hands in the air to express frustration or giving themselves a gleeful hug if they receive good news. Corianders are people to enjoy!

When they're positive, Corianders are full of imagination and very creative. To say they do their own thing would be a bit of an understatement and whatever they're involved in, it'll be different. Take their home, for example; it might be minimalist in the extreme – white and totally empty except for a futon, or they might have a shocking pink dining room with a plastic fish hanging from the ceiling. The radiators might be decorated with sparkles or sequins, or there might be so many objects around the place you have difficulty finding a seat. Corianders definitely do things their own way!

This personality has a quite extraordinary memory, and they're able to recount an event that happened years ago in precise detail, repeating conversations word for word that you or I would have long forgotten. It can all be very unnerving! They remember not only words, but the expressions people used when they said them and their tone of voice – all of which provides a great store of information for those who become actors and actresses. If there was an animal equivalent to this personality it would be the chameleon, and only very close friends will be able to ignore the different characters they take on every day and see the real person underneath. This is not to say these people have multiple personalities, it's just that they can adopt different looks and behaviour patterns at a moment's notice, and discard them just as easily. All this makes them very stimulating people to be with – providing you can keep up the pace! Corianders will accept your faults and foibles with perfect, nonjudgemental tolerance.

I once had a secretary who did not fit what might be the stereotype, because she'd come to work in quite outlandish clothes . . . sometimes! This was in the early days of punk and one day she came in with shocking pink hair and Vivienne Westwood clothes. A week later she walked in with short black hair and a suit that would have looked at home in the law courts. She was *amazing*, there is no other word for it. She laughed a lot and everyone liked her, plus she was good at her job. I was pregnant during this time and she fulfilled my strange dietary requirements without saying a word. If I'd asked her for a coal and cinnamon sandwich, I swear she wouldn't have batted an eyelid! She'd just ask 'with or without mayonnaise?'

Corianders are passionate in whatever they do, even if it just takes a minute, and it can be very confusing (not to say exhausting) to the uninitiated. The person who gets involved with a Coriander will never quite know who they are meeting. As one lover of a Coriander told me 'I'm left breathless but captivated'. They eventually drift into jobs where their talent is recognized, but may start out in a different field altogether.

When they're negative, Corianders can be very uncooperative, questioning everything. They will sulk and become very vulnerable to criticism, sometimes having a weariness upon them which makes you wonder if they can carry on. They become almost childlike in the sense that they have no confidence or self-esteem. This is particularly noticeable if they're in show business or in any type of job that involves daily contact with the public, such as sales. As they start to doubt their abilities, Corianders become nervous and if they're actors or actresses will develop bad stage fright and lose their memory for lines. This can be a truly terrifying experience for them. Mesmerized into inactivity, it can take the negative Coriander a very long time to recover and, sadly, some performers never do.

If a Coriander falls into negativity, they'll need their family and friends to rally round and slowly coax them back into life. The knocks will show and although they'll be bright and breezy, they'll adopt an air of caution for a while – until something new and wonderful happens, which recharges their batteries and they're off again!

Nicole Perez, MIFA Reg., aromatherapist and tutor:

'Coriander begins with "C" as in Confidence and it often takes confidence and courage to allow the experience of life to move and release our deepest feelings. Its scent pervades, giving a feeling of being slightly drunk and, as with alcohol, it frees the senses from inhibition and brings out our sensuality but it can also stir our libidinous self.'

CYPRESS
LEAFIE/WOODIE
Cupressus sempervirens

CHARACTER
Protective, Righteous, Wise, Direction

USE TO COUNTERACT THESE NEGATIVE ATTRIBUTES
Grief, Sorrow, Self-loathing, Pressurized, Being dominated, Opinionated, Jealous, Lethargic, Weak-willed, Fearful, Timid, Emotional turmoil, Unbalanced, Isolated, Inconsolable, Frustrated, Unable to speak up for oneself, Emotionally tired, Emotionally unstable, Tearful, Loss, Regret, Distracted, Lack of concentration, Absentminded, Uncontrollable passions

USE FOR THESE POSITIVE ATTRIBUTES
Strength, Comfort, Change, Direction, Assertion, Control, Understanding, Balance, Sensitivity, Generosity of spirit, Contentment, Stillness, Confidence, Inner peace, Wisdom, Purity of heart, Stability, Patience, Trust, Incorruptibility, Structured, Softly powerful, Direct, Willpower, Straightforward

CYPRESS PERSONALITY PROFILE

Cypress represents the strength within. Its character is wisdom, strength and uprightness. It stands proud, only slightly swaying, always forceful and direct. Cypress is a symbol of eternity that directs itself to the heavens, answering to no-one but the great spirit. The human counterpart of cypress is very similar. They tend to be forceful, outspoken, and firm in their views – if perhaps at times a little dogmatic. The air of an authoritarian can often disguise the subtle undercurrent of sensitivity that wells in sympathy to sorrow and loss.

There is never an excuse not to be straightforward with this type. In fact, they demand it, along with your respect in every-thing, not expecting to be crossed nor, at times, disobeyed. But their wisdom in sorrows of the heart, grieving and loss, often allows them to give the best advice to people, as does their tendency to see both sides of the story – even if they dis-approve of one of them. People will turn to them in times of extreme distress, usually when there is no other path to travel for advice and comfort.

People perceive Cypress to be powerful and able to sort out most problems. If they are not a person's first choice of con-fidante, it is perhaps because they see them as proud, and even arrogant. This is because of their air of honesty, lawfulness and their unbending search for truth – even if this isn't always authentic. The Cypress personality doesn't always tread the straight and narrow, sometimes using their air of credibility for their own advantage. These are clever types, and will have the edge where matters of money or finance are concerned.

Often, Cypress doesn't see the need for earthly pleasures – including spending money on what could be considered frip-peries, considering that there are more lofty pleasures to pur-sue. They may feel drawn to the role of clergyman, or become active in religious sects, and other very masculine areas such as Masonic orders and so on. A Cypress will be the head-teacher you dread bumping into when skipping school, but will care enough to ask why you skipped school in the first place. A female Cypress will be in charge of the household and may be considered domineering, although always ready to physically help when someone's world starts to crumble.

Cypress make great grandparents because children always know the boundaries and feel comfortable in their presence, while Cypress loves the children's free spirits. As the children get older, discipline and respect will be expected, while

Cypress will be in the forefront of defending the family. This personality often dwells on spiritual matters, and has no fear of death. Once Cypresses have found their pathway, wherever it may lead, they can become unbending in their attitudes and fixed in their ideas, which can be difficult for other, freer, minds to bear. Cypresses have an air of knowing, but are sympathetic to less structured minds. They help balance the unstable, and patch up the holes.

Jan Kusmirek, MIFA Reg., MDDH, MED, LLFA, LCSP, DM, aromatherapist, medical herbalist and lecturer:

'Cypress . . . I see it or sense it as reliable, clean, upright yet with the warmth and comfort of masculinity. Not stern or cold like some pines, more solemn or even soothing. It is strangely astringent (personality) so helps to withstand pressure, reduces fear of one's peers, etc. It tightens up and centres.'

EUCALYPTUS
LEAFIE/WOODIE
Eucalyptus radiata

CHARACTER
Energizing, Stimulating, Balancing, Sheltering

USE TO COUNTERACT THESE NEGATIVE ATTRIBUTES
Exhaustion, Heated emotions, Mood swings, Lack of concentration, Cluttered thoughts, Temper tantrums, Irrational thoughts, Explosive nature, Argumentative

USE FOR THESE POSITIVE ATTRIBUTES
Emotionally balanced, Concentration, Logical thought, Centred, Rationality, Composed, Predictable, Cooling

EUCALYPTUS PERSONALITY PROFILE

Just as there are many species of eucalyptus tree, so there are many variations on the Eucalyptus personality. Here, we are talking about the *Eucalyptus radiata* personality, which I shall simply refer to as 'Eucalyptus'. For the most part Eucalyptus are very calm, rational people. They don't have any special abilities and wouldn't stick out in a crowd. Everyone seems to know one. Eucalyptus remains calm in a storm and, when they're in positive mode, try not to make a fuss, preferring to sort things out for themselves. They don't gossip and can keep a secret.

In general, the Eucalyptus personality is content and well-balanced. Some people might call them dull but they're a refreshing change from some of the more dynamic personalities and they do have an adventurous spirit, which takes the form of planning a project and quietly getting on with it. They don't make plans just for the sake of it; we're talking action. It should come as no surprise when Eucalyptus suddenly announces that they're off on an adventure holiday trekking across swampy marshes. Being highly suspicious people, they won't divulge a great deal about their plans to anyone, and will just tell you what you need to know. For them, that is sufficient. After all, they reckon, it's their business, not yours. You could say they're too secretive but they just don't think anyone should be interested in what is a private matter. This can be very annoying to the more outward types such as Fennels, who will share their every thought. Generally eucalyptus is a stable personality, able to diffuse an argument simply by being in the room. They have the coolness not to argue back, unless in negative mode – but that's another matter. Eucalyptus appears cool, logical and, at times, calculating, and it seems as if everything must have an explanation or be proven before they'll consider it. Although this personality is very laid back, they can have an exhilarating effect on others, instilling enthusiasm and confidence with logical reasoning – which gives the more imaginative personalities a good basis from which to launch their ideas and creativity.

Eucalyptus types go in for the sciences and are often found in the medical professions – such as doctors, nurses and pharmacists – but they're also quite likely to be accountants, bankers and solicitors. The professions that suit them are those that don't require much creative thought and have strict guidelines to which they must adhere. Even as scientists, they will never make any earth-shattering discoveries unless they have a fair proportion of a more imaginative personality within them. Basically, they're happy knowing that two plus two make four and four plus four make eight.

In their private life, Eucalyptus is very similar – choosing carefully where they live and who they have as partners. Sometimes, but not often, you find they choose a floral partner, but this is not a good match for them as their cooling nature tends to put out the flames of the passionate florals and it all ends in tears. Eucalyptus is very predictable in love, making a list of the potential partner's good and bad points and going for the one who complements him or her in some way or other, and who won't rock the boat too much. As partners, Eucalyptus is entertaining and can make one laugh.

A negative Eucalyptus is another matter. They can store up resentments and slights, taking them all on board until one day they snap, becoming explosive. As they never let on to anyone that they've been feeling hurt and disillusioned, when the explosion comes it can be very heated – and you'd better run for cover! A barrage of verbal abuse comes out as they release years of pent-up feelings. Others may stare in surprise, unable to believe that Eucalyptus could go so obviously over the edge. However, it's all over as quickly as it started and they'll apologize with, 'Sorry about that, I don't know what came over me', embarrassed that anyone should have seen them with their guard down.

It's not good for anyone to keep things bottled up and if Eucalyptus doesn't find some regular means of release it can lead to nervous exhaustion, temper tantrums and, eventually, burn-out. If this happens it can take a long time to get them back on their feet because they feel they were indulgent to release their emotions in that way and to sink into such a state. They are easily addicted to anything that relieves their emotional discomfort and it can be difficult for them to be weaned from whatever it is.

Eucalyptus are good, solid characters, often shy, who believe in reasonable behaviour. They can be very willing to help others, not expecting thanks or praise and, indeed, would probably be embarrassed if it's offered.

EUCALYPTUS CITRIODORA (LEMON)
LEAFIE/WOODIE
Eucalyptus citriodora

CHARACTER
Vital, Harmonious, Stimulating, Comforting

USE TO COUNTERACT THESE NEGATIVE ATTRIBUTES
Sluggishness, Emotional crisis, Emptiness, Confusion, Disillusionment, Restlessness, Fear, Despondency, Loneliness, Unable to let go

USE FOR THESE POSITIVE ATTRIBUTES
Concentration, Enthusiasm, Upliftment, Vitality, Understanding, Creativity, Regeneration, Optimism, Encouraged, Empathy, Freedom, Expressiveness, Soundness, Trusting

EUCALYPTUS CITRIODORA PERSONALITY PROFILE

This personality is fresh, alive, and loves freedom. Eucalyptus citriodora is like the youngest member of the eucalyptus family, constantly expressing new ideas and full of vitality and laughter. Indeed, expressiveness and enjoying life to the full is what this personality is about. What excites them is new things and new ideas and anything which catches their imagination and is inventive. Citriodoras will be the whizz kids on the latest computer games, and they'll invent a gadget if they find one is needed – a capacity made possible by their tremendous imagination. When you're around a Citriodora, you feel as if you're on the edge of making a new discovery – which you very possibly are!

The one thing Citriodora cannot stand is being tied down or feeling hemmed in. They love, and indeed *need*, freedom – freedom to express themselves, freedom to move wherever it pleases them to go, and freedom to be who they really are. This can be quite disconcerting if you're in a relationship with a Citriodora because they'll only want to see you (and be really happy to do so) when they want to (although they may agree to compromise!). This 'on-off' quality can make having a relationship with them seem rather like having a relationship with a roller coaster, especially if you're a home-loving Marjoram.

Citriodoras have a freshness and exuberance which they bring to everything they do, whether this is in a relationship, at home or at work. In the workplace they are a veritable dynamo, very dynamic and go-getting, yet they're also very sound and trustworthy. They abhor disharmony and will often try through humour to bring about a balance. Secrets are very safe with this personality and you can have absolute faith they will not exploit any weakness they may discover in you or anyone else. If you're going through an emotional crisis, Citriodora will be a tower of strength, listening attentively, never criticizing or judging, or even remarking on any aspect of your behaviour that others would call pathetic. For all their love of freedom, Citriodoras are very sound people.

When Citriodoras get downhearted, it's usually because there is just too much to do, too many ideas to process, too many places to visit, and too many people to see. Will Citriodoras ever be able to do it all in one lifetime? This question bothers them and they are often drawn to the idea of re-incarnation, if only because it gives them the opportunity to get more done. People disillusion Citriodoras, rather than events, and they can feel empty and lonely if they somehow forget (in the rush) to include love and romance on their agenda. Instead, they leave it all to fate. They can become sluggish and apathetic, fearful of situations which otherwise would not bother them.

Judy is a typical Citriodora in that she is bright, funny, and encourages and comforts everyone. Whenever she sees her friends she boosts them up so they can forge ahead or take that vital risk which moves them closer to their goal. This is one of the reasons why Citriodoras are so well-loved. When there are steps to be taken into the unknown, Judy is always willing to hold her friends' hands – when she's around. And there's the rub because, like any Citriodora, Judy begins to feel uneasy and trapped after a while, and must put on her wings and fly! Her friends would get a postcard from India or Australia once in a while and then, knock, knock, she'd be on the doorstep again – as if four years hadn't even passed. However, she started to feel lonely as if she'd missed out on meeting Mr Right by being constantly on the move but, eventually, so I'm told, Judy married an Orange type personality on top of the Andes mountains, and they are now living happily in Brazil.

Overall, Citriodoras are fun people, creative and enthusiastic and, if you can handle friends who knock on the door at two o'clock in the morning for a cup of coffee after not seeing them for two years, great friends.

FENNEL, SWEET
SEEDIE
Foeniculum vulgare dulce

CHARACTER
Clearing, Resolute, Enlightening

USE TO COUNTERACT THESE NEGATIVE ATTRIBUTES
Mental blockages, Emotional blockages, Boredom, Unable to adjust, Fear of failure, Hostile, Overburdened, Lack of creativity

USE FOR THESE POSITIVE ATTRIBUTES
Enlivened, Motivated, Fortitude, Clarity, Forceful, Perseverance, Courageous, Reliable, Confident, Assertive

FENNEL PERSONALITY PROFILE

The highly active Fennel personality will take brisk walks, regular exercise, and be a member of a sports' club. At school they will love athletics, be on a sports team, and they may even receive a sports' scholarship. Fennels are constantly active and always on the move. They don't walk – they hurry along – leaping up the stairs rather than waiting for a lift. Fennels buy exercise tapes to use at home, they belong to swimming clubs and probably play squash at the weekend. They excel at any type of competition – at work as well as at play.

Fennel is a very assertive personality, invigorating and determined. They'll decorate the house while everyone else is only thinking about it, redesign the garden over a weekend, and change the furniture around on a whim – and still find time to visit friends! They're very kind people, and will help their neighbours or friends if they can't find anything else to do at home. As children, they'd willingly walk the dog, run errands and generally be helpful, getting bored easily and preferring to do anything rather than sit still.

Emotionally too, Fennels are very active, moving from one emotion to another – crying one minute and laughing the next. It's very easy for Fennels to build a brick wall to hide their emotional pain, and it can take for ever to knock it down and get to know them deeply. They'll talk for hours and hours about themselves and then you realize – they actually told you nothing! Nothing important, anyway. Not that these are super-ficial people, although at times it may seem that way. Although apparently easygoing, they're actually shifting gear constantly, so you can't really catch who they are. They're not big on pro-found relationships, thinking they may hold them back in life, and often end up alone if they can't find someone who can fit into their plans. Fennels can be very tiresome because you never get a straight answer, even to a simple question like, 'Which day shall we go to the movies?' This personality is just too frightened of commitment. But, although sometimes exas-perating, Fennels are never dull.

Fennels are very intelligent people, quick-witted and creative and needing a lot of mental stimulation. The partner should be an equal, rather than one who simply complements their personality. Provided that you don't need to understand how they tick, and don't want to dig too deeply into their motives for doing things, Fennels make terrific friends. Being intellectually sharp, Fennels are often ahead of the game – as if they have inside knowledge.

This personality makes good stockbrokers and financiers because they love the risk element in making a deal which might make them, or lose them, ten million pounds. Money is very important, and they enjoy making it, so they also make good entrepreneurs – whether male or female. Fennels are assertive and know what they want and 'go for it', but not at the expense of others – unless it really can't be avoided!

When they're being negative, it's a complete reversal – Fennels will become what can only be described as a slob, and slump in a chair, not bothering to see friends. Activities fly out the window as Fennels lose their competitive edge, not really bothering about anything – which can be a disaster if they have a job that involves quick thinking. The only race they think about will be the one on TV. The more negative they become, the sharper their tongue becomes and anybody who passes them on the success ladder will be ridiculed and become the subject of sarcasm.

Unless something snaps them out of this negative mode, Fennel will get more guilt-ridden. For their family and friends it'll be like watching the *Titanic* go down, a horrifying loss of potential. It takes a brave person to attempt to budge them, and the best thing is flattery. Once they're roused, it will be painful to watch them try to repair the damage to their health and business contacts. Fennels, meanwhile, will be totally perplexed as to how they allowed all this to happen.

FRANKINCENSE
RESINIE
Boswellia carteri

CHARACTER
Elevating, Spiritual, Meditative, Wisdom

USE TO COUNTERACT THESE NEGATIVE ATTRIBUTES
Fears, Grief, Blockages, Over-attachment, Burn-out, Exhaustion, Insincerity, Panic, Anxiety, Disconnection, Repression, Resistance, Self-destruction, Apprehension, Despair

USE FOR THESE POSITIVE ATTRIBUTES
Comfort, Healing, Emotional stability, Enlightenment, Protective,
Introspection, Courage, Resolution, Fortitude, Acceptance,
Inspiration

FRANKINCENSE PERSONALITY PROFILE

Frankincense people are compassionate and interesting and
something of an enigma in that they often display an air of
mystery and secretiveness, even hinting at an understanding of
the nature of the universe. There is a driving forcefulness
about this personality, a strength and fortitude supported by
maturity, conscientiousness, confidence and efficiency. At the
same time, Frankincense can be impetuous, compulsive and
generous.

Frankincense personalities are often geniuses and may well
have invented practical contraptions for use around the
home and at work. They don't rely on others to do things for
them, preferring to use their own initiative, and are sometimes
called eccentric. Frankincense will drive fast on dangerous mountain roads, ski down runs nobody else would dare, and swim
in shark-infested waters without turning a hair. It's not that they're
reckless but they believe they are protected in ways that the rest
of us are not.

The Frankincense personality has what one might call para-
psychological tendencies – they're very sensitive to atmospheres, sensing unhappiness or evil in a room or house,
although this wouldn't necessarily be mentioned if they didn't
think you would understand. Although no particular personality has more psychic experiences than another, some *notice*
them more than others, and Frankincense notices the most.
They also sense the intentions of other people, which is a very
useful tool for them to have.

Frankincenses are very steady, upright citizens and are often
found in jobs that command respect and even honour. In business, their ability to sense accurately whether a deal will turn
out well or be a waste of time is a very useful tool for them to
have. Although this profile may make them seem rather cold,

Frankincenses are very kind, warmhearted personalities with a knack of making people feel both confident and secure. They'd make good counsellors as their advice is often very down-to-earth and practical, not impossible for mere mortals to carry out.

The Frankincense person may not think of themselves as religious and may avoid places of worship, but they carry a profound love of God in their hearts. Frankincenses question things in terms of good and evil and have a love of all things spiritual, which gives them a deep wisdom. They are often excellent speakers, clear and eloquent, but are inclined to be somewhat blunt.

If they're negative, the Frankincense personality can be destructive and bitter, full of scepticism and cynicism, inclined to become guilt-ridden, insecure and uncertain, liable to suffer anxiety attacks and stress, also becoming short tempered and agitated. However, this is such an enlightened personality they soon realize what's going on and make a concerted effort to change direction – into positivity! Frankincense is a well-balanced personality and remarkably gifted. They are terrific communicators and are friendly, warm and loving.

Maureen Farrell, MRPharmS, FRSH, MIFA Reg., MISPA, aromatherapist and tutor:

'Frankincense – the traveller, the pilgrim on the Way of Life – a steadfast companion in a journey through grief and in letting go of fear or suppressed emotions. For me, the resins and resinoids, most frequently used in aromatherapy, come into the category of Wounded Healer.'

GERANIUM
HERBIE
Pelargonium graveolens

CHARACTER
Harmonizing, Healing, Comforting, Cushioning

USE TO COUNTERACT THESE NEGATIVE ATTRIBUTES
Anxiety, Depression, Acute fear, Extreme moods, Inner child,
Abuse, Confusion, Rigidity, Instability, Worry, Moodiness,
Lack of self-esteem, Insecurity, Over-sensitivity, Tension, Stress,
Hurt, Crisis, Apprehension, Aggression, Irrationality,
Discontent, Heartache

USE FOR THESE POSITIVE ATTRIBUTES
Consoled, Flexible, Elevated, Regenerated, Humour, Friendliness,
Balanced, Soothed, Secure, Assured, Shielded, Mothered, Stable,
Tranquil, Steady

GERANIUM PERSONALITY PROFILE

The Geranium personality is friendly and comforting,
although not in any way extroverted or over-talkative. This is
one of the mothering type of personalities, always taking care
of someone or something, just getting on with things, allowing
everyone the freedom to have their own thoughts and never
interfering unless you want them to. This personality seems to
be able to create a feeling of security and stability wherever
they go. This doesn't mean they're boring, far from it, but they
just seem to have the knack of making everything all right
again. Say, for example, you feel frustrated and hurt about
something and need to make a phone call to sort it out,
Geranium will make you a cup of tea, settle you in a chair and
make the call for you. Your tension is relieved because you
don't have to make the unpleasant call and you feel cared for
(and about three years old!).

Geraniums never consciously look for thanks or appreciation but get it naturally, which makes it a pleasure to give to

this personality. They have the ability to wash away your tension and stress just by being there, and caring a great deal for their family and friends – which are very valuable to Geraniums. However, they tend to take on too much, and don't leave enough space for themselves and, unfortunately those who are helped may not even notice that help may sometimes be needed in return.

Geraniums are seldom eccentric, outlandish characters prone to great strokes of genius, just steady and stable, but they often do have the most bizarre friends and companions, flamboyant and colourful – the complete opposite to themselves. This feature makes them even more popular. This personality has interesting dinner parties, interesting house guests, and their homes are always full of people – not because Geranium is the most sensational cook, nor because they are sparkling conversationalists; what attracts people to Geranium is their marvellous ability to make people feel worthy and wanted.

Geraniums may be surrounded by fascinating people but fascinating people are often too full of their own self-importance to think about lending a hand. Geranium will lay the table, cook the meal, clean up, wash the dishes and glasses and if someone asks, 'Oh, do you want a hand?' they'll offer knowing that, more often than not, Geranium will say 'You sit down, I'll do it' (unlike Jasmine, who'll leave the washing-up for someone else to do).

Within the family, this generosity of nature can really be exploited and Geraniums will continue to do their children's laundry twenty years after they left home, mind the grandchildren, and take on the chore of washing and repairing the entire football team's kit. Unless they occasionally shout 'Stop!' very loudly, they can easily become the dogsbody. Geranium is the ultimate personality for being taken for granted, never really getting their due but they astound friends and family in middle age by suddenly packing a bag and going in search of personal happiness. If not appreciated, Geraniums can get very anxious and depressed and may find their heart being broken many times over, by thoughtless friends and family.

Negative Geraniums have devised a ten-point plan to inflict guilt on their families and refer to it at every opportunity, and if that doesn't work, there's always the medical dictionary of imaginary illnesses to work through, another way to ensure people provide the (much-deserved) attention. Unfortunately, this often has the opposite effect, and drives people away. Geraniums in general cannot be said to be passive people, but some can be very mean. These personalities may have suffered emotional abuse as a child and feel they somehow have to make up for what they perceive to be their faults.

Geraniums are a much under-valued personality who generously comforts those who suffer, those with broken hearts, the grieving and the stressed-out. Whether male or female, Geranium is a warm, kind and generous personality, which deserves to be appreciated for the very special person they are.

GINGER
ROOTIE/SPICIE
Zingiber officinale

CHARACTER
Warming, Strengthening, Encouraging

USE TO COUNTERACT THESE NEGATIVE ATTRIBUTES
Sexual anxieties, Lack of direction, Purposelessness, Unfocused, Apathy, Burn-out, Confusion, Fatigue, Loneliness, Sadness, Resignation

USE FOR THESE POSITIVE ATTRIBUTES
Confidence, Warmth, Fortitude, Empathy, Courage

GINGER PERSONALITY PROFILE

The Ginger personality is often called the strong, silent type because with them, actions speak louder than words. If you think of a large, gentle giant, you'll get the picture. This doesn't mean Ginger types will be either large or gentle but explains the largesse and warmth this personality exudes. Ginger types couldn't be described as being sedative – they are stimulating and lively company with a very wicked sense of humour, definitely everyone's favourite uncle.

This personality can be very masculine, forceful, and profound, able to sort out problems philosophically without relying on anybody else. The personal space of people around is respected and Gingers never crowd you or become possessive. That's something the Tuberose personality finds hard to take, whether a member of the family or in another type of relationship with Ginger but, in fact, these two match quite well, balancing out each other. Ginger's lack of possessiveness is part of their charm and they don't expect to have interdependence – Gingers expect you to do your own thing, just as they expect you to leave them alone to do theirs.

Ginger personalities make good listeners but bad conversationalists and prefer jobs that don't entail much conversation. As their caring nature often needs expression, they're good in one of the caring professions that involve listening – counselling, psychology, probation officers, social workers and so on. They also seem to do well as farmers dealing with animals and will be more inclined towards natural farming methods. Animals respect their quiet strength and Gingers make good vets and veterinary nurses, partly too because they have the ability to comfort the owners. Perhaps though, the ideal job for this independent soul would be looking after the animals in an African game park.

Although Gingers don't invite people into their homes very often – they like their privacy too much – they will be welcoming when people call by. Although they believe their door is always open, others can sense that actually Ginger wants to be left alone.

In love, Gingers will dedicate their lives to the loved one, even though they don't often say the magic words 'I love you'. Because they allow their partner freedom, this is often misunderstood. But don't think freedom means infidelity, it doesn't. Ginger expects fidelity along with respect from partners, parents, children, friends and business partners – and if they don't get it, their Ginger temper really becomes apparent. Don't cross a Ginger, or you'll be sorry. They'll hunt you down and that temper, once roused, will make sure you pay for any wrongs against them or their loved ones – and beware, grudges can be held for years and years.

Gingers have a very sexual nature and love making love, choosing a mate who shares their enthusiasm. This is one way in which Gingers can express themselves perfectly. They exude a powerful sexuality rather than sensuality, which can be unnerving to more timid profiles, but it explains why florals are often drawn to them.

Negative Gingers are just awful. They withdraw into a silent world of sulking, and appear confused, apathetic and with no memory of who they were formerly. They will not get depressed as such, but can lose their purpose and joy in life, becoming directionless as if resigned to whatever fate has in store for them. Great bouts of loneliness can engulf them, no matter how many people are around.

After knowing the warm, positive Ginger, this drop into sadness seems profound indeed. They're liable to be unstable at times, particularly if unemployed or passed over for promotion. It's not that they seek power, they do not, it's already built into them, but they'll be upset that they haven't been treated with the respect they deserve, whether for work or some other achievement. They don't like 'losing face', as the Chinese say.

Gingers may suffer in silence from emotional burn-out – quite a common trait of this personality, which often results in their sex drive diminishing, which is devastating to a Ginger. Luckily, the Ginger personality has remarkable powers of recovery and although these negative bouts may come often, they can go away very quickly too. Ginger is a great friend or relative to have around you because they'll always listen to your problems with patience, sincerity and kindness. Just don't forget sometimes to ask them about theirs!

GRAPEFRUIT
FRUITIE
Citrus paradisi

CHARACTER
Radiating, Cheering, Joyful, Liberating, Boosting

USE TO COUNTERACT THESE NEGATIVE ATTRIBUTES
Depression, Dependency, Sadness, Grief, Apathy, Mental pressure,
Mental exhaustion, Emotional violence, Self-doubt, Self-criticism,
Aggravated, Frustration

USE FOR THESE POSITIVE ATTRIBUTES
Joyful, Positive, Confident, Clarity, Balanced, Attuned, Alert,
Inspired, Generous, Uplifted, Emotionally purified, Spontaneous,
Co-operative

GRAPEFRUIT PERSONALITY PROFILE

The Grapefruit personality is about freshness and newness.
These are happy, warm people who are usually bursting with
energy – even when they're sitting down – with a wonderful
radiation of pure energy that gives light to everything they do.
Even in the poorest countries, where you might think everyone
is weighed down with daily problems of survival, the
Grapefruit personality can be found with a big smile on their
face, cheerfully helping a neighbour.

The Grapefruit personality has a very deep concern for
humanity, and the direction the world is taking. They can't
really understand why we allow people with no consciousness
or consideration for their fellow man to take over the controls,
and why we do nothing about it. Grapefruits are not particularly concerned about money, although they're not blind to its
importance in allowing us to get through life. Being 'comfortable', to them, doesn't mean having lots of money, instead
'comfort' equates with being contented.

Grapefruits love people and they dislike seeing someone not
fulfilling their potential. They become great motivators, the

'get up and go' people, although not overbearing, not saying 'do something worthwhile with your life', rather, they give out subtle, discreet suggestions which the recipient doesn't realize were intended to give them confidence or motivation.

Infused with happy joyfulness, Grapefruits sing and laugh the loudest and are not in the least self-conscious. They might have difficulty toning all this down, however. Having no fear of other people, no matter how illustrious they may be, Grapefruits are able to see clearly unspoken intentions and innermost thoughts. Other people are often unaware of this ability of Grapefruit, seeing only the superficial, jolly exterior.

Grapefruits are very clear thinkers. They make wonderful healers because, if nothing else works, the placebo effect of their infectious enthusiasm creates well-being and because Grapefruits are attuned to their spiritual selves, and have an affinity with the unseen realms. Because they have a global perspective and care very strongly for the future of the planet, Grapefruits are very good in jobs concerned with the environment. It's almost as if they've been put on this earth as guides to light and happiness for the rest of us and would make very good leaders, if goodness were a prerequisite for leadership. It is a pity that they are often ignored in favour of the more ambitious personalities. As group leaders they can instil enthusiasm on a grand scale, but may tend to overdo it.

Grapefruits make thoughtful, caring partners and lovers and very good parents but they may mentally (never emotionally) neglect their own children as they spend so much time trying to save the children of the world. This can lead to resentment and discord. It's fairly easy for a Grapefruit to become bogged down with work or other responsibilities, or to get emotionally overloaded with the problems of this planet, weighed down with the inhumanities human beings can commit against each other. It all becomes just too much. Tired and irritable with those nearest and dearest, an overwhelming sadness can rest on their shoulders like a mantle.

Happily, a Grapefruit's light is not easily extinguished and it's always there, ready to be rekindled. When they're on form, Grapefruits are warm, generous and very cleansing, mentally.

Grapefruit is tempted by the prospect of being able to make a clean sweep, and helps many people to do just that.

HELICHRYSUM
(Immortelle or Italian Everlasting)
FLORAL
Helichrysum angustifolium, H. italicum, H. orientale

CHARACTER
Gentleness, Harmonizing, Caring, Warming, Meditative

USE TO COUNTERACT THESE NEGATIVE ATTRIBUTES
Abuse, Stress, Tension, Emotional crisis, Depression, Lethargy, Mental exhaustion, Emotional exhaustion, Tiredness, Overwork, Emotional blockages, Disorientation, Loneliness, Insecurity, Hypersensitivity, Grief, Addiction, Negative inner child

USE FOR THESE POSITIVE ATTRIBUTES
Calm, Accepting of change, Buffered, Dreams, Energy, Patience, Idealism, Understanding, Perserverance, Inner strength, Acceptance, Awareness, Positive inner child

HELICHRYSUM/IMMORTELLE PERSONALITY PROFILE

The Immortelle profile is one of quietness, introversion and youth, with a quiet knowing that comes from being sure of the spirituality of all things, and the understanding that there are greater things in heaven and earth than we can see. Fragile innocents in a harsh world, Immortelles are frequently called naive because of their compassionate nature and understanding of the frailties of others. This type can easily accept changes of any sort as they're not fixed in their ideas or thoughts.

The Immortelle person is spiritually highly evolved and often seems almost fairy-like, having high consciousness and mental agility. If wronged, they can forgive quickly, and do not bear grudges, but will not encourage the company of anyone who does commit a wrong against them. This cold shoulder can be difficult for the persons concerned, who often don't realize what it is they have done wrong.

This personality has a dry, cheeky, kooky sense of humour and is great fun to be with. Friendship is very precious to an Immortelle who, with an inner strength and genuine love, is always encouraging and helpful. Immortelles are always able to see other people's points of view, even if they don't agree with them, and accept other people's way of doing things. Immortelles always try at least to understand other ways of thinking and doing.

Because of their inner strength and open heart, Immortelle is willing to see new points of view and loves exploring new ideas, walking new pathways, and heading in new directions. They can easily leave people and problems behind, and don't worry about the past. Having a strong sense of what is right and wrong, Immortelles have a willingness to develop and can learn life's lessons very quickly, developing ideas as they go along, learning from everyone and everything, from mistakes as well as successes.

This personality may have suffered abuse as a child – either emotional, verbal or physical. The sensitivity felt by Immortelle is partly due to their caring, in a corner of their heart, for a child hurt a long time ago. The neglect as a child may have taken the form of lack of love or emotional warmth in the home, and Immortelle may have had difficulty in understanding why they were feeling hurt. Rejection is a very powerful emotion that can be carried throughout life – whether that rejection comes from parents, peers, teachers, or siblings. They carry the emotional wounds very deeply (as does a Chamomile Roman type, but in a slightly different way). Immortelles may always be searching for the comfort needed to assure them that everything is all right. The Immortelle personality often appears guarded, as if protecting themselves emotionally, but this is an inaccurate judgement because it's just that they feel no need to externalize and express their emotions to everyone. Sometimes a crisis of identity will occur if Immortelles did not receive enough nurturing love as a child or young person. They have no difficulty in acknowledging the child within themselves, just as they can acknowledge unseen forces, such as guardian angels or God, but just don't always tell you!

Ever young at heart and youthful in appearance, Immortelles will have the air of eternal youth about them, even in the last stages of their journey on this earth. They're very emotional and will cry like a baby at sad movies, being able to identify with the dramatized sorrow as if it were their own. Immortelles are often very shy but if they could overcome that shyness, would become the world's greatest actors and actresses because they've got such good empathy with other people, are exemplary speakers of truth, outspoken and direct – representative of people, animals and plant life.

Immortelles can get very apathetic and tired – both emotionally and mentally – often in middle age. When depressed, they cannot be consoled and will often be irrational and irritable, preferring to shut themselves off from the world, just hiding in bed or lying on the sofa, refusing to accept help. They can also become disoriented and confused and lose their valued friendships through simple things like never phoning, missing meetings, being late and standing people up – and through a host of other annoying but not life-threatening faults.

For all this, the Immortelle personality is a floral who loves beauty, delicacy and joy – all qualities which they carry within their beautiful open heart. These are sensitive, caring and loving people and their idiosyncrasies should easily be forgiven.

HYACINTH
FLORAL
Hyacinthus orientalis

CHARACTER
Gentle, Trusting, Soothing, Enlightening

USE TO COUNTERACT THESE NEGATIVE ATTRIBUTES
Instability, Stress, Repression, Apathy, Lovesick, Dejection, Distress, Grieving, Sorrow, Powerlessness, Regret, Unforgiving, Naiveté, Dependency, Apprehension

USE FOR THESE POSITIVE ATTRIBUTES
Calming, Forgiving, High self-esteem, Perseverance, Equilibrium,
Trust, Faith, Courage

HYACINTH PERSONALITY PROFILE

The Hyacinth personality is forgiving and trusting, and this personality's gentleness and good nature is apparent in everything they touch. They love beauty and beautiful things and can decorate a room exquisitely simply by using their ingenuity and artistry and a few pots of paint, taking immense trouble over every little detail. When you come for lunch the table will look fabulous with little pretty touches to catch the eye. Of course, there will be flowers! That goes without saying. Indeed, Hyacinths are happiest when they are tending gardens and plants and taking care of animals (who don't talk back).

Having an unshakeable belief in people, Hyacinths think that good will always triumph over evil. Needless to say, they are often disappointed. Their faith in the human race is a virtue that is easily taken advantage of, particularly by those with no scruples. Time after time, sweet Hyacinth will be drawn into plans with which they don't really want to be involved and schemes that are detrimental to their well-being. Relationships are just the same, and Hyacinth is just the personality to choose the wrong man or woman to be their life partner – one who will strip them of all their emotions, and their money! They try to make the best of it because that's how they are!

Hyacinths are very mindful of other people's feelings and love to be privy to their secrets. They don't *mean* to pass them on, but do, sometimes thinking other people won't repeat what they say. Hyacinth never seems to understand that some people live vicariously through others and *need* interesting titbits of information to keep their lives exciting, and Hyacinth likes talking too. So, innocently, Hyacinth inadvertently passes on secrets, not realizing that they may be the subject of discussion at a dozen social events before running out of steam!

Hyacinths never have any trouble talking about their own problems, usually to do with the opposite sex and no matter how naive, gentle and caring they are, they can drive the more assertive types, like Bergamot, to distraction. Hyacinths can take on almost any job provided that the circumstances are right. For example, they make good salespeople only so long as they have faith in the product; they make good secretaries and assistants so long as the boss is honest with them and the job doesn't entail any underhand dealings. They'd be marvellous at animal breeding and any job involving flowers and plants. Although they love music, dance and theatre, these professions, even on the administrative side, are much too cutthroat for Hyacinth.

Negative Hyacinths often emphasize their fragile, delicate nature to get sympathy if all else fails, creating the illusion of a tragic personality, and can act out this role to the full, particularly if they find it working to their advantage. However, tension, stress and stress-related disorders are invariably genuine, common to this personality type.

Hyacinths make good Samaritans – listening to people in trouble and, being basically very charitable, would be happy working in any capacity in the charity field. Being very intuitive and known as 'sensitives', these are nice, gentle, soft people who need space to breathe and be who they are – without any interference.

JASMINE
FLORAL
Jasminum officinale, J. grandiflorum, J. sambac

CHARACTER
Euphoric, Sensual, Welcoming, Intuitive, Soothing

USE TO COUNTERACT THESE NEGATIVE ATTRIBUTES
Depression, Anxiety, Pessimism, Tension, Indifference, Repression, Bitterness, Jealousy, Low self-esteem, Guilt, Emotional frigidity, Emotional abuse, Emotional violence

JASMINE PERSONALITY PROFILE

From the top of their head to the tip of their toes, the Jasmine
personality is pure femininity. We're talking womanhood in
full bloom. Jasmine is a no-holds-barred personality, the
passionate seductress, gentle and charismatic, bewitching all
who come into her presence. Before all the men reading this
go rushing out to find one, let me say that ultimate femininity
can dwell in the heart of most women but only the true
Jasmine has the courage to expose it to the world.

Jasmines are beautiful from within, whether they're a girl
on the cover of a western magazine, or a tribeswoman in the
Amazon. Their beauty has the ability to transcend the daily
battles of existence; it's a glimpse of the archetypal female,
Mother Earth – giver of all life. Jasmines are the mermaids
that touch the hearts of man, the petal that drifts gently by on
the breeze. No wonder that this personality, like the perfume,
has enchanted the world since time began.

Jasmines are joyful, happy people, comfortable with who
they are. They have no wish to stop enjoying the sensuality of
their surroundings or fabulous objects, and have no wish to
become part of an androgynous society. They enjoy all the
things that are generally considered, in the western world, to
be essentially feminine – fragile silk underwear, perfume, the
touch of cashmere against their skin, or the sweet smell of a
new-born babe. If they can afford it, they'll dine on straw-
berries and champagne and, whatever their financial status,
will enjoy the sight and aroma of flowers. Jasmines have no
intention of forsaking these pleasures for anyone.

Jasmines won't stand for sexual harassment and anyone
bold enough to attempt it with them will receive a barrage of
abuse powerful enough to blast them on to another planet, but
are flattered when someone suggests they are looking nice,

and enjoy old-fashioned courtesies and thoughtfulness – which they also give to others. Whether they're brunette, blonde, black or red-headed, whether they're nine hours or ninety years old, whether they're pretty or ugly by conventional standards, Jasmines will have people queuing up just for a smile. They have a wonderful ability to really listen and the time and attention given to others instils confidence in them. Past lovers will remember Jasmine with a smile, and Jasmine will remember every lover and friend they've ever had. Usually independent, these are intelligent, assertive, confident people.

Having a great sense of humour, Jasmines are great fun to have as friends – imaginative and alive. There'll be no dull moments with them. They're the kind of friend you can call at midnight after a dreadful day, without worrying whether they'll be upset that you bothered them so late. Jasmines are passionate lovers and understand the spirituality of sex, enjoying it without guilt or hang-ups. It doesn't matter to them whether the soulmate is rich or poor, just as long as they're right for each other.

Jenny is a Jasmine personality, a social worker who fights for her clients in court, not missing a trick as she presents an argument, then sends the sweetest smile across the room to the magistrates. She wears perfume and exquisite fabrics and somehow manages to get her way every time, without realizing how she's done it. The charm of the Jasmine personality is in-born, and subconscious most of the time. This is what is so attractive to other people.

The male Jasmine personality is charming, charismatic and at ease with his femininity. He is devastatingly attractive to the opposite sex, as Jasmine females are to men. He'll be able to hold his peers spellbound as he recounts tales, about his latest passion, over lunch. The male Jasmine uses his sensuality to get what he wants more consciously than the female, and can flirt with both sexes. Jasmines can be very unnerving if you're not used to them – particularly at work. After a heated debate they may storm out of the room but, disconcertingly, almost surreally, will find time to touch the petal of a particularly beautiful flower as they pass. This personality is found in every kind of job although they're happiest in those in which they can use their instinctive intellect and behaviour. They'll be unhappy as an accountant, but will enjoy the challenge of physics. They also make good designers, artists and gardeners.

Jasmines can become depressed at the discord in today's life, and be self-destructive. Indeed, negative Jasmines can be lethal to themselves. Passionate jealousy can become a serious problem and, as they turn their passion inward, can become addicted and obsessive. Of course, this affects everyone around them, which makes things worse, and Jasmine can become paranoid, miserable and prone to emotional illness. The depths of emotion that Jasmine can reach can only be truly understood by another floral, also delicately balanced between the conscious and subconscious. In negative mode, Jasmines can make everyone's life hell on earth, and can easily destroy their own careers and relationships. It takes a long time for them to pull themselves out of the mire, and they require a lot of help. Fortunately, nearly always, they have generated many friendships and, in these times of stress, the chaff is separated from the wheat. After they recover from a negative phase, Jasmines will carry an air of fragility and melancholy. This doesn't affect their passion, however, and it even makes them more desirable to some.

This joyful personality is often attacked by those who don't understand just how fragile they may be feeling, and this can lead to all kinds of problems. However, if you want warmth and gentleness, with passionate benevolence, there is no other personality quite like the true Jasmine.

Nicole Perez, MIFA Reg., aromatherapist and tutor:

'The character of Jasmine is represented by the two Js – as in Jasmine for Joy. This, to me, is the true character of Jasmine. Jasmine has the most uplifting and beautifying effect on people. It elevates us to higher spheres; it is also renowned for increasing sensuality as well as personal charisma.'

JUNIPER
FRUITIE
Juniperus communis

CHARACTER
Cleansing, Purifying, Sacredness, Visionary

USE TO COUNTERACT THESE NEGATIVE ATTRIBUTES
Nervous exhaustion, Emotional exhaustion, Lack of self-worth,
Guilt, Dissatisfaction, Anxiety, Abused, Listlessness, Weakness,
Transience, Emptiness, Conflict, Defensive

USE FOR THESE POSITIVE ATTRIBUTES
Self-worth, Spiritually supported, Peace, Inner vision, Uplifted,
Strength, Vitality, Cleansed, Meditative, Conviction, Sincerity,
Enlightened, Wisdom, Humility

JUNIPER PERSONALITY PROFILE

The Juniper personality is radical in that they have no concern
for human authority, preferring to be directed by their intuition or religious belief. They have a reverence for anything
sacred and will inevitably take a spiritual path through life –
whatever form that may take. As children, they may be drawn
to church or other spiritual places, without knowing why and
even if their parents never go to them. One young man I had
as a patient always had the desire to go to church but was
never taken by his parents so joined the local church youth
centre held in the church hall and would pop into the even-
song service every day on his way home from college – and
his parents never knew a thing! The Juniper personality
doesn't consciously seek out spiritual places, but just seems
drawn to them. The Juniper personality has a profound spiritual
ease, which is obvious to all who come into contact with them.
This doesn't mean they are religious fanatics, in fact they may
never tell you how they feel about spiritual matters, apparently feeling this is a private matter between them and God.

This spiritual thread runs through everything Juniper does through life.

Juniper is also a personality of Spring – of things fresh and new. To others, it sometimes appears that Junipers are immature because they take such a delight in new experiences and knowledge. This is a misjudgement, however, because Junipers are simply not afraid to enjoy themselves in a way that expresses their delight. They rejoice in simple pleasures like meeting new people, taking a trip to the country, having a drink with friends or lunch with the family. Although these things would have been experienced many times before, each time is like the first to them, fresh and new. This is actually a very endearing quality because it shows Juniper's appreciation of the uniqueness of each occasion and the fleetingness of the moment, and their ability to live in the present time. Junipers always have time for other people. They'll invite you along to whatever activity they may be going to not out of obligation, but because genuine pleasure is taken in sharing your company.

When they're negative, Junipers appear very vulnerable, as if their very soul is being attacked. They become uneasy among other people and disquieted by all manner of things. Anyone used to their usual easy-going nature may sense the disquiet that is being generated. During these bouts of doubt and anxiety Junipers can become very weak-spirited, depressed and exhausted – as if they've fought an enormous battle. Their faith never falters though, which is a great strength. No matter what life throws at them Juniper will always pull through and once again laugh and believe in themselves and others.

Junipers are best suited to professions which allow them freedom of thought and speech. They don't take kindly to authority or to being the underdog, and are best suited to jobs in which they can be left on their own to carry out the work in their own way although they can have a wishful nature, approaching things in ways that are not always practical or efficient. This type of person has difficulty choosing romantic partners because they need someone who understands why they need to withdraw into themselves for inner reflection, without feeling excluded. There are many personalities Juniper is not compatible with and they often wrongly feel that they will never find their soulmate or true love.

Teddy Fearnhamm, IScB France, MRQA, aromatherapist and tutor:

'Definitive personality; Peter Pan/Juvenescence. Clears and detoxes the mind as well as the body – promising a fresh vitality and promoting the desire to live up to our expectations and the dreams we had when we were very young.'

LAVENDER
FLORAL/HERBIE
Lavandula angustifolia, L. officinalis

CHARACTER
Harmonious, Calming, Healing, Caring, Embracing

USE TO COUNTERACT THESE NEGATIVE ATTRIBUTES
Anxiety, Irritability, Stress, Tension, Mental exhaustion, Panic, Hysteria, Shock, Apprehension, Fears, Nightmares, Insecurity, Lost inner child, Restlessness, Moodiness, Distracted, Addiction, Obsessional behaviour, Trauma, Conflict, Emotional violence, Agitation, Jitteryness, Depression, Psychosomatic illness, Nervousness, Worry, Over-excitedness, Burn-out

USE FOR THESE POSITIVE ATTRIBUTES
Secure, Gentle, Compassion, Balanced, Reconciled, Vital, Clarity, Comforted, Acceptance, Inner peace, Relaxed and alert, Rested, Aware, Emotionally balanced, Spiritual growth, Meditative, Visualization, Rejuvenated

LAVENDER PERSONALITY PROFILE

Lavender could be called the mother, or grandmother of essential oils, able to care for a multitude of physical and psychological problems and, like a mother, accomplishing several jobs at the same time. Lavender is the most useful essential oil and is usually the first that any student of aromatherapy learns about. It is the preferred essential oil of the nursing professions, who use it more for its calming and sedative properties rather than for its anti-infectious ones. Lavender is the most commonly used essential oil in aromatherapy treatments and aroma-psychology research. There are several species of lavender which are distilled to make essential oil, and there are subtle personality variations between them, but here we are looking at the personality of *lavandula officinalis* or *angustifolia*, the most commonly used species.

Lavender is the perfect balance between the masculine and feminine traits that are within us all, and that all *grande dames* exhibit boldly. Lavender is completely mothering in its personality – electric, formidable, yet gentle and kind, and the perfect embodiment of Mother Earth. Embracing Lavender is direct, pure of thought, brave and humble. It makes men gentle, and women strong.

Even in times of hardship a Lavender personality bravely continues overcoming obstacles that are placed in their way, having the ability to give generously of themselves – caring for others, often with gentleness and sacrifice. This type will be the first to offer to hold the baby to lull it to sleep, and the first to come to the rescue in times of trouble when help is needed. Lavenders seem to have an inexhaustible amount of energy to call upon, which their own calm exterior belies, and are the ones who will sit and talk to your plants or feed your cats when you go away, and who'll do the shopping for sick neighbours, and are always ready to listen.

The Lavender personality loves the earth, the flowers and trees, and will fill their homes with living things if they can. True Lavenders have an in-built correctness and spirituality. Nurses, buddies and foster parents are just some of the roles taken on by people who have a fair proportion of Lavender in their make-up. They're also often found fighting for a cause, but one usually nearer home than the rain forest – such as for facilities for nursing mothers, or the physically disadvantaged. Whatever they put their campaigning energies into, it will be for a home issue, in one form or another. Lavender types are often subject to flights of fancy and are happy to search for the elusive solution to life's problems – which is an aspect of mothering to a certain extent. A male Lavender is often drawn to the Ghia principle and New-Ageism, and will go looking for the goddess within himself, or may go into farming where the mothering instinct can have expression in the care of animals and crops. Whether male or female, Lavenders are very versatile, and if stuck in a city job they'll be drawn to volunteer jobs such as helping the homeless and otherwise disadvantaged.

A negative Lavender will be highly strung, wound up, and absorbing energies off everyone, never discharging them. They won't disclose their problems or troubles to anyone as they believe they must always care for others, overdoing it, never resting or sleeping properly. Unexplained headaches and migraines are conditions which afflict this personality, along with aches and pains – which go away as soon as everything returns to normal.

Lavenders are gentle men and women. These intelligent people often become teachers but whatever they do, they will be kind-hearted, benevolent, humane, worthy and valuable.

LEMON
FRUITIE
Citrus limonum, C. medica

CHARACTER
Purifying, Stimulating, Directional, Versatile

USE TO COUNTERACT THESE NEGATIVE ATTRIBUTES
Resentful, Depressed, Bitter, Touchy, Apathetic, Lethargic, Humourless, Indecisive, Bad attitudes, Distrust, Mental blocks, Stress, Mental fatigue, Turmoil, Irrationality, Fear

USE FOR THESE POSITIVE ATTRIBUTES
Joy, Emotional clarity, Direction, Awareness, Calm, Concentration, Lively, Conscious, Strength, Clarity of thought, Memory, Emotionally invigorated

LEMON PERSONALITY PROFILE

The sweet Lemon is like a breath of fresh air on a summer's day, positively wonderful to have around. Lemon-types are lively and casual – not too bothered by the struggles and strains of living, able to take it all quite calmly, dealing with each problem as it comes along. They have a sense of energy about them and are very active people. Lemon-types sparkle, full of life, with a very positive approach, in the form of an unshakeable confidence in everything they do. Even if this personality has never attempted a particular job before, they categorically believe it can be done, with success. This 'never doubt yourself' attitude can rub off on other people around, which is a blessing for personalities who have difficulty starting or finishing projects. Lemon's enthusiasm just seems to roll off on to those around, with subtle and permanent effect.

The Lemon personality type can be sweet, sour, or confusingly balanced between the two. Even sweet Lemons can be sharp, and these people are inclined to be rather critical, not understanding why everyone doesn't strive for perfection as they do. So work colleagues often come in for harsh words, while the mistakes of Lemon's children are not always easily tolerated.

Although Lemons have no difficulty in concentrating or being engrossed in a job, it has to be one they like otherwise they won't be interested. It's no good trying to get a Lemon involved in a business deal, no matter how much money it could make, if the project isn't interesting. As Lemons often reach the top of their chosen profession they are much sought after on the work front, but do better owning their own business, where it is easier to set the pace of the work and where Lemon's originality and intuition can be put to good use. Lemons are workaholics who, if they enjoy their work, will let it dominate their lives – but always with a casual air about it. If a business deal is lost, Lemon will not fret but go out for a nice lunch with someone whose company they enjoy.

In relationships, Lemons can be wonderful as they always have an answer for all life's problems. As lovers, Lemons can be thoughtful, original and very energetic – as they are in most things when in positive mode. Positive Lemons never seem to have any illnesses, and germs just seem to pass them by – a fact which often makes other people wonder what their secret is. These are athletic people who love sport and competition, often playing amateur or professional sports or becoming sports teachers or trainers; while those who make their living in commerce or industry usually take up sport in their spare time. Whatever the sport, Lemons often become the captain of the team.

Lemons do not usually bear grudges unless in negative mode, when you had better watch out! That carefree manner can become scornful, sarcastic and sharp-tongued. A negative Lemon can be scattered, selfish, arrogant, uncompromising and a bully. Lemons can turn to negative mode if they're unable to express themselves either in the workplace or during outside activities. Burn-out and overwork are other situations which can propel them into negative mode, although these can quickly be readjusted with a holiday in the sun, under clear blue skies.

Lemons who are oscillating between positive and negative can be very confusing as they smile one minute and scowl the next. Workaholics as Lemons are, they're inevitably under stress and when the crunch comes, everyone is in the firing line. Their mood swings come very fast, confusing those around them, as positivity turns to deceit.

LINDEN BLOSSOM
FLORAL
Tilia vulgaris

CHARACTER
Consoling, Serenity, Security, Patience

USE TO COUNTERACT THESE NEGATIVE ATTRIBUTES
Nervousness, Anxiety, Nervous tension, Emotional debility, Hysteria, Over-excitement, Insecurity, Emotional blockages, Possessiveness, Jealousy, Anger, Stress, Irritability, Mood swings, Guilt, Lovelorn, Over-sensitivity, Indecision

USE FOR THESE POSITIVE ATTRIBUTES
Relaxed, Calm, Soothed, Self-confident, Secure, Balanced,
Structured, Stable

Linden Blossom

LINDEN BLOSSOM PERSONALITY PROFILE

The sweet perfume of linden blossom gives a clue to the character of this profile – sweet, calm, gentle and very feminine – whether the person is male or female. If male, he will be in touch with his feminine side, appearing to understand women – a 'new man', one might say. If female, she will be 'womanly'. This profile has a calmness about them that affects other people deeply. Usually these types have very rounded personalities. They stand no nonsense from anyone and are happy and content with themselves. Confident with who they are from an early age, Lindens will be determined to follow the path they have set for themselves, carrying on regardless of any opposition to their plans. These are open and up-front people, helpful when the mood takes them. They're a very interesting personality as they can change and wear many guises.

Lindens are perfectly happy to reside in the shadow of their partner or family, nurturing their growth and encouraging their ambitions, perhaps hoping to win a large amount of cash so they will never have to work again ... or leave the home domain. When arriving back from a holiday, Lindens say, 'It's good to be home, I don't know why I bothered to go away.'

Lindens love nothing better than being at home with their family, and, if possible, often have large families. This personality can cook up a meal out of practically nothing in a minute, get the grass stains out of your clothes, and could write a book full of useful hints about running a home efficiently and taking good care of a family. Guests are welcome but will not get preferential treatment over a Linden's family – who always come first. In return, Lindens expect their family to adore them.

Due to lack of ambition, Lindens are often found in jobs which do not suit their temperament. They tell themselves this is a temporary measure but once in a familiar routine, will be reluctant to change, enjoying the train route, or the people they work with, or the way in which the company is run. These are people who will stay in a job for ever provided that it pays them sufficiently, the work is moderately satisfactory, and they're not expected to sacrifice too much. Workmates like Lindens because they're calming when a panic is on – when a deadline has to be reached, for example. (Just don't expect them to stay late!) Lindens are by no means timid, however, and will not suffer fools gladly.

A Linden woman can flirt outrageously just because it's fun, and with no ulterior motive – like trying to catch somebody else's man. She flirts like a three-year-old on her father's knee, all fluttering eyelashes and coy expression – with the milkman and the office clerk – yet rarely suffering sexual harassment, perhaps because of a child-like innocence. Linden males also flirt and will be quite surprised when it's taken for anything other than a little bit of fun. In fact, they don't know they're doing it and it can quite often lead to trouble – particularly when they try it on a Tuberose personality.

Many Lindens find that their idealized perfect partner simply doesn't exist so they end up with people who are inevitably less than perfect in their eyes. Although drawn to people similar to themselves, this is a disastrous partnership decision for them. They aim to partner successful people, and this can take many forms, not necessarily financial. Indeed, money is not the Linden's measure of success. Once in a relationship, infidelity never crosses their minds, and they would be hurt if anyone thought otherwise.

In love, Lindens can act more like a parent than a lover and will want to be in touch every moment of the day, just to make sure their loved one is all right. Being incurable romantics, in the first stages of romance Lindens will send poems, love letters, flowers, chocolates and all the traditional lover's gifts. This phase does wear off and then they'll wonder why there's no romance in their lives. In fact, this lack of romance is often due to a poor choice of partner and Lindens often turn to daydreaming.

If not satisfied with their lot, at some stage in life Lindens will look back on the past with regret and this can turn into recrimination, aimed at whoever they're with at this stage. This is when other activities start to take an interest, particularly as the children start to leave the nest. Lindens never get nervous or excited and are unlikely to shout in temper or anger. Instead, they sulk – which is not always good for their psyche.

In negative mode, Lindens are possessive – of their partner or children – always reminding everyone of what could go wrong. They become the worriers, the 'what if ?' type – 'what if the world blows up?', 'what if you have an accident, or there is no work, or I get the sack?' Negative Lindens half-expect to get mugged on the way home. If anyone is more than half an hour late, they'll wait by the phone getting more anxious by the moment. Lindens can easily end up having anxiety attacks over things they cannot possibly control while their families are caused to have tremendous guilt, and children may find it difficult to cut the ties that bind them.

Lindens hoard papers, books, old toys, clothes and furniture until the house is full of junk. Negative Lindens can easily start to envy others their possessions, blaming everyone around them for their lack of money, success and recognition, easily falling into the 'nobody cares if I live or die' type of speech to get sympathy. If all this becomes a regular occurrence, Lindens can drive friends away, children out of the home, and the partner insane. 'I gave up everything for you' will be heard, along with 'you never really loved me' – and selfishness will rule supreme. Luckily, before this happens, a bit of praise (a lot actually) coupled with reassurances and continual expressions of love, will put Lindens back on their feet.

MANDARIN
FRUITIE
Citrus reticulata, C. nobilis

CHARACTER
Gentle, Peaceful, Revitalizing, Sympathetic

USE TO COUNTERACT THESE NEGATIVE ATTRIBUTES
Anxiety, Depression, Grief, Inner child, Abuse, Dejection, Emptiness, Dwelling on the past, Over-excitable, Desolate, Emotional trauma

USE FOR THESE POSITIVE ATTRIBUTES
Calm, Uplifted, Refreshed, Inspired, Soothed, Sprightly, Integrity, Tranquility

MANDARIN PERSONALITY PROFILE

The Mandarin personality is sweet, gentle, kind and loving – one of the softest personalities. Their kindness is extended to all living, breathing things including plants, fish, animals, humans, and to inanimate objects like the teddy bear that was precious to them as a child, and still is. They'll have boxes full of letters from old friends, photos, dried flowers, and champagne corks kept from rendezvous long ago. Everything is lovingly protected. Gentle in everything, the Mandarin personality has a meek manner but this doesn't mean their spirit is meek – which is a mistake many people make.

Mandarin personalities are childlike in that they need love and protection and, not consciously, they draw out protectiveness in others with an air of needing to be looked after, even if they don't actually need it. Women want to 'mother' male Mandarins, knitting them sweaters and cooking them dinner, while men find themselves carrying shopping for the female Mandarin, helping with chores and protecting them from the wicked world. Mandarins don't complain about all this attention, and rather like it, but to be constantly cosseted in this way can get on the nerves of even the gentlest, sweetest person and Mandarin will feel at some point the need to break free. This they will eventually do, after some diplomatic scheming – the last thing a Mandarin would do is hurt somebody's feelings or bruise their ego.

Mandarins are very uplifting and, as the saying goes, can 'gladden the old man's heart'. They often take care of the older generation, who appreciate their courtesies. The fact that the Mandarin personality can spend much of life caring for other people shows they are quite tough, despite their childlike qualities. This toughness becomes apparent when Mandarins are left entirely on their own to fend for themselves. They manage better than most of us – proving what a paradoxical and complex character they are. With careful nourishing, they bloom and outlive everyone, still carrying on when stronger types have fallen by the wayside. Perhaps nature looks more kindly on the docile and cautious!

Actually, Mandarin might have drifted into this personality just for the sake of peace and that becomes a problem when their true selves break free of whatever restrictions have been built up. Friends and family can't believe what's happening, as Mandarins shed their meek personality like a snake skin. The Mandarin personality is sometimes adopted as a result of childhood trauma, in one of its many forms – from actual physical abuse to unkind words overheard and taken into the subconscious. The child decides it's better to be meek, gentle and caring as a protection mechanism, so they might avoid getting more of the same.

Mandarins love children and will protect them fiercely, ever watchful and mindful of what dangers could befall them. This constant awareness of potential dangers can make Mandarins reluctant to have children but, when they do, the children complain of the lack of freedom. Hopefully, they won't choose a partner who repeats the patterns they suffered as a child – they need someone who won't take advantage of their good naturedness and kindness, and who helps them become more assertive and carefree.

A negative Mandarin can become hysterical at the slightest thing, and compulsive – usually about cleanliness, both personal and domestic. They have night terrors and experience fear out of all proportion – afraid to meet people, afraid of life – and will be nervous, jumpy and full of unnecessary grief. When their emotional sanity is so shot to pieces they can become quite uncontrollable, like creatures much too fragile to walk this earth.

One typical Mandarin personality who came to me as a patient was Jennifer, who had reached the age of sixty without ever having thought of doing anything for herself. She came from a household that forbade any extrovert behaviour, with a very authoritarian father, and escaped at the age of seventeen into a loveless marriage to a man ten years older, who needed someone to care for him, rather than a loving relationship. For over forty years she cooked and cleaned, doing everything for him and their children, constantly at everyone's beck and call. She went to work as a school cook and handed her wages over to the husband at the end of the week. Everyone thought she was contented, driving the kids back and forth to their activities, and her husband to his rotary club or for a night out with the boys. Only her best friend, another meek Mandarin type, knew how boring she found it all.

When her husband died suddenly as a result of an accident, Jennifer realized she didn't even know where her husband banked their money! She got furious with herself, with her parents and especially her husband for leaving her like this.

Jennifer had to become assertive. Enjoying her new independence, she sold the house and eventually moved to France where she fell in love for the first time, and started a new life. Finally, she said, she had found herself. Of course the children said 'what about us?', and the rest of the family thought she'd gone completely mad, but Jennifer was happy at last – with someone who realized how precious her kindness and gentleness were; a true partner.

MARJORAM, SWEET
HERBIE
Origanum marjorana

CHARACTER
Comforting, Soothing, Warming, Strengthening

USE TO COUNTERACT THESE NEGATIVE ATTRIBUTES
Anxiety, Hysteria, Hostility, Withdrawn, Mental strain, Tantrums, Anger, Irritability, Overactivity, Weak will

USE FOR THESE POSITIVE ATTRIBUTES
Calm, Balanced, Direct, Self-assured, Integrity, Courage, Confidence, Focus, Perseverance, Restored, Sincere

MARJORAM, SWEET, PERSONALITY PROFILE

The Marjoram personality is warm and friendly, always ready to offer comfort and solace under their wing. These people make really good friends and are solid, calm, steady, organized, and potentially strong and straightforward. Although they generally prefer to watch events from the sidelines, they can be outspoken if necessary. It's quite difficult to gauge their feelings because emotions are rarely shown, and are certainly never over-dramatized. Generally, Marjorams keep themselves to themselves and will not intrude upon another person's privacy unless asked to. The steadying influence of Marjoram is often mistaken for dullness or lack of imagination but this is a mistake soon recognized once you get to know them. They do enjoy life, but choose to show it in caring.

Marjorams are great animal lovers. They'll take in any stray cat or dog and look after the neighbour's hamster when they go on holiday. Indeed, Marjorams often feel more in tune with animals than with people and are often found in jobs relating to animals, such as vets, veterinary nurses, animal rescue teams, animal wardens and the like. Although not active campaigners, they are quite likely to be found working in the offices of organizations concerned with saving whales and dolphins or, if they have the money, will send donations to help the cause.

Marjorams don't hang on to money for long, not because they spend it on themselves, but because it goes on family or friends. It'll be the Marjoram who lends the Jasmine personality the money to buy a new outfit for a hot date, and the Marjoram who will stock up the fridge with goodies to please the Cardamon. These things are done out of the kindness of Marjoram's heart, with no thought of reward but, because Marjoram is so generous, they are often taken advantage of. Sadly, because Marjorams don't expect any rewards, they often don't even receive a courteous 'thank you'. This can make Marjoram very depressed actually, because all they really want is for people to appreciate their kindness and when they realize they're being taken advantage of can become irritable, withdrawn and, apparently, emotionally cold.

Marjorams often find that people drop into their houses as if it were their natural right, which is all very well except that people often forget to invite Marjoram around to their place in return. Relationships can be very one way. Often, Marjorams don't get invited to parties, not because they weren't intended to come, but because they were simply forgotten! They're like the toothbrush you use several times a day but forget all about when you're not using it – an essential but invisible part of life. If Marjorams are romantically teamed up with a Floral you can expect sexual disharmony because although Marjorams are gentle, kind people, they aren't very sexy, much preferring to curl up with a good book in front of the fire, than share a candlelight bath with their partner.

Marjorams can quite happily live in a house that is tumbling down around their heads, with a threadbare carpet and doors that don't shut properly . . . because they're just not bothered. The same goes with appearance. Old, comfortable clothes are preferred and Marjorams will stick with the style adopted in their thirties right through to old age, never changing. They cannot see the need to buy anything new, thinking that if you already possess something why throw it out and, indeed, take pleasure in making things last for as long as possible. This attitude can cause problems with the family, who are also expected to make do with what they've got.

Marjorams are good people, not necessarily the go-getters, but needed to stabilize and 'ground' the more flamboyant types. They are sincere, having great courage, stamina and perseverance.

MELISSA
HERBIE
Melissa officinalis

CHARACTER
Calming, Supportive, Sensitive, Fostering

USE TO COUNTERACT THESE NEGATIVE ATTRIBUTES
Nervous tension, Stress, Anxiety, Irritability, Over-excitement, Restlessness, Melancholy, Sadness, Grieving, Sorrow, Depression, Emotional crisis, Mental exhaustion, Lethargy, Negativity

USE FOR THESE POSITIVE ATTRIBUTES
Strength, Revitalized, Happy, Gentle, Spiritual growth, Relaxed, Peaceful, Positive, Progressive, Cheerful

MELISSA PERSONALITY PROFILE

The Melissa personality is bubbly, fizzy, full of energy and usually delightful, with a multitude of interests and activities. This personality finds time to go to yoga class, attend interest-

Melissa

ing talks, and will know about all the events worth seeing, listening to, or being part of. Not only that, they find time to do it all as well as hold down a full-time job and, possibly, take care of a family. Melissas never forget to phone home, feed the cat, walk the dog or make sure the essential groceries are in the house. How do they do it? The fact is that Melissas are not only highly organized, like the Grapefruit personality for example, but they have such a love of life that even one second is, to them, too precious to waste. Melissa doesn't waste time thinking *'Shall* I do it?', but just muddles through without giving it much thought, doing things because they *want* to.

Melissa has a youthfulness, and a revitalizing effect on just about everyone they meet, so is very much in demand. You can find many imitations of the Melissa personality but a true Melissa is unmistakable. Their house is full of things, but this is not collecting for collecting's sake; they gather things around them that they need for some reason, that are relevant to them at a particular time. For example, they might purchase an Indian art object without any particular purpose but then discover in it something they feel a connection with, and go on to collect many Indian art pieces. When they no longer feel connected to whatever it was that appealed to their soul,

Melissa will dispose of the collection and go on to something else.

When Melissas come to look after their health they throw themselves into a quest of knowledge as if it were their vocation. No stone will be left unturned. Melissa will read everything available on the subject, and discuss it with everyone, gleaning more information all the time. However, this knowledge will not be used on themselves. It's almost as if by absorbing all the information about a particular disorder, the actual treatment is no longer required.

Melissas are very enthusiastic and like to try new and exciting things. Some people might accuse them of being 'over the top', but this is unfair – there's nothing wrong with having an open mind and being positive about things. Some people find them frivolous and perhaps not serious enough, again this is unfair because Melissas are actually very serious people and are usually born with a good sense of judgement, sometimes bordering on that of the sage.

Because they bubble with so much enthusiasm, Melissas are not usually thought of as candidates for meditation or other solitary practices but they do indeed excel at receiving insight and truths, which are lost to others who are not so open to all that life has to offer. Melissas live very much in the here and now, although they have respect for the past and thought for the future.

Partners who cannot let go of the past are very bad for Melissas, dragging them into the negative vortex. The soft-hearted Melissa cannot absorb this fundamentally opposing view. Melissa wants to get on with life and anyone harping on about the past prevents them doing that. Indeed, Melissa cannot take the weight of unnecessary guilt or emotional baggage and if forced to take it on board will crack, and become negative. They can become anxious and lose interest in life, stop their many activities and just sit in front of the TV, never going out and seeing friends. The wrong partner can turn these bright effervescent people into zombies, and the sad thing is that Melissa may not even notice this process happening, until it's too late. The shocking thing is that their partner and friends may welcome this change because it means there is more time for them. At least if Melissa is at home on the sofa, one knows where to find them! Parents are usually the first to recognize what's going on and, sadly, can welcome the change with 'good, they've slowed down, more time for me to visit and get attention'.

Melissas attract jealousy and spitefulness and unadventurous souls, who feed off their vivacious, outgoing nature, and admire their control of life. The trouble is, these people want to *tame* Melissa and make her (or him) more like themselves. Throughout it all, however, Melissa will always try to find the good side in people. Melissa is a very sweet-natured personality and, despite the attempts of negative people to make them otherwise, essentially independent.

Elizabeth Jones, OBE, MCSP, DRE, MIFA Reg., MISPA, physiotherapist and aromatherapy tutor:

'Uplifting, joyous, quickens the spirit, having a subtle, piquant character, unlike the more direct citrus note of lemon. A "happy" oil.'

NARCISSUS
FLORAL
Narcissus poeticus

CHARACTER
Hypnotic, Empowering, Mesmerizing, Sagacious

USE TO COUNTERACT THESE NEGATIVE ATTRIBUTES
Hysteria, Nervousness, Irritability, Tension, Grief, Addictions, Withdrawal, Loneliness, Illusions, Disillusionment, Longings, Hopelessness, Obsessions, Trauma, Emotional wounding, Misery, Anguish, Emotional analgesia

USE FOR THESE POSITIVE ATTRIBUTES
Inspired, Creative, Stillness, Meditative, Inner vision, Aspirations, Idealistic, Sensuous, Visionary, Discovery, Truthfulness

NARCISSUS PERSONALITY PROFILE

Before saying anything about the Narcissus personality, I must first dispel any preconceived associations that may be made with the personality trait 'narcissism'. This word comes to us from the ancient Greek tale of a young man, Narcissus, who fell in love with his own reflection and eventually pined away. Narcissism thus means to have a morbid self-love or self-admiration. In fact, by strange coincidence, the very next word in my dictionary is 'narcosis', meaning 'the production of a narcotic state' and it is this which more accurately reflects the quality of narcissus, the flower and essential oil, the aroma of which can achieve mystical effects on the emotions and mind. Indeed, it was probably the hypnotic effect of the plant narcissus which induced the person Narcissus, so long ago, to transport into another, unreal world – a world in which he could so detach from himself, he thought he was someone else! So, while the fragrance of narcissus is most certainly a hypnotic, it would be quite wrong to think that the Narcissus personality suffers from self-admiration and love.

The Narcissus personality is one of closeness, of clandestine moments, poised between the conscious and subconscious. This is the personality of the seeker of truth – no matter how deep or painful that journey may be. Narcissus is deep and thoughtful so people often refer to them as old souls that have been reincarnated. There is nothing carefree about them although being masters of camouflage they're very often able to give the opposite impression. Narcissus is found at the trendiest parties, laughing and joking, and at the art event or reception of the year, pursuing someone who may give them a contract. They enjoy being involved in the most 'happening' events – and this can lead to the impression of superficiality. In fact, they are quietly weighing up the objectives of everyone and subtly rooting out dark secrets, while sensing the place of everything, as well as everyone, in the room.

Because the Narcissus personality is ever changing, it's not easy to get to know them intimately. They change the colour and cut of their hair, their clothing style, their friends, lovers, houses and even the country in which they live. Like many other free, creative people, Narcissus is often misunderstood. It is wrong to accuse Narcissus of not having any passion, or for not being understanding, but the accusation of delving into things too deeply may sometimes be justified.

Narcissus points out other people's mistakes and notices potential dangers at work or play – and 98.9 per cent of the time they're correct. It is precisely this ability to see what's ahead, their precognitive faculty, which infuriates others and leads them to mistrust Narcissus. But, through it all, Narcissus has complete trust in their own judgement, which is excellent. Being a friend of Narcissus is an experience in itself – once they feel comfortable with you, you'll see that they can be hilariously funny, with a wicked, dry sense of humour.

This personality type is always impeccably dressed, with clean pressed clothes and mended, polished shoes. Loving fine things that have been crafted with sweat and tears, Narcissus will fondle a piece of carved wood as if actually identifying with the pain and sacrifice of the tree from which it came. Not only that, they can tune in to the feelings of the man or woman who carved the wood and even imagine the chips of wood that fell to the ground in the process. Everything is experienced in the round, totally – beyond three dimension.

The presence of Narcissus is inspiring – a mystical transference of self-confidence and assurance. They're very kind in their words, even if they are not always genuine, saying 'it does no harm to be graceful', and are invariably found in jobs which match their abilities – anything that requires creativity, inspirational actions and intuitive behaviour. They make great composers, writers, painters, architects and scientists and are often black-balled for ideas that seem to be 'off the wall' but which will, in time, become accepted theory.

Narcissus personalities have freedom of mind and consciousness and there are no ties which can bind them down or hold them back. This is irritating for others, even their family. But they make great parents, never questioning their offspring's motives for doing anything, just accepting them for who they are – independent beings. This, in turn, gets Narcissus into trouble because people accuse them of having no interest in anyone other than themselves, of being arrogant and too involved in their own affairs to worry about their children (or anyone else). But of course they worry about other people. Indeed, they've probably had premonitions and think about them more than anyone could ever guess.

Narcissus personalities are what one might call 'relaxed passionates'. In love they'll be both tender and passionate and love both physically and spiritually, seeing no point to love unless a spiritual bond can be forged with the partner. However, if they become negative their love can indeed turn inwards and, preferring their own company and thoughts, all overtures of love will be rejected. Being distant and withdrawn is used as a protection from more hurt and thoughtlessness. Those who have the capacity of loving unconditionally, like Narcissus, need to withdraw sometimes as a self-protection mechanism. If, as a child, they were subjected to emotional trauma, Narcissus could retreat into a shell and may never emerge unless coaxed out by gentleness and love, such as can be given by the Rose Otto type of personality. Any early trauma will be carried over into adulthood, ready to resurface at times of stress.

It seems that the Narcissus personality needs acclaim, kudos and even exaltation, when in negative mode; this is when their egos become very fragile and Narcissus becomes self-effacing, self-limiting and doubting of the intuition they previously trusted. No longer listening to their inner dialogue, Narcissus can turn to new ways to seek truth – such as using drugs.

Generally, however, Narcissus-type people are gentle souls, much misunderstood. They seem to have brought knowledge forward from past lives, knowledge which gives them both anguish and pleasure. But only Narcissus will know the extent of all this because they will never tell anyone the whole story.

Vivian Lunny, MD, MBBS, MDMA, MIFA Reg, MISPA, RQA, aromatherapist and tutor:

'Narcissus has a spiritual quality and a flair for dissolving different boundaries, breaking through mental and spiritual blockages. This personality can be very persuasive, seductive and broadminded. It despises pettiness, while loving freedom, joy, laughter and fun. It clears away low self-esteem.'

NEROLI (Orange Blossom)
FLORAL
Citrus aurantium, C. brigaradia, C. vulgaris

CHARACTER
Spiritual, Pure, Loving, Peaceful

USE TO COUNTERACT THESE NEGATIVE ATTRIBUTES
Anxiety, Stress, Tension, Shock, Emotional crisis, Sadness,
Longing, Panic, Grief, Inner child, Abused as child,
Abused as adult, Depression, Hopelessness, Fear

USE FOR THESE POSITIVE ATTRIBUTES
Lightness, Lifting of sorrows, Spiritual, Connected, Completeness,
Joy, Understanding, Guided, Calm, Stable, Regenerated, Peaceful

NEROLI PERSONALITY PROFILE

Neroli, also known as Orange Blossom, is one of the most spiritual personalities – another angel, like Chamomile Roman. Whatever their age, there is an in-built wisdom that extends far beyond that of worldly knowledge. Neroli is another personality that seems to have found a way to be ageless, forever young in a Spring-like way. This is not the rashness of youth, but the fresh enjoyment of everything from the smallest flower to the tallest tree.

The Neroli personality is not a cynic, and will always be

able to find happiness in something, acknowledging the imper-
fections in people but easily bypassing them to find the good.
This is not a blind judgement. This personality is fully aware
of the evil that exists in the world, just as the Frankincense
personality is, and will be quite open about it, possibly recognizing it in people before others do, but in charity will say
'something has to make a person like that'. If nasty gossip is
heard about someone they will be the first to point out the
person's good points, reminding the scandal-mongers of things
of merit that the person may have done.

In today's aggressive world Neroli's good intentions may
seem misplaced, and they get mistaken for being daft or
stupid, easily taken in by people. But Nerolis like to give,
within reason, their fellow man every possible chance. This
personality has high morals – and will not lie, cheat, steal,
murder or harm anyone or anything. Apart from that, anything
goes! Being a floral, they can understand overwhelming
passion but will not condone extra-marital affairs – yet not
condemn them either. Always giving credit where credit is
due, Nerolis are altogether good people.

If you have a lover or friend who fits this personality they
will never crowd you, sensing when you need to be alone, but
be ready to have fun when you are. Unfortunately, Nerolis can
easily be taken advantage of by people they love. Friends and
family get so used to being put first, it often leads to Neroli
types having their own needs go unrecognized, yet they do not
bear grudges or resentments.

Neroli strongly believes that no-one on this planet has any
right to dictate how they should think, feel and act. This can
sometimes get them into hot water. They respect authority as
necessary for an orderly life but all other matters are between
God and themselves – so you'd better not interfere. This basic
respect of authority can mutate into a strong sense of injustice
as this sensitive personality battles with the understanding that
some people in power are not as honest as they portray themselves to be. Neroli can have a hard time grappling with the
fact that not all people on this planet realize that you can't take
it with you when you go, so why be greedy now?

Neroli types are happiest when searching the mysteries of

life as a hobby. Saddened by the lack of understanding in the world today, they can turn to being supersensitive souls. This can be tricky if you work for a Neroli or have one as a partner because, half the time, you won't understand what it is you did wrong.

Neroli can be very deep emotionally, and if in a negative frame of mind, are easily angered, usually with the 'you just do not understand' kind of line. They can stray from reality, and be unaware of it, and may be inclined to dismiss many of the facts of living today, just because the ideas don't fit into their philosophy. It is at this point Neroli may become withdrawn and timid, and refuse to enter into the physical world, deciding it's just too bad out there – prone to dark, deep depressions, feeling that the world is against them. These types may say they are communing with angels, have visions, and so on, and who can say they are not? But they can get drawn in by tricksters during these negative periods and start to mistrust their own inner feelings and knowledge.

Nerolis are good in jobs that do not have to deal with any of the things they abhor, particularly deviousness, so won't do well in politics or law, nor will they want to take jobs which deal exclusively with money. They are good in professions that are fairly straightforward, such as crafts, carpentry, electronics, engineering, conservation and teaching. They are very good with children and make great playleaders or, because of their empathy, carers for the physically and mentally challenged. Many Nerolis are found to be florists or gardeners, and may choose to become spiritual counsellors of one kind or another, playing an active role in their chosen religion or belief. They're clear-sighted and calm, with a peaceful air, seemingly quite balanced emotionally – and between their male and female sides, believers in great love for all.

ORANGE
FRUITIE
Citrus sinensis

CHARACTER
Warming, Happy, Resolute, Energizing

USE TO COUNTERACT THESE NEGATIVE ATTRIBUTES
Depression, Hopelessness, Sadness, Apathy, Resignation,
Withdrawn, Self-consciousness, Anxiety, Emotional violence,
Emotional abuse, Worry, Selfishness, Obsessions, Addiction,
Burn-out

USE FOR THESE POSITIVE ATTRIBUTES
Joy, Uplifted, Sunny, Balanced, Lighthearted, Regenerated, Strong,
Creative, Positive, Self-confident, Sympathetic, Courageous

ORANGE PERSONALITY PROFILE

There can be very few people who dislike the smell and
taste of the orange fruit, and there are very few people who
wouldn't fall under the spell of the cheerful, optimistic orange
personality. These sunny people are a joy to be with. They're
open-hearted, witty, funny, honest, and embrace ideas and suggestions as easily as they embrace people. The Orange personality is never shy and loves to touch, giving a quick cuddle
if you need it. Luckily, their personality doesn't lead people to
think they have ulterior motives, which is a good thing
because they're inclined to touch a lot – children, adults, family, friends, workmates and strangers.

What people notice first about the Orange personality type
is their great sense of humour. They have an easy, friendly
smile, an amused look in their eyes, and openness and understanding seems to exude from every pore in their body. What
a pity there aren't more Orange personalities in the world!
They're quite often found mixed with elements of the Neroli
or Petitgrain personalities, complicating the matter of recog-

nition. The Orange type is warm, sweet and sensuous, and has a positive effect on everything and everyone – not in an over-bearing way, but in a gentle, harmonizing effort to make everything all right.

Oranges are found in all walks of life and are very adapt-able, although particularly in any sort of job that needs kind-ness and an empathetic approach. They enjoy working in areas which utilize their natural flamboyance, such as show-business and, if successful, will devote time to charity work. They make good supervisors and administrators, being good organizers who won't stand for any nonsense. Any job close to negativity or human suffering affects their sensitivity, and disillusionment and burn-out will eventually result.

Negative Oranges become despondent and emotionally dis-torted. They're liable to be the receivers of emotional abuse and violence, particularly if the wrong partner is chosen. Because of their deep faith in the human race, Oranges can become victimized if they're not careful, or are unbalanced, and can quite often resort to obsessive behaviour such as con-tinually washing their hands, checking they've locked up over and over again, and so forth. They tend to put their feelings of unhappiness aside and do not recognize the harm they are doing to themselves. This is further aggravated by the fact that other people don't see the sadness and hopelessness and when they do, it may be too late.

When you're so used to seeing someone always in positive mode, happy and optimistic, you'd think it would be easy for people to recognize depression when it comes along. Not so. Orange's family and friends are likely to say 'what's wrong with you?' or 'cheer up, it's not like you to be this down' but replying 'I'm fine' with a smile, poor Orange may be sinking further down each day. Not only does Orange refuse to recog-nize that they need help, other people get so used to Orange being so cheerful and helpful, they just don't see that Orange can have problems too.

Oranges make marvellous parents and are popular with all children, including their own. They are like the mothers in situation comedies who keep the family together through end-less dramas, work themselves to the bone, and are sunny and funny while they do it. Oranges can be loud, over-confident and, because of the amount of energy they have, exhausting. An inner radiance gives them incredible beauty, and their vitality makes them very thoughtful, considerate and fun lovers and, when single, they'll have prospective partners queuing up to take them out.

ORMENIS FLOWER
(Chamomile Maroc)
HERBIE/FLORAL
Ormenis multicaulis

CHARACTER
Unhurried, Composed, Mindful, Mystic

USE TO COUNTERACT THESE NEGATIVE ATTRIBUTES
Stress, Tension, Anxiety, Dread, Overactive mind, Highly strung,
Impulsive, Indecisive, Confused, Abused, Bad temper,
Emotionally controlling, Emotional blockages, Fearful

USE FOR THESE POSITIVE ATTRIBUTES
Calm, Empathetic, Courageous, Earthed, Relaxed, Mindful,
Able to let go, Attentive, Meditative, Consoled, Soothing

ORMENIS FLOWER PERSONALITY PROFILE

Ormenis Flower has long been mistaken for and used as Chamomile when it cannot be said to be anything like it, not having the chemical constituents of Chamomile – although it does come from the same botanical family. Its use in aromatherapy derives from the fact that it has long been sold as Chamomile, and is far cheaper. Over the years, the qualities of Ormenis have been hidden behind this mis-naming but its true personality is easy to smell! Ormenis is rich and balsamic with hidden depths that are unmistakably alive and very vibrant.

The Ormenis profile is of the secret person, one who always likes to keep their true selves hidden. They are masters of disguise in everything they do, and very efficiently hide their emotions and true intentions. Ormenis is a slow, dilatory type of person, who takes everything at their own pace, with no hurrying, rushing or rashness in their movements. Everything will have a motive, and every step will be a deliberate one. Although they may have been planning something for weeks Ormenis can make it seem unplanned and fateful, but in fact, this type never leaves anything to fate. Everything is carefully planned and calculated.

Ormenis personalities may talk for hours and hours about a project they intend to start, but it may never get off the ground. 'Why hurry?' they'll ask, 'there is plenty of time to sit, think and talk about it.' Laid back isn't the word for it and to Grapefruit personalities, for example, Ormenis types can be infuriating but, in fact, some projects do actually make it off the drawing board.

Ormenis people like to be in charge and like to be thought of as thinkers – wise men or women not in the medicinal sense, but in metaphysical *knowing*! Secrets are safe with them so don't tell an Ormenis if you want a rumour spread, but take them for an ally. You can unload your problems on to this personality but be prepared for a long speech advising and counselling you, and you'll be expected to carry it all out. They tend to have an answer for everything, and if they haven't, they know a man who does. Ormenis types are full of wonderful and exotic stories and experiences and make wonderful story-tellers. As a family member, and with friends, Ormenis is always able to calm explosive situations.

It's difficult to see when Ormenis is in negative mode because most of the time they appear to be in control, although paradoxically passive, and being in control is what their negativity is about. But negative Ormenis types can be very controlling, expecting to be obeyed no matter what, without question and immediately. They can cut you dead in the street, or be abusive, and may stop talking to you one day and never speak to you again. This type do not listen to reason easily (except their own), and may be very patronizing and condescending towards others when in this negative mode. They seem to have a coldness of emotion completely in contrast to their normal warm selves. Ormenis types appear more male in character than female, although this personality is very much attuned to the earth's ways. Ormenis seems to be an adaptogen between the male and female parts of us. It brings a warmth that the Chamomiles can never bring, and is the personality of the wise person who values the earth and all its treasures.

PATCHOULI
LEAFIE
Pogostemon cablin

CHARACTER
Grounding, Soothing, Unruffled, Assured

USE TO COUNTERACT THESE NEGATIVE ATTRIBUTES
Depression, Anxiety, Indecision, Lethargy, Sluggishness, Egotistical, Stress, Tension, Mood swings, Touchiness

USE FOR THESE POSITIVE ATTRIBUTES
Invigorated, Restored, Reasonable, Lucid, Astute, Stimulating, Persistent

PATCHOULI PERSONALITY PROFILE

Patchouli is well balanced between the earth and the sky, grounded yet able to lift up and reach for the unattainable. As this type are grounded, they often have that effect on people around, giving the impression, perhaps, that they are slow or sluggish – which couldn't be further from the truth. There is an elderly quality about Patchouli, ancient and steady, no matter how old they may be. Patchoulis are born aged forty!

As a child, Patchouli may seem dull compared with their hyperactive siblings, and parents may worry that they never seem to want to play with the other children, being perfectly happy on their own. But by the time Patchouli reaches the teens, they'll be further advanced than their peers – both emotionally and intellectually, which may find them having older friends. Patchoulis will convince the family that they have ambition, strength and courage to attain their dreams, even if

Patchouli

they don't have the talent for it, but because they have the determination. It is Patchoulis' ability to stick at a thing, and be tenacious, that in most cases will allow them to succeed. Once a course has been determined, Patchouli will strive hard to reach the highest positions.

This personality is very astute, never missing a trick, always ready when a good opportunity presents itself. Not that Patchouli is opportunistic, it's just that they happen to be in the right place at the right time, so why let the chance go to somebody else? Patchoulis stand their ground and when at school or university will be a strong member of the debating society.

Activities which might be considered slightly oddball will appeal to Patchouli, who may very well end up being an intrepid explorer. They also enjoy delving into the psyche and, with their gift of being able to draw people out of their shells, make good psychologists. Intensely interested in all sorts of obscure subjects which other people may find boring and irrelevant to life (like how long it takes a snail to cross a road compared to a worm) once Patchoulis get hooked on a subject, they'll keep exploring, over and over again, until fully satisfied that they have an answer to their questions. This personality gets indignant and outraged by all manner of things going on in society and is inclined to send letters to newspapers or television companies, not for publicity, but both as a way of protesting and using their right to do so. Patchoulis do not have a lot of friends, nor do they encourage the family to invade their personal territory – whether this is one room or a mansion, being perfectly happy on their own and quite capable of seeking out the company of others when desired.

The Patchouli personality can do well in science or related professions where his or her powers of reason can be put to good use. As Patchoulis have the power to be able to convey a complicated message in a more easily accessible form, they make good commentators and would do well in journalism, particularly of the investigative kind, or as a documentary film maker. Indeed, these people will do well in any job that requires reasoning and is intellectually stimulating, from librarianship to cabinet-making.

Patchoulis are not boring people and can be found burning the candle at both ends – until they burn themselves out! Being so grounded, it never occurs to them that they are just as fragile as other personalities and need to watch their health too. But when they do become ill, Patchoulis will become immobilized, unable to function or even think clearly; be tetchy and trying. Until they can get back on their feet again, depression often follows illness, and this personality may become even more negative as time goes on, as if rooted to the spot, unable to move.

In relationships, Patchouli likes to be in charge and will seek a partner who is able to take a passive role. The same goes for friendships. As the years go on, Patchouli seems to go into reverse, appearing younger in spirit and more adventurous, seeking out new experiences and relationships. Patchouli is a mysterious personality and you can never be quite sure how their lives will develop. Warmhearted, but slightly overbearing at times, they tend to hang on to people as if afraid to let them go, yet still want to be alone. This paradox is all part of the personality that is Patchouli.

Anna Marie Joyeux, MIFA Reg., aromatherapist:

'I see Patchouli as a link between the spiritual and the physical level. It is grounding, but at the same time can awaken the spiritual side of a person or balance it if they are feeling confused on the spiritual level.'

PEPPERMINT
HERBIE
Mentha piperita

CHARACTER
Clarifying, Awakening, Stimulating, Penetrating

USE TO COUNTERACT THESE NEGATIVE ATTRIBUTES
Mental fatigue, Shock, Helplessness, Overwork, Sluggishness, Lethargy, Apathy

USE FOR THESE POSITIVE ATTRIBUTES
Regenerating, Emotionally refreshed, Self-acceptance, Concentration, Vitality, Vibrancy

PEPPERMINT PERSONALITY PROFILE

The Peppermint personality is difficult to forget once you have met one as they cause an immediate reaction: either you like them or you can't stand them. There are no half measures. Some timid souls find them brash and overpowering, but they are never dull. Peppermint has an almost fearless spirit and this spills over into their relationships with people and animals. Unusual things will surround Peppermints, who are drawn to bright colours, loud clothes and even louder friends. They are very quick thinkers – the salesmen of life – alert to opportunities, excellent speakers with a quick intellect. On a good day Peppermint can remember the names of a whole gang of people they haven't met for years.

Peppermint's swiftness and quick thinking, combined with a good sense of humour, makes them witty, and they'd certainly make good stand-up comedians. Whatever the work, they are usually dynamic, and if working for someone else will charm them with wit, agility and adaptability. Jobs which are totally involving, both physically and mentally, suit this personality well. It might be flying a plane, sailing a ship or doing a stressful driving job, but whatever it is, it must combine mental agility and physical stamina to truly satisfy this type.

Peppermints are friendly people, who are quite concerned about the fate of others, even though they do like to be the centre of attention. They are not always thought of as honourable, but are, and can be quite old-fashioned about it – particularly if out to impress members of the opposite sex, who flock around them. This personality type enjoys mixed company more than that of their own gender. As friend or lover, be prepared to take a back seat to Peppermint's life.

Peppermints will be very loyal in relationships – no matter how stormy, but confusions often arise because the partner doesn't always know what the game-plan is. The younger males are inclined to brag as they're sure to get an audience that way. As an older person, Peppermint becomes the parent who always plays the clown at the PTA school play – 'a jolly good person', you hear people say about them.

A negative Peppermint is inclined to struggle between highs and lows, sadness and happiness. These swings can be quite severe and if they continue Peppermint will start to get sluggish, dull and lethargic, forget about everything and become intolerant and frustrated. At this point the fridge might become the focus of comfort eating and Peppermints can put on weight, get depressed and, eventually, become mentally incapacitated.

Positive Peppermints are often found as healers because

they have an empathy and sympathetic approach to life and, surprisingly perhaps, are quite able to stay calm and still enough for the healing to flow. They are popular in this profession because they can charm the client and make them feel at ease. These are sparky people who often act as a catalyst, inspiring others to get up and go.

PETITGRAIN
LEAFIE/WOODIE
Citrus aurantium, C. brigaradier

CHARACTER
Revitalizing, Balancing, Restoring, Clarifying

USE TO COUNTERACT THESE NEGATIVE ATTRIBUTES
Disharmony, Confusion, Difficulties, Depression, Mental fatigue, Nervous exhaustion, Insomnia, Sadness, Disappointment, Rigidity, Betrayal, Anger, Irrationality, Introversion, Pessimism

USE FOR THESE POSITIVE ATTRIBUTES
Harmonized, Uplifted, Joyful, Relaxed, Inner vision, Strength, Self-confidence, Stability, Optimism, Expressiveness

PETITGRAIN PERSONALITY PROFILE

Petitgrain, the orange leaf person, is often closely associated with the Neroli and, to a lesser extent, Orange personalities. This isn't surprising as all three essential oils are distilled from different parts of the orange tree and one person might have elements of all three personalities, which can make them difficult to categorize or recognize. At first, the Petitgrain personality may seem somewhat subdued or overshadowed by the more flamboyant Orange, or the more spiritual Neroli but in fact Petitgrain feeds the ego of Orange and balances the spirituality of Neroli. Petitgrain is like the first-born in a family, often carrying responsibility for the siblings, but not overloaded by them, because Petitgrain has copious amounts of energy, which can be equally distributed between various activities, and is apparently in tune with the rhythm of life. A link between sun and earth, Petitgrain personalities are the providers of comfort and emotional nourishment.

This personality appears to be in control, capable and never fazed, but are often underestimated and their qualities are not always given the recognition they deserve. Petitgrain may serve on a committee for years, gently guiding and counselling, doing all the work while others take the credit. They are respected at work and deemed responsible and steady.

But Petitgrains are by no means dull and can make stimulating company if given the chance, being good conversationalists and interested in other people's opinions – at least they give that impression, being too polite to do otherwise. Petitgrain will be totally taken with anyone who is not quite of such a responsible nature and one often wonders if they wouldn't secretly be happier if they themselves let go a bit. This isn't to say that Petitgrains aren't happy. At least, they always appear contented, no matter what, and they'd never admit to being otherwise – it would be, to them, 'terribly bad form'.

Petitgrains are the keepers of the small niceties that stop this world from going out of control – they're the maiden aunt who insists on tea at four o'clock or the middle-aged father who wants to give his children a sense of decency. Petitgrain parents will take the time and effort to point out both the good and bad and will try to present as many sides to a story as possible. They often feel that the world is toppling off its axis and that things need to be balanced and harmonized, but remain basically optimistic and can stimulate others into change.

Being optimistic doesn't stop Petitgrains being the providers and making sure there's money in the bank for a rainy day and a roof over their head. This personality isn't usually very well off, however, because promotions at work are given to whizz kids instead – not because Petitgrains aren't capable but because they are the anchors of the workplace and are just too valuable to move on upwards. Jobs that involve something other than making money for the shareholders interest these people (although if able to afford them, they'll have a few shares themselves), such as governmental office or a profession associated with care, hospital administration and the like. Petitgrain may dream of being an adventurer or film-star but wouldn't even try to pursue something so ambitious.

In a relationship, Petitgrain will only be as attentive as necessary and may have difficulty expressing how deeply they feel about a person. But when they fall in love they fall very hard and very deep and this can be a disaster for them if the relationship doesn't continue because their trust (more so than their heart) will have been broken. As lovers, Petitgrains wouldn't set the world on fire and although they have a warm nature it is not fiery or passionate. Because Petitgrain doesn't like to take risks, and may not feel they've met the right person, a long-lasting romantic relationship often eludes them.

When they're negative, Petitgrain gets very disillusioned with the general lack of concern for human life that is expressed in this world and often tries to alleviate these feelings by doing something positive themselves, no matter how small. Although often mistaken for being snobbish and cold, they are far from this; but can't be gushing or sentimental, which seems to them somewhat intrusive. Negativity makes Petitgrain irritable and their energy level goes right down so they may appear ill, and become very fixed in their ideas. This is especially the case when they want advancement but find their way blocked. If this happens Petitgrain can become quite eccentric, preferring their own company to anyone else's – cutting themselves off from human beings in general. You can still find them sitting in the sun, feeling the earth beneath them, and talking to the flowers or admiring the architecture, but they'll have no time for people. They'll become impatient, ill mannered and rude in an effort to get people out of their life – but this only happens when they've been deeply hurt. Indeed, Petitgrain becomes impossible when negative, particularly for their partners. They become snappy and find fault in everything, their nurturing instincts gone out of the window, despair having come in its place. Confusion, pessimism and rigidity can set it.

Generally, however, Petitgrains are stimulating and can harmonize the most fraught situation. They have a calm that transposes people, giving them the confidence to go out and do things for themselves. These are complex characters with profound spirituality and wisdom; however, they will not belong to any particular religious group because their conception of a deity is completely universal.

PINE
WOODIE/LEAFIE
Pinus sylvestris

CHARACTER
Acceptance, Understanding, Patience, Self-forgiveness

USE TO COUNTERACT THESE NEGATIVE ATTRIBUTES
Regrets, Guilt, Self-blame, Dissatisfaction, Self-critical, Worried, Overly responsible, Unconfrontational, Self-reproach, Unworthiness, Exhaustion, Masochistic, Miserable, Shameful, Feeling rejected, Unsympathetic, Feeling inadequate

USE FOR THESE POSITIVE ATTRIBUTES
Humility, Simplicity, Assured, Buffered, Forgiving, Perseverance, Sharing, Mindful, Trusting, Directness, Direction, Exhilarated, Acceptance of love, Tenacity, Confident

PINE PERSONALITY PROFILE

Although one would think that, like the Cypress, the Pine personality would be upright, direct and sometimes self-righteous, it is not, being like no other in that it is the child betrayed. Pine persons are the soft, gentle types who often go through life afraid to make a sound, or a mistake, and when they do will always say it was their fault. This personality can be self-critical, full of guilt, and constantly apologizing for everything and everyone. Never mind that it isn't their fault. The pine type is invariably 'wrung out' – you cannot carry the world on your shoulders and not feel exhausted.

Pine people are never satisfied with themselves, their work, or play, and then blame themselves for not having tried harder.

Pines are often the workaholic who has forgotten that it's OK to play sometimes – the sky won't fall in on them if work stops for five minutes.

Pines do not accept that anything can change, and may not wish it to, thus perpetuating the negative aspects of their life. However, there is a lighter side to Pine, who is capable of giving love in enormous quantities, and they're fearfully protective of their family and any causes which have caught their imagination. Pines can have large amounts of energy and are often able to help people in a similar situation to themselves without realizing it, becoming a home from the storm for troubled souls. Pines can help you see through the mists, and become clearer and calmer.

Because the Pine personality can be rather masochistic it is important that they recognize this tendency so that any guilty feelings can be transformed into a positive look at what is really happening, and in this way Pine learns to accept love instead of just giving it. They need to learn to understand their needs and desires, accept that it's OK to have them, and reach out to obtain them; it's OK to want to receive love – and you don't have to be passive about it. Using Pine essential oil can help put back the clear-sightedness needed to take a good, hard look at what you need, and it helps you slowly to put into practice the art of striving for it without setting unrealistic goals for happiness and life. Like a good walk in an alpine forest, Pine can help you make important decisions calmly and confidently.

Molly is typical of those who fall into the trap Pine personalities set for themselves. She got engaged on her sixteenth birthday, left school and became an apprentice hairdresser. By eighteen she had been talked into marriage and felt obliged to help her young husband build up his career as an electrician, spending every evening after work placing the adverts, doing the books, washing his overalls and tidying up the electrical equipment which he left all over the living-room floor, on the sofa, in the bedroom and on the kitchen table. She gave up her dream of owning her own salon, and concentrated on her husband's needs, and her growing family of four children. After all, she said, he was trying to make a good life for them all and she shouldn't moan.

When her husband started to buy second-hand equipment that also ended up all over the house, Molly would patiently clear it up, making a little space for herself, apologizing every time she moved something. Although it irritated her like mad, and she grew to hate her home, and avoided it whenever possible, she still carried on telling herself that it would all be all right one day. After all, she said, they needed the money. The children had to be fitted in around the wires, plugs, soldering irons and various boxes of tiny screws – a difficult thing with small children, who kept moving things about, for which she got the blame.

Gradually the strain became too much and Molly snapped. She had a breakdown which, of course, she thought was her fault. Wherever she went, others would burden her further with their own horror stories and tales of abuse but somehow, listening to others locked out her own problems. When she came out of hospital, with the help of various therapists, she started to look at what she wanted. It was a long, slow process during which her husband left her – taking his mess with him. Molly learned to take walks in the countryside, enjoy her children, and found she could say what she felt, and that she was a lovable human being.

ROSE MAROC
FLORAL
Rosa centifolia

CHARACTER
Passionate, Harmonious, Reassuring, Comforting

USE TO COUNTERACT THESE NEGATIVE ATTRIBUTES
Grief, Bitterness, Fear of letting go, Fear of love, Fear of sexuality, Jealousy, Resignation, Passivity, Deception, Vengefulness, Lack of ambition/motivation, Self-destruction

USE FOR THESE POSITIVE ATTRIBUTES
Motivated, Inner vitality, Revived, Confident, Passionate, Co-operative, Sense of freedom, Fulfilled, Forgiving, Sensual

ROSE MAROC PERSONALITY PROFILE

Just as Rose Otto represents the gentleness of spirit, Rose Maroc represents passion of the spirit. This is the passionate Rose, with a deep, hypnotic personality – vivacious and alive. The Maroc personality is deeply erotic in nature, and their lives are full of excitement and emotion.

The Rose Maroc is alive in every sense of the word. They love dramas – other people's, because Roses have no room in their own life for such time-wasting, life is too short for that. Everything this personality does is done with great fervour, delighting friends with sensuality and appreciation of life's pleasures. Imagine a flamenco dancer – that is Rose Maroc: very erotic, fully aware of their sexuality – and of the effect it can have on others. Many of the traits of Rose Otto are in the Rose Maroc personality too, the difference is that Rose Otto does everything with gentleness, while Maroc is soft but purposeful. This spiritual personality appreciates all life's sensual pleasures, so long as their enjoyment is not causing detriment to others.

Rose Marocs can comfort the deeper emotions and affect the souls of others. These Roses often become artists, poets, composers, musicians, singers, dancers, cooks, bodyworkers, or become involved in film, photography, journalism or design. They tend to wilt in any profession that does not allow them free rein of expression yet, like many people, may not have the choice.

When in negative mode, Rose Marocs can be overbearing and deceptive. They often unwittingly become involved in power struggles. If truly wronged and hurt, these are the Rose personalities that could become jealous and vengeful – particularly if someone hurts a member of their own circle. For themselves, they never worry and just accept the hurt and pain.

If the more spiritual side is neglected, Rose Maroc can become controlling and impatient, and when driven to succeed, can even become self-destructive. Although they get accused of bullying and always knowing best, nothing is done out of malice, but out of concern for the individual. They'll seek out the truth in all things, and won't tolerate lying or cheating, prudery or puritanical morality.

Marocs are often the power behind the throne of great men and women (and the not so great – which is why they need Rose Maroc). Parents can be charmed just as much as lovers and friends, and Rose gives unconditionally to everyone if deserving of their attention. Growing older, Roses can become eccentric and, if totally negative, impossibly cantankerous. But the younger generations love older Rose Marocs because of their wild stories and charming tolerance.

ROSEMARY
HERBIE
Rosmarinus officinalis

CHARACTER
Vigorous, Strengthening, Restorative, Centring

USE TO COUNTERACT THESE NEGATIVE ATTRIBUTES
Loss of memory, Learning difficulties, Lethargy, Disorientation, Fatigue, Indecision, Nervous exhaustion, Overburdened, Overworked, Strain, Emotional exhaustion, Sluggishness

USE FOR THESE POSITIVE ATTRIBUTES
Energy, Upliftment, Confidence, Creativity, Clarity, Structured, Concentration, Stabilized, Fortified, Sincere, Purified, Aware

ROSEMARY PERSONALITY PROFILE

Rosemarys are young at heart and seem to have found the elixir of youth. These are imaginative, happy, sensitive people, quite determined at times, but quite gentle souls, who are free of mental restrictions. They can be very creative and have quite a refreshing approach to the eternal problems of love and happiness.

Rosemary enjoys security and will aim to be in a secure position in love and in life because it's within a secure environment that they can express themselves fully. Nevertheless juggling things around is a feature of this

Rosemary

personality, who can easily balance two jobs, four hobbies and many friends. With a knack of putting things in order and well able to manage time and negotiate with people, Rosemary can achieve a great deal and will never do so by intentionally manipulating others.

Rosemary has a spirit that vibrates at an astonishing level, and some other types may find it difficult keeping up the pace. This vibrancy extends to their mental states, and to their ability to organize and concentrate on the many tasks they set themselves. Rosemarys have high ideals and like to think of themselves as slightly above the cut of others – not consciously arrogant, it's just their way. Challenges and new activities are welcomed, especially if they involve travelling. Their lighthearted approach can get them into trouble because others can take offence. Rosemarys judge things by the head, rather than the heart, and in general are open and trustworthy and make great mates. However, be prepared to be dragged out on cold, wet mornings to join in with the latest enthusiasm.

Rosemarys are usually very ecology conscious, and vegetarian – or at least trying, believing in animal rights and so on.

They don't want to be leaders but will be found going on marches or lobbying parliament or in jobs concerned with green politics, conservation or gardening, and would suit politics, trade unionism and teaching.

If they find themselves in jobs to which they are unsuited, Rosemarys will develop their negative traits. A lack of sincerity shows first, then they become surly, withdrawn and temperamental. In a relationship that is not altogether alive, they tend to become reproachful and have unaccountable traumas and dramas becoming, as they sink further into reproachfulness, very sharp tongued and quite unlikeable.

Rosemarys like beauty and their eyes may tell them to choose a gorgeous, drop-dead-for type – usually a Floral – and this might be fine while flirting and playing mind-games, but no good when it moves to the bedroom. Rosemarys are not the greatest lovers, being much more interested in why humans have a sex drive, than in sex itself. It can be difficult to be intimate with a Rosemary, although you would never believe it at first. Either male or female, they can also be abusive – turning their sexuality into anger. As young people they'll have lots of affairs, trying to find out just exactly what it is that interests everybody so much, but as they get older, will look for a secure relationship that doesn't ask too much of them in terms of romance – a good buddy rather than a lover.

Rosemarys remain happy into old age, and even when injustices befall them they feel invincible, protected by the gods. You can call on Rosemarys to help clear out old ghosts and memories from your cupboard, and clean the dark secrets out of your life.

ROSE OTTO
FLORAL
Rosa damascena

CHARACTER
Loving, Harmonizing, Comforting, Happy, Caring, Euphoric,
Gentle, Peaceful

USE TO COUNTERACT THESE NEGATIVE ATTRIBUTES
Depression, Sadness, Grief, Anger, Anxiety, Bitterness, Emptiness,
Fear of loving, Fear of not being loved, Broken heart, Guilt,
Shyness, Jealousy, Touchiness, Emotional crisis, Resignation,
Inexpression, Hopelessness, Despair, Abused, Emotional violence,
Hurt inner child

USE FOR THESE POSITIVE ATTRIBUTES
Comforted, Contentment, Devoted, Motivated, Inner vision,
Revival, Joy, Happiness, Inner freedom, Acceptance,
Completeness, Wisdom, Spirituality, Patience, Love,
Sensuality, Purity

ROSE OTTO PERSONALITY PROFILE

The Rose epitomizes the floral characteristics of the truly
feminine personality – both the positive and negative sides.
Although all Roses come under the same banner there are
subtle differences between the Rose Otto from Bulgaria,
Turkey, France or India, and as more species are distilled and
become available, such as the Rose di Mai, so other slight
variations will be noted. However, generalization does suit the
Rose personality as all Rose types are only a slight variation
on a theme – except for the absolute of the Rose Maroc.

The Rose Otto personality is one of gentleness and apparent
perfection. Although thought of as mainly feminine, the Rose
is also the feminine in the male. Some males carry more of this
type than others, and surprisingly perhaps the negative Rose
personality is often detected in males. Bulgarian Otto of Rose

is more suited to the feminine while Turkish Otto of Rose is more masculine.

Whatever the species, Rose is perfection personified. It's the ultimate female – one who can give unconditional love. This, and spirituality, is what the Rose personality strives for in themselves and others. The Rose is charming and lovely, an exquisite person. They will be well-mannered, ever-mindful of any hurtful phrases that may utter from them, caring, gentle and joyful. Roses are able to laugh at themselves, admit their silly actions and wrong deeds with no self-recrimination, or ego, always accepting full responsibility for their actions. Roses have the wisdom to know that there are far greater things in the universe than them, and that humans do make mistakes. Indeed, their presence and understanding is so peaceful, you'd think they were angels.

The pure-hearted generosity that Rose extends to other people is often misunderstood, but Rose seems to understand this as their fate and just continues anyway. Others are drawn to them, perhaps in the hope that some of their spirituality and inner vision might rub off. Bewitchingly lovely, Rose's words will be well-chosen, often soothing and peaceful.

However much the Rose personality might seem like the ultimate spiritual human being, they live in the real world and are real people, fighters who won't tolerate anyone undermining their efforts at work or at play. Full of confidence, they tend to play a lot, and are another Floral who use the sensuality to get what they want – although this is often subconscious, just part of their sensual selves. On form, Roses can be the ultimate lovers – full of sexual confidence, sensual and aware of their partners' needs, fully understanding of the spiritual elements in love and sex. People with a Rose profile enjoy life as it is, but you can't shackle this type if you try, in marriage for example. They'll be gone. However, this type never seem to bear grudges and will always consider themselves your friend.

The Rose personality loves co-operation, and unco-operative people shatter their rose-coloured world and may find it diffi-cult to understand why everyone doesn't operate on the same level as they do. Self-indulgence is enjoyed without guilt, whether this is reading a book when they should be at work, or playing in the park with a child when the car needs washing. Serving humanity is a trait of the Rose provided that it doesn't interfere with the pleasures and pathways of life – their life. If you get in the way, you could be on your way! Roses can be very blunt at times, and hate to lie – and see no point in it. If a Rose tells you to pack your bags, that doesn't mean they don't love you any more, just that they have to move on.

The Rose personality is found in jobs where the appreciation of fine, sensual things can be utilized. They are the silk merchants and art dealers, the models in fine gowns, the filmmakers and photographers, the artists and sculptors, composers and musicians, the writers, philosophers and spiritual counsellors. Places of spiritual worship hold a fascination for this personality, who may experience *déjà vu*, prophetic dreams, insight, and the all important *knowing*.

When Rose is in a negative mood everything becomes fate. Interest disappears and complete apathy takes over, along with moodiness, feelings of abandonment and resignation to their situation. They seem barely to exist in this world, all life drained out of them, as if stuck for eternity in a slow whirlpool of emotions with no exit. Only their sensuality remains.

Rose will blame outside influences for how they feel – not another person, but illness or job failure. It isn't always easy to see this side of Rose because to the outside world they appear much the same – concerned with others, caring and considerate. But the spark will be gone and eventually Rose will become boring company. People will leave them, and it becomes self-perpetuating. You hear 'I wonder why nobody visits me any more?' When ambition is thwarted, it becomes worse. The more sensitive Rose can just give up on life altogether. They will still love their friends, and give love, but they'll shut themselves off from receiving love – and a Rose without love shrivels up and dies.

If a loved one dies before Rose they'll be inconsolable, often dying of a broken heart. The Rose type doesn't grieve a little, they will grieve through to their very soul, for a very long time. As Rose's love touches the spiritual in the loved ones, the loss will be profound. Even if a brave face is shown to the world, the grief will still be there deep inside.

SANDALWOOD
WOODIE
Santalum album

CHARACTER
Enlightenment, Meditative, Balancing, Connecting

USE TO COUNTERACT THESE NEGATIVE ATTRIBUTES
Anxiety, Nervous tension, Possessiveness, Manipulating,
Unforgiving, Obsessive, Lonely, Accepting, Cynical, Insecurity,
Recurrent nightmares, Selfishness, Distressed, Uneasy, Hasty,
Aggressive, Irritable, Dwelling on the past

USE FOR THESE POSITIVE ATTRIBUTES
Warm, Comforted, Sensitive, Serene, Trusting, Harmonized,
Peaceful, Wise, Sensual, Expressive, Good self-esteem, Open,
Insightful, Unity

SANDALWOOD PERSONALITY PROFILE

The Sandalwood personality is serene and in charge of their
emotions, fully aware of their direction in life, even anticipating the rocky sections ahead. Their inner calm is like that of an
old soul, and Sandalwoods are certainly familiar with the concept of reincarnation. Their laid-back, philosophical attitude
mistakenly leads to them being accused of detachment.
Sandalwoods are very still people who listen more than they
talk, sizing you up – which they are very good at. This personality never consciously strives to be ahead of anyone else
in their thinking or deeds, but usually are, so invoke a lot of
jealousy.

The Sandalwood personality has a direct line with the universal telephone exchange and instinctively knows when
something is missing or not quite right. They leave no stone
unturned in the search for truth and are sometimes mistaken
for being terribly serious, which they can be *but* they're also
able to laugh at themselves and other people without any

malicious intent. The Sandalwood personality is supportive to people trying to pick up the pieces of their lives but tends to ignore their own problems, only handing out solutions to everyone else! Sandalwoods can be quite tactile people, in a gentle sort of way, depending on the mores of the culture in which they live. At times, they may long for the answer to life, appealing to the heavens to reveal just a little bit more. Understanding humanity so well, Sandalwoods make good healers.

Sandalwoods are very sensuous and sex is important to them and they may even have studied the secrets of Tantra, the ancient Indian cult of ecstasy, and will be amused by the antics in the Kama Sutra. These people are not afraid of their sexuality and will view it as one of the precious gifts we've been given here on earth to help us through this lifetime. Sex is never thought of simply as a means of procreation, or used for any ulterior motives – like making contacts or getting money. The Sandalwood personality is easy-going and comfortable, making them self-assured, calming people to be with, at ease with both genders.

On the negative side, Sandalwoods can be possessive of their knowledge, manipulating, bossy, controlling, and unable to admit mistakes. They may be prone to fits of anguish about their plight, and unforgiving. It has also been known for Sandalwoods to cut people out of their lives completely – as if they never existed. If negativity strikes, Sandalwood can be prone to sleepless nights because of stressful dreams, and become irritable, unco-operative and dissatisfied.

As partners, Sandalwoods expect an equal relationship, and continual support. If they don't get it, the partner will be changed. When Sandalwoods fall desperately in love they can become intolerant of any company other than the loved one. Sandalwoods make good parents and their children's friends will usually spend more time at their house than their own, particularly as teenagers, when Sandalwoods are ready to answer questions about life, love and sex.

Sandalwoods are good in any job that needs direct communication and ingenuity, otherwise they'll become bored easily. They make good artists, writers, theologians, psychologists, counsellors and buyers for companies but also seem to have leanings towards botany and archaeology, and make good members of management teams. In fact, they'll make a serious effort in most professions, so long as it engages their intellect.

Elizabeth Jones, OBE, MCSP, DRE, MIFA Reg., MISPA, physiotherapist and aromatherapy tutor:

'Infinitely soothing qualities. Deep, woody, subtle, in no way overpowering. Has a timeless, soporific character.'

THYME LINALOL
HERBIE
Thymus vulgaris, sp linalol

CHARACTER
Gently empowering, Invigorating, Assisting

USE TO COUNTERACT THESE NEGATIVE ATTRIBUTES
Lack of direction, Intellectual or physical exhaustion, Weakness, Over-reactive, Nervous debility, Blockages

USE FOR THESE POSITIVE ATTRIBUTES
Fortified, Balanced, Tolerant, Courageous, Supportive, Decisive, Alert, Focused, Concentration, Warming

---

THYME LINALOL PERSONALITY PROFILE

These charming, intelligent, proud people pride themselves on being honest and straightforward and in having command over their actions and deeds. Thyme Linalols have an exuberance and freshness about them which transfers to almost everything they do and they are always full of new ideas and projects. This isn't always apparent at first because they like to hold back a little until a person is well known. The Thyme Linalol

Thyme Linalol

personalities seem able to command attention although they don't ask for it. They're considerate, thoughtful and discreet.

Thyme Linalols have an in-built genius which allows them to look at things in fresh and unique ways, bringing life to any project in which they become involved; forging forward in everything they do, leaving others behind. Thymes have a vivacious spirit, inner strength and fortitude which far out-weighs any weakness they may have. This isn't brute strength but gentle persuasion, and Thymes can be very supportive. The great affinity this person has with children of all ages is probably due to the fact that children feel confident with them, going to them with troubles and worries. This protectiveness extends to members of the family, who can always rely on Thyme's assistance and support. This personality falls in love easily, partly perhaps because they spend so much time alone, so when they do fall, it's hook, line and sinker, becoming prone to bouts of love-sickness and emotional trauma.

Thyme Linalols are the strong, silent types but when in neg-ative mode, are quick to anger. They're prone to nervous prob-lems, and if they push themselves too hard Thyme may suffer nervous exhaustion, even nervous breakdown. This person-ality can become hypersensitive and may occasionally retreat from the world. As children, Thymes often seek solitude, per-haps playing with an imaginary friend, even if they have brothers and sisters. As an adult, Thymes are at ease with their own company, sometimes preferring the chance to be peaceful and reflective.

Thyme Linalols often have a revolutionary outlook and are colourful characters. They're honest, open people who ultimately believe that the world is a good place. Because they go where angels fear to tread they make good, easy-going travellers and their unique ways of looking at old problems gives them an inventive streak, helpful in science. Because of their ability to understand difficult moral situations and their capacity to relate to events happening to other people, this personality can do well in personnel, counselling or spiritual leadership.

TUBEROSE
FLORAL
Polianthes tuberosa

CHARACTER
Transformative, Spontaneous, Extroverted, Centring

USE TO COUNTERACT THESE NEGATIVE ATTRIBUTES
Stress, Irritability, Emotional conflict, Over-sensitivity, Jealousy, Bitterness, Anger, Confusion, Disorientation, Hostility, Insincerity, Resentment, Selfishness, Falsity

USE FOR THESE POSITIVE ATTRIBUTES
Motivation, Enthusiasm, Encouraged, Expansive, Sensuous, Sensitive, Spontaneous, Expressive, Frank

TUBEROSE PERSONALITY PROFILE

The Tuberose personality is daring, attractive, hypnotic, charming and good company. They love gossip but beware, if you do tell them your deepest, darkest secrets, they are not above blackmail! This inclination is further compounded by the fact that the Tuberose personality loves danger and will

Tuberose

take huge risks for the sake of excitement. Tuberoses have an obsessive nature – whether they lament the losing of a lover or the fact that they didn't have the opportunity this morning to spend their usual ten minutes chanting under a tree. Their addictive nature often gets them into hot water.

The Tuberose personalities will use all their skills of seduction to get exactly what they want. Their physical appearance is extremely important to them and they'll always be nicely dressed, with manicured nails and well-groomed hair. If female, she wouldn't contemplate opening the door to let the cat out unless she was fully made up or wearing dark glasses! Looking good and being desired are Tuberose's number one priority, important because physical attraction can be used to gain power – sexual, economic and political. Tuberose *loves* power of any kind, and they'll use lovers to gain money, fame or prestige. The age of their lover is immaterial to them. Older lovers are taken for the prestige they can confer, while younger lovers are taken for their prowess. An older Tuberose personality will go through younger lovers like a bag of toffees – discarding the wrappers without a care.

The male Tuberose is often overly fussy in his dress – to the point of obsession. If he doesn't have the money to buy his own designer suits, he'll borrow a friend's. He's a born flirt and will flirt with both women and men. In love, he'll find himself in intriguing or difficult situations and will avoid people of his own age if he doesn't find them challenging enough. He's often found with an older lover, so long as they have power and money – the things he loves more than anything (or anyone)! Tuberose is ruthless – in business as in play.

Just as the Tuberose personality gets a kick out of being 'close to the edge', they enjoy putting people in that situation too. They'll charm a cobra out of a tree, telling you it won't bite, and then as you approach and get closer to it, they'll suddenly 'remember' that it does in fact bite and tell you a milli-second before you get within attacking distance. No personality loves the dark side of the paranormal or mysterious more than Tuberose. The dark side of human nature may repel this Floral type but at the same time, it holds an almost unhealthy fascination for them.

Shelly is a typical Tuberose personality. She'd married rather young to a nice handsome man who was a kind father to their two daughters but, and this drove her crazy, he had no ambition. So when she started work as a secretary in the office of the chairman of a large manufacturer, and found that he was single, she set out to catch him. Being naturally charming and employing her feminine wiles to the full, Shelly became his lover within three months. She didn't stop there of course. Pretty soon Shelly and her two daughters were living in her boss's luxurious mansion, divorce proceedings were in hand, and Shelly was enjoying her new life of designer clothes, expensive jewellery, health farms and the tennis club.

For the first few years Shelly was happy, sweet, charming, obliging and attentive to her lover. Her children were now in private schools, holidays were spent at the villa in Spain, and Shelly thoroughly revelled in her new-found status. Then boredom set in. She started being ridiculously extravagant, treating her friends to endless expensive meals, evenings at the theatre and nights out clubbing, with Shelly lapping up the kudos that came with being lady bountiful. However, she still didn't love the man and gradually became bitter and vindictive towards him, 'paying him back' by taking a stream of young lovers who, in exchange for expensive gifts, told her they loved her. For several years this pattern continued, and by this time Shelly was also taking any drugs she could lay her hands on.

Eventually, of course, the man became aware of what was going on and took a younger and prettier lover himself. Shelly found out and, at the same time, realized that because they didn't have any children together and weren't married, she wasn't actually in a very secure position. Still, she continued to lie and cheat on him and one day got caught *in flagrante*, as they say, and was promptly thrown out on the street. The man continued to house the children and pay their school fees and the children, who were quite happy to stay where they were, were used by Shelly as tools for gaining sympathy. Her ploy didn't work, however, and Shelly was homeless, jobless and broke – although still bejewelled.

At their best, Tuberoses are warm, seductive and hypnotic. Their most challenging lesson in life is to learn to love genuinely, to forget the superficialities and appreciate people for their good qualities. They also need to learn to love themselves – without make-up! If they can do that, the charm and warmth shines through.

VETIVER
ROOTIE
Vetiveria zizanoides

CHARACTER
Grounding, Centring, Visionary, Wisdom

USE TO COUNTERACT THESE NEGATIVE ATTRIBUTES
Fear, Anxiety, Obsession, Overwork, Agitation, Intellectual fatigue,
Hurt, Scattered thinking, Irritability, Anger, Emotional burn-out,
Mental exhaustion, Unworthiness, Instability, Loss of purpose,
Emotional weakness, Addiction, Disconnection, Fantasizing,
Emotional blockages, Neurotic behaviour, Disorientated

USE FOR THESE POSITIVE ATTRIBUTES
Spiritual calmness, Growth, Integrity, Mind-body connection,
Strength, Honourable, Protected, Self-esteem, Grounded

VETIVER PERSONALITY PROFILE

Vetivers are often strong and intellectual, with a strong sense
of reality and awareness of what is happening around them,
embodying the relationship between mind and body. The
essential oil of vetiver is obtained from the root of the plant
and has a vitality and energy associated with it which is earthy,
and this personality certainly feels a connection with Ghia.
This is an earthy kind of person, ready to laugh out loud at
risqué jokes, not easily embarrassed. Vetivers are very comfortable with their sexuality, seeing sex very much as pure
vitality and energy. They're also very likely to experiment, and
their sensuality does have a deep, mysterious side.

Although the fragrance is often associated with the masculine, the Vetiver personality – whether male or female – will be
perfectly balanced between their masculine and feminine
sides. There is nothing delicate or ethereal about the Vetiver
profile, it's very much of the here and now. Often gentle and

wise in spirit, friends turn to Vetivers for advice, which will be blunt and straight.

The Vetiver type will be very interested in the esoteric side of life, particularly the journeys of the shamans and voyages to uncover the earth's mysteries, and may be visionaries. Green issues, such as pollution and the depletion of the rain forests concern them, and they'll very likely become disillusioned with the world as it is. Although not the best travellers, this personality will follow the quest for idealism and a place to be. They may travel with groups of people but as they get older, will search for their roots. Vetivers are not exactly restless; they could settle down anywhere if they ignored the call of the wild. Remote villages in so-called Third World countries hold an attraction for them – the raw elements of the earth and nature appeal to them.

Vetivers revel in the sensuality of life, very much the person who holds and touches things to appreciate fully all aspects of the object, but they are also often very academic and philosophical, sometimes teachers. However, Vetiver's academic associates may have lost touch with themselves through too much 'living in the head' and can't understand why, when there are intellectual problems to be solved, Vetiver should prefer to indulge his or her attraction to the opposite sex, or other earthly matters. At the same time, these people *need* Vetiver precisely because this personality helps them to be drawn into their own bodies.

Jan Kusmirek, MDDH, MED, LLFA, MIFA, Reg. LCSP, DM, aromatherapist, medical herbalist and lecturer:

'It is a hidden oil to do with the dark recesses and the potential for life and energy. There is an earthy fragrance with spice overtones, warmth and comfort as on a sun-drenched day. Tenacious with a sense of belonging and grounding. Its personality is one of renewal, ripeness and maturity, excellent for all those who have "lost touch" with something.'

YLANG YLANG
FLORAL
Cananga odorata

CHARACTER
Euphoric, Sensuous, Stimulating, Unifying

USE TO COUNTERACT THESE NEGATIVE ATTRIBUTES
Depression, Anxiety, Tension, Stress, Frustration, Irritability,
Emotional guilt, Resentment, Jealousy, Selfishness, Impatience,
Irrationality, Stubbornness, Obstinacy, Shyness

USE FOR THESE POSITIVE ATRRIBUTES
Self-confidence, Warmth, Awakened, Uplifted, Calm, Joyful,
Enthusiastic, Meditative, Sensual, Soothed

YLANG YLANG PERSONALITY PROFILE

The Ylang Ylang personality is intensely feminine. She has a
passionate nature, tempered by a calm and balance many find
unnerving. Ylang Ylangs are the *femmes fatales*, the
Casanovas, the mistresses and the lovers. They are people who
delight in the erotic and sensual. No shrinking violets here!

Neither male nor female Ylang Ylangs are happy alone,
flourishing best when they have an audience to applaud their
achievements or commiserate with their failures. Ylangs are
usually charismatic, bewitching, gracious and delightful company, and their incredible fantasy life makes great entertainment for their friends. However, this type rarely enters the
world of entertainment themselves, much preferring to be
friends or lovers of famous people, particularly people with
power. Power is an aphrodisiac to these types, male or female,
who are good companions in these relationships because they
have a balancing quality about them, and will relieve the stress
that often goes with powerful positions.

It's difficult to handle a true Ylang Ylang because they often
live in a dream world where they are king or queen and nothing will ever harm them, where they always come out on top.

Often these dreams are impossible to achieve, as is wealth, for the majority of Ylang Ylangs. The female Ylang Ylang may resort to older men who indulge her image of herself, who enjoy her sexuality and power over younger men. She will be worn like a trophy until she leaves, bored and frustrated. This is not what Ylang Ylang women are intended for!

These passionate people live for love. As men, they love the thrill of the chase and conquest, and as women they delight in obtaining the unobtainable and having secret rendezvous. Ylang Ylang has a fiery, passionate nature, intensely sweet, and would sacrifice everything for love, and I mean *love* – at the time, at least, because this personality falls in and out of love easily.

Ylang Ylangs are found in jobs that give expression to the aesthetic side of life – those dealing with beautiful fabrics, cosmetics, hairdressing and anything that entails love, a designer of bridal wear for example. They could also be involved in any profession involving exciting physical pursuits – such as racing cars.

Ylang Ylangs enjoy creating a mountain out of a molehill and look for excitement continually. They scream and shout, and know how to let rip with anger if crossed, and of course, to get their own way. The daredevils of life are often Ylang Ylang types who will try anything once, for the experience. There is insecurity in this personality though, and this often manifests itself in dislike of their looks, or feeling acutely any lack of money. A male Ylang will need to have money to survive and may lose himself searching for it. He likes fast cars, expensive clothes, exotic locations and beautiful women.

A negative Ylang Ylang will be neglectful of their appearance, not bothering with hair and clothes, careless of the impression they are making on others. As the neglect extends beyond themselves, Ylangs frequently lose interest in their work, so in the end they'll become depressed and downhearted, with no self-confidence and, barely living, they'll hide away from the world. Other Ylangs will become frustrated, extremely nervous and irritable, losing all interest in life and love. Which, if in a partnership of any kind, can lead to untold problems – just compounding the myth they have created about themselves being unlovable. Whatever relationship Ylangs may or may not be in when negative, they can be angry and jealous, and in need of rebalancing.

Love conquers all, so they say, and with Ylang Ylang that is certainly true – love can brighten up the morning and dispel the darkest clouds, giving Ylangs a new lease of life. If on form, Ylang Ylang can balance the two extremes of their character very well. They have a soft side to them and are joyful and fun, good friends, who will never be dull company.

CHART 14.1

QUICK REFERENCE AROMA-GENERA ESSENTIAL OIL CHART

FOR MIND, MOOD AND EMOTION

Basil *Ocimum basilicum*   **HERBIE**

Character Uplifting, Awakening, Clarifying, Stimulating

Use for these positive attributes

Positivity, Purposefulness, Concentration, Assertiveness, Decisiveness, Straightforwardness, Trust, Integrity, Enthusiasm, Clarity, Cheerfulness, Strength.

Use to counteract these negative attributes

Indecision, Mental fatigue, Mental exhaustion, Negativity, Lack of direction, Fear, Burn-out, Confusion, Intellectual fatigue, Apathy, Bitterness, Resentment, Addiction, Conflict, Fear of intimacy, Shame, Doubts, Melancholy, Sadness.

Bergamot *Citrus bergamia*   **FRUITIE**

Character Joyous, Refreshing, Uplifting, Encouraging

Use for these positive attributes

Concentration, Confidence, Balance, Strength, Joy, Motivation, Good cheer, Harmony, Completeness.

Use to counteract these negative attributes

Depression, Anxiety, Helplessness, Apathy, Bitterness, Burnout, Despondency, Emptiness, Exhaustion, Grief, Hopelessness, Sadness, Loneliness, Stress, Tension, Emotional imbalances.

Black Pepper *Piper nigrum*   FRUITIE/SPICIE

Character Security, Comforting, Directional, Endurance

Use for these positive attributes

Comfort, Stamina, Endurance, Motivation, Changeability.

Use to counteract these negative attributes

Emotional blockages, Compulsions, Confusion, Disorientation, Fatigue, Begrudging, Indecision, Irrationality, Anger, Frustration, Emotional coldness, Apathy, Mental exhaustion.

Cardamon *Elettaria cardamomum*   FRUITIE/SPICIE

Character Clarifying, Stimulating, Encouraging, Enthusiastic

Use for these positive attributes

Clarity, Concentration, Direction, Motivation, Straightforwardness, Enthusiasm, Confidence, Courage, Fortitude, Purpose.

Use to counteract these negative attributes

Mental stress, Apathy, Confusion, Inflexibility, Judgemental, Intolerance, Unreasonableness, Burn-out, Suspicion, Sluggishness, Self-pity, Bewilderment, Rigidity.

Carnation *Dianthus caryophyllus*   **FLORAL**

Character Secretiveness, Stillness, Originality, Liberating

Use for these positive attributes

Self-worth, Communication, Radiating, Creativity, Independence, Tenderness, Nurturing, Encompassing, Cushioning, Openness, Releasing.

Use to counteract these negative attributes

Disregard, Neglect, Detachment, Cynicism, Disorientation, Doubt, Mental loneliness, Aloneness, Emotional domination, Emotional solitude, Neglect, Self-criticism.

Cedarwood *Cedrus atlantica*   **WOODIE**

Character Grounding, Strengthening, Dignified, Powerful

Use for these positive attributes

Focus, Concentration, Strength, Confidence, Balance, Stability, Comfort, Persistence, Fortitude, Nobility of spirit.

Use to counteract these negative attributes

Scattered thoughts, Thoughtlessness, Fixation on past, Anxiety, Obsessions, Mental strain, Irrationality, Emotional sensitivity, Touchiness, Gloomy thoughts, Worry, Fear, Too analytical, Paranoia, Selfishness.

Chamomile German *Matricaria recutita*
                                        HERBIE/FLORAL

Character Strong, Peaceful, Healing, Cooling

Use for these positive attributes

Communicative, Relaxed, Understanding, Organized, Soothing, Empathy, Patience, Calm.

Use to counteract these negative attributes

Nervousness, Frayed nerves, Anger, Frustration, Emotional

dramas, Emotional tension, Irritability, Temper, Tenseness, Over-sensitive, Moodiness, Stormy, Bitterness, Resentment, Indifference, Deep emotional baggage.

Chamomile Roman *Anthemis nobilis*   **HERBIE/ FLORAL**

Character Harmonizing, Peaceful, Soothing, Spiritual

Use for these positive attributes

Stillness, Calm, Softness, Gentleness, Relaxed, Serene, Spiritually aware, Emotionally stable, Inner peace, Understanding, Co-operative.

Use to counteract these negative attributes

Nervousness, Irritability, Temper, Anger, Depression, Hysteria, Fear, Anxiety, Exhaustion, Worry, Stress, Tension, Grief, Emotional imbalance, Broken heart, Grumpiness, Moroseness, Discontent, Impatience, Short temper, Over-sensitive, Melancholy, Spiritual disconnection.

Cinnamon *Cinnamomum zeylanicum*   **LEAFIE/SPICIE**

Character Warming, Secular, Fair-minded

Use for these positive attributes

Invigorated, Steadfast, Benevolent, Strength, Practicality, Energized, Realistic, Direct.

Use to counteract these negative attributes

Instability, Severity, Bleakness, Malice, Spitefulness, Coldness, Fear, Nervous Exhaustion, Debility, Introversion, Superficiality.

Clary Sage *Salvia sclarea*   **HERBIE**

Character Euphoric, Restoring, Harmonizing, Warming

Use for these positive attributes

Calm, Soothed, Confidence, Grounded, Regenerated, Inspired, Tranquil, Revitalized, Uplifted, Balanced, Strength, Relaxed, Restores equilibrium.

Use to counteract these negative attributes

Nervousness, Stress, Tension, Changeability, Worried, Anxious, Claustrophobic, Compulsive, Depression, Nightmares, Hostility, Hyperactivity, Lethargy, Obsession, Panic, Mental strain, Fear, Paranoia, Melancholy, Burn-out, Delusions, Emotional debility, Absent-mindedness, Weepiness, Guilt.

Coriander *Coriandrum sativum*   **SEEDIE/SPICIE**

Character Enlivening, Motivating, Encouraging

Use for these positive attributes

Creativity, Imagination, Good memory, Confidence, Motivation, Optimism, Sincerity, Expressiveness, Enthusiasm.

Use to counteract these negative attributes

Emotional tiredness, Weariness, Irritability, Nervousness, Stress, Nervous debility, Doubt, Fear of failure, Sulkiness, Being unco-operative, Vulnerability.

Cypress *Cupressus sempervirens*   **LEAFIE/WOODIE**

Character Protective, Righteous, Wise, Direction

Use for these positive attributes

Strength, Comfort, Change, Direction, Assertion, Control, Understanding, Balance, Sensitivity, Generosity of spirit, Contentment, Stillness, Confidence, Inner peace, Wisdom, Purity of heart, Stability, Patience, Trust, Incorruptibility, Structured, Softly powerful, Direct, Willpower, Straightforward.

Use to counteract these negative attributes

Grief, Sorrow, Self-loathing, Pressurized, Being dominated, Opinionated, Jealous, Lethargic, Weak-willed, Fearful, Timid, Emotional turmoil, Unbalanced, Isolated, Inconsolable, Frustrated, Unable to speak up for oneself, Emotionally tired, Emotionally unstable, Tearful, Loss, Regret, Distracted, Lack of concentration, Absent-minded, Uncontrollable passions.

Eucalyptus *Eucalyptus radiata* LEAFIE/WOODIE

Character Energizing, Stimulating, Balancing, Sheltering

Use for these positive attributes

Emotionally balanced, Concentration, Logical thought, Centred, Rationality Composed, Predictable, Cooling.

Use to counteract these negative attributes

Exhaustion, Heated emotions, Mood swings, Lack of concentration, Cluttered thoughts, Temper tantrums, Irrational thoughts, Explosive nature, Argumentative.

Eucalyptus Citriodora (Lemon) LEAFIE/WOODIE

Character Vital, Harmonious, Stimulating, Comforting

Use for these positive attributes

Concentration, Enthusiasm, Upliftment, Vitality, Understanding, Creativity, Regeneration, Optimism, Encouraged, Empathy, Freedom, Expressiveness, Soundness, Trusting.

Use to counteract these negative attributes

Sluggishness, Emotional crisis, Emptiness, Confusion, Disillusionment, Restlessness, Fear, Despondency, Loneliness, Unable to let go.

Fennel, Sweet *Foeniculum vulgare dulce* **SEEDIE**

Character Clearing, Resolute, Enlightening

Use for these positive attributes

Enlivened, Motivated, Fortitude, Clarity, Forceful, Perseverance, Courageous, Reliable, Confident, Assertive.

Use to counteract these negative attributes

Mental blockages, Emotional blockages, Boredom, Unable to adjust, Fear of failure, Hostile, Overburdened, Lack of creativity.

Frankincense *Boswellia carteri* **RESINIE**

Character Elevating, Spiritual, Meditative, Wisdom

Use for these positive attributes

Comfort, Healing, Emotional stability, Enlightenment, Protective, Introspection, Courage, Resolution, Fortitude, Acceptance, Inspiration.

Use to counteract these negative attributes

Fears, Grief, Blockages, Over-attachment, Burn-out, Exhaustion, Insincerity, Panic, Anxiety, Disconnection, Repression, Resistance, Self-destruction, Apprehension, Despair.

Geranium *Pelargonium graveolens* **HERBIE**

Character Harmonizing, Healing, Comforting, Cushioning

Use for these positive attributes

Consoled, Flexible, Elevated, Regenerated, Humour, Friendliness, Balanced, Soothed, Secure, Assured, Shielded, Mothered, Stable, Tranquil, Steady.

Use to counteract these negative attributes

Anxiety, Depression, Acute fear, Extreme moods, Inner child,

Abuse, Confusion, Rigidity, Instability, Worry, Moodiness, Lack of self-esteem, Insecurity, Over-sensitivity, Tension, Stress, Hurt, Crisis, Apprehension, Aggression, Irrationality, Discontent, Heartache.

Ginger *Zingiber officinale*   ROOTIE/SPICIE

Character Warming, Strengthening, Encouraging

Use for these positive attributes

Confidence, Warmth, Fortitude, Empathy, Courage.

Use to counteract these negative attributes

Sexual anxieties, Lack of direction, Purposelessness, Unfocused, Apathy, Burn-out, Confusion, Fatigue, Loneliness, Sadness, Resignation.

Grapefruit *Citrus paradisi*   FRUITIE

Character Radiating, Cheering, Joyful, Liberating, Boosting

Use for these positive attributes

Joyful, Positive, Confident, Clarity, Balanced, Attuned, Alert, Inspired, Generous, Uplifted, Emotionally purified, Spontaneous, Co-operative.

Use to counteract these negative attributes

Depression, Dependency, Sadness, Grief, Apathy, Mental pressure, Mental exhaustion, Emotional violence, Self-doubt, Self-criticism, Aggravated, Frustration.

Helichrysum *Helichrysum angustifolium*   FLORAL
(Immortelle or Italian Everlasting)

Character Gentleness, Harmonizing, Caring, Warming, Meditative

Use for these positive attributes

Calm, Accepting of change, Buffered, Dreams, Energy, Patience, Idealism, Understanding, Perseverance, Inner strength,

Acceptance, Awareness, Positive inner child.

Use to counteract these negative attributes

Abuse, Stress, Tension, Emotional crisis, Depression, Lethargy, Mental exhaustion, Emotional exhaustion, Tiredness, Emotional blockages, Disorientation, Overwork, Loneliness, Insecurity, Hypersensitivity, Grief, Addiction, Negative inner child.

Hyacinth *Hyacinthus orientalis*   **FLORAL**

Character Gentle, Trusting, Soothing, Enlightening

Use for these positive attributes

Calming, Forgiving, High self-esteem, Perseverance, Equilibrium, Trust, Faith, Courage.

Use to counteract these negative attributes

Instability, Stress, Repression, Apathy, Lovesick, Dejection, Distress, Grieving, Sorrow, Powerlessness, Regret, Unforgiving, Naivete, Dependency, Apprehension.

Jasmine *Jasminum officinale*   **FLORAL**

Character Euphoric, Sensual, Welcoming, Intuitive, Soothing

Use for these positive attributes

Uplifted, Confident, Sexual, Assertive, Relaxed, Optimistic, Open, Sensitive, Harmonized, Aware, Profound, Inspired, Joyful.

Use to counteract these negative attributes

Depression, Anxiety, Pessimism, Tension, Indifference, Repression, Bitterness, Jealousy, Low self-esteem, Guilt, Emotional frigidity, Emotional abuse, Emotional violence.

Juniper *Juniperus communis* **FRUITIE**

Character Cleansing, Purifying, Sacredness, Visionary

Use for these positive attributes

Self-worth, Spiritually supported, Peace, Inner vision, Uplifted, Strength, Vitality, Cleansed, Meditative, Conviction, Sincerity, Enlightened, Wisdom, Humility.

Use to counteract these negative attributes

Nervous exhaustion, Emotional exhaustion, Guilt, Lack of self-worth, Dissatisfaction, Anxiety, Abused, Listlessness, Weakness, Transience, Emptiness, Conflict, Defensive.

Lavender *Lavandula angustifolia* **FLORAL/HERBIE**

Character Harmonious, Calming, Healing, Caring, Embracing

Use for these positive attributes

Secure, Gentle, Compassion, Balanced, Reconciled, Vital, Clarity, Comforted, Acceptance, Inner peace, Relaxed and alert, Rested, Aware, Emotionally balanced, Spiritual growth, Meditative, Visualization, Rejuvenated.

Use to counteract these negative attributes

Anxiety, Irritability, Stress, Tension, Mental exhaustion, Panic, Hysteria, Shock, Apprehension, Fears, Nightmares, Insecurity, Lost inner child, Restlessness, Moodiness, Distracted, Addiction, Obsessional behaviour, Trauma, Conflict, Emotional violence, Agitation, Jitteriness, Depression, Psychosomatic illness, Nervousness, Worry, Over-excitement, Burn-out.

Lemon *Citrus limonum* **FRUITIE**

Character Purifying, Stimulating, Directional, Versatile

Use for these positive attributes

Joy, Emotional clarity, Direction, Awareness, Calm,

Concentration, Lively, Conscious, Strength, Clarity of thought, Memory, Emotionally invigorated.

Use to counteract these negative attributes

Resentful, Depressed, Bitter, Touchy, Apathetic, Lethargic, Humourless, Indecisive, Bad attitude, Distrust, Mental blocks, Stress, Mental fatigue, Turmoil, Irrationality, Fear.

Linden Blossom *Tilia vulgaris*   FLORAL

Character Consoling, Serenity, Security, Patience

Use for these positive attributes

Relaxed, Calm, Soothed, Self-confident, Secure, Balanced, Structured, Stable.

Use to counteract these negative attributes

Nervousness, Anxiety, Nervous tension, Emotional debility, Hysteria, Over-excitement, Insecurity, Emotional blockages, Possessiveness, Jealousy, Anger, Stress, Irritability, Mood swings, Guilt, Lovelorn, Over-sensitivity, Indecision.

Mandarin *Citrus reticulata*   FRUITIE

Character Gentle, Peaceful, Revitalizing, Sympathetic

Use for these positive attributes

Calm, Uplifted, Refreshed, Inspired, Soothed, Sprightly, Integrity, Tranquility.

Use to counteract these negative attributes

Anxiety, Depression, Grief, Inner child, Abuse, Dejection, Emptiness, Dwelling on the past, Over-excitable, Desolate, Emotional trauma.

Marjoram, Sweet *Origanum marjorana*   HERBIE

Character Comforting, Soothing, Warming, Strengthening

Use for these positive attributes

Calm, Balanced, Direct, Self-assured, Integrity, Courage, Confidence, Focus, Perseverance, Restored, Sincere.

Use to counteract these negative attributes

Anxiety, Hysteria, Hostility, Withdrawn, Mental strain, Tantrums, Anger, Irritability, Overactivity, Weak will.

Melissa *Melissa officinalis*   HERBIE

Character Calming, Supportive, Sensitive, Fostering

Use for these positive attributes

Strength, Revitalized, Happy, Gentle, Spiritual growth, Relaxed, Peaceful, Positive, Progressive, Cheerful.

Use to counteract these negative attributes

Nervous tension, Stress, Anxiety, Irritability, Over-excitement, Restlessness, Melancholy, Sadness, Grieving, Sorrow, Emotional crisis, Depression, Mental exhaustion, Lethargy, Negativity.

Narcissus *Narcissus poeticus*   FLORAL

Character Hypnotic, Empowering, Mesmerizing, Sagacious

Use for these positive attributes

Inspired, Creative, Stillness, Meditative, Inner vision, Discovery, Truthfulness, Idealistic, Sensuous, Visionary.

Use to counteract these negative attributes

Hysteria, Nervousness, Irritability, Tension, Grief, Addictions, Withdrawal, Loneliness, Illusions, Disillusionment, Longings, Hopelessness, Obsessions, Trauma, Emotional wounding, Misery, Anguish, Emotional analgesia.

Neroli *Citrus aurantium*   **FLORAL**
(Orange Blossom)

Character Spiritual, Pure, Loving, Peaceful

Use for these positive attributes

Lightness, Lifting of sorrows, Spiritual, Connected, Completeness, Joy, Understanding, Guided, Calm, Stable, Regenerated, Peaceful.

Use to counteract these negative attributes

Anxiety, Stress, Tension, Shock, Emotional crisis, Sadness, Longing, Panic, Grief, Inner child, Abused as child, Abused as adult, Depression, Hopelessness, Fear.

Orange *Citrus sinensis*   **FRUITIE**

Character Warming, Happy, Resolute, Energizing

Use for these positive attributes

Joy, Uplifted, Sunny, Balanced, Light-hearted, Regenerated, Strong, Creative, Positive, Self-confident, Sympathetic, Courageous.

Use to counteract these negative attributes

Depression, Hopelessness, Sadness, Apathy, Resignation, Withdrawn, Self-consciousness, Anxiety, Emotional violence, Emotional abuse, Worry, Selfishness, Obsessions, Addiction, Burn-out.

Ormenis Flower *Ormenis multicaulis* **HERBIE/FLORAL**
(Chamomile Maroc)

Character Unhurried, Composed, Mindful, Mystic

Use for these positive attributes

Calm, Empathetic, Courageous, Earthed, Relaxed, Mindful, Able to let go, Attentive, Meditative, Consoled, Soothing.

Use to counteract these negative attributes

Stress, Tension, Anxiety, Dread, Overactive mind, Highly strung, Impulsive, Indecisive, Confused, Bad temper, Emotionally controlling, Emotional blockages, Abused, Fearful.

Patchouli *Pogostemon cablin* **LEAFIE**

Character Grounding, Soothing, Unruffled, Assured

Use for these positive attributes

Invigorated, Restored, Reasonable, Lucid, Astute, Stimulating, Persistent.

Use to counteract these negative attributes

Depression, Anxiety, Indecision, Lethargy, Sluggishness, Egotistical, Tension, Stress, Mood swings, Touchiness.

Peppermint *Mentha piperita* **HERBIE**

Character Clarifying, Awakening, Stimulating, Penetrating

Use for these positive attributes

Regenerating, Emotionally refreshed, Self-acceptance, Concentration, Vitality, Vibrancy.

Use to counteract these negative attributes

Mental fatigue, Shock, Helplessness, Overwork, Sluggishness, Lethargy, Apathy.

Petitgrain *Citrus aurantium* **LEAFIE/WOODIE**

Character Revitalizing, Balancing, Restoring, Clarifying

Use for these positive attributes

Harmonized, Uplifted, Joyful, Relaxed, Inner vision, Strength, Self-confidence, Stability, Optimism, Expressiveness.

Use to counteract these negative attributes

Disharmony, Confusion, Difficulties, Depression, Mental fatigue, Nervous exhaustion, Insomnia, Sadness, Disappointment, Rigidity, Betrayal, Anger, Irrationality, Introversion, Pessimism.

Pine *Pinus sylvestris*   **WOODIE/LEAFIE**

Character Acceptance, Understanding, Patience, Self-forgiveness

Use for these positive attributes

Humility, Simplicity, Assured, Buffered, Forgiving, Perseverance, Sharing, Mindful, Trusting, Directness, Direction, Acceptance of love, Tenacity, Confident, Exhilarated.

Use to counteract these negative attributes

Regrets, Guilt, Self-blame, Dissatisfaction, Self-critical, Worried, Over-responsible, Unconfrontational, Self-reproach, Unworthiness, Exhaustion, Masochistic, Shameful, Feeling rejected, Unsympathetic, Miserable, Feeling inadequate.

Rose Maroc *Rosa centifolia*   **FLORAL**

Character Passionate, Harmonious, Reassuring, Comforting

Use for these positive attributes

Motivated, Inner vitality, Revived, Confident, Passionate, Co-operative, Sense of freedom, Fulfilled, Forgiving, Sensual.

Use to counteract these negative attributes

Grief, Bitterness, Fear of letting go, Fear of love, Fear of sexuality, Jealousy, Resignation, Passivity, Deception, Lack of ambition/motivation, Self-destruction, Vengefulness.

Rose Otto *Rosa damascena*   **FLORAL**

Character Loving, Harmonizing, Comforting, Happy, Caring, Euphoric, Gentle, Peaceful

Use for these positive attributes

Comforted, Contentment, Devoted, Motivated, Inner vision, Revival, Joy, Happiness, Inner freedom, Acceptance, Completeness, Wisdom, Spirituality, Patience, Love, Sensuality, Purity.

Use to counteract these negative attributes

Depression, Sadness, Grief, Anger, Anxiety, Bitterness, Emptiness, Fear of loving, Fear of not being loved, Broken heart, Guilt, Shyness, Jealousy, Touchiness, Emotional crisis, Resignation, Inexpression, Hopelessness, Despair, Abused, Emotional violence, Hurt inner child.

Rosemary *Rosmarinus officinalis*   **HERBIE**

Character Vigorous, Strengthening, Restorative, Centring

Use for these positive attributes

Energy, Upliftment, Confidence, Creative, Clarity, Structured, Concentration, Stabilized, Fortified, Sincere, Purified, Aware.

Use to counteract these negative attributes

Loss of memory, Learning difficulties, Lethargy, Disorientation, Fatigue, Indecision, Nervous exhaustion, Overburdened, Overworked, Strain, Emotional exhaustion, Sluggishness.

Sandalwood *Santalum album*   **WOODIE**

Character Enlightenment, Meditative, Balancing, Connecting

Use for these positive attributes

Warm, Comforted, Sensitive, Serene, Trusting, Harmonized,

Peaceful, Wise, Sensual, Expressive, Good self-esteem, Open, Insightful, Unity.

Use to counteract these negative attributes

Anxiety, Nervous tension, Possessiveness, Manipulating, Unforgiving, Obsessive, Lonely, Accepting, Cynical, Insecurity, Recurrent nightmares, Selfishness, Distressed, Uneasy, Hasty, Aggressive, Irritable, Dwelling on the past.

Thyme Linalol *Thymus vulgaris, sp linalol*   **HERBIE**

Character Gently empowering, Invigorating, Assisting

Use for these positive attributes

Fortified, Balanced, Tolerant, Courageous, Supportive, Decisive, Alert, Focused, Concentration, Warming.

Use to counteract these negative attributes

Lack of direction, Intellectual or physical exhaustion, Weakness, Over-reactive, Nervous debility, Blockages.

Tuberose *Polianthes tuberosa*   **FLORAL**

Character Transformative, Spontaneous, Extroverted, Centring

Use for these positive attributes

Motivation, Enthusiasm, Encouraged, Expansive, Sensuous, Sensitive, Spontaneous, Expressive, Frank.

Use to counteract these negative attributes

Stress, Irritability, Emotional conflict, Over-sensitivity, Jealousy, Bitterness, Anger, Confusion, Disorientation, Hostility, Insincerity, Resentment, Selfishness, Falsity.

Vetiver *Vetiveria zizanoides*   ROOTIE

Character Grounding, Centring, Visionary, Wisdom

Use for these positive attributes

Spiritual calmness, Growth, Integrity, Mind-body connection, Strength, Honourable, Protected, Self-esteem, Grounded.

Use to counteract these negative attributes

Fear, Anxiety, Obsession, Overwork, Agitation, Intellectual fatigue, Hurt, Scattered thinking, Irritability, Anger, Emotional burn-out, Mental exhaustion, Unworthiness, Loss of purpose, Emotional weakness, Addiction, Disconnection, Fantasizing, Emotional blockages, Neurotic behaviour, Instability, Disorientation.

Ylang Ylang *Cananga odorata*   FLORAL

Character Euphoric, Sensuous, Stimulating, Unifying

Use for these positive attributes

Self-confidence, Warmth, Awakened, Uplifted, Calm, Joyful, Enthusiastic, Meditative, Sensual, Soothed.

Use to counteract these negative attributes

Depression, Anxiety, Tension, Stress, Frustration, Irritability, Emotional guilt, Resentment, Jealousy, Selfishness, Impatience, Irrationality, Stubbornness, Obstinacy, Shyness.

CHART 14.2

QUICK REFERENCE AROMA-GENERA CHART

POSITIVE EMOTIONAL STATES

This list is by no means comprehensive, in that it does not include all the essential oils that could be used for the listed purpose. Those in italics are those used in classical aromatherapy; the others have been adopted for these uses in more modern times.

Ability to let go

ormenis flower, *coriander, lemon, peppermint, pine, tuberose*

Acceptance (general)

frankincense, grapefruit, lavender, pine, rose otto, helichrysum

Acceptance (of love)

pine, *rose otto, chamomile*

roman, melissa

Acceptance (self)

peppermint, *cypress, helichrysum, petitgrain*

Accepting (of change)

grapefruit, helichrysum, *geranium, lemon*

Alertness

grapefruit, lavender, thyme, *basil*, bergamot, black pepper, cardamon, cinnamon, coriander, eucalyptus citriodora, *grapefruit*, juniper, lime, *peppermint*, petitgrain, pine, *rosemary*, thyme linalol

Assertion

jasmine, fennel, *basil,*

cedarwood, cypress, sweet fennel, frankincense, ginger, patchouli, *ylang ylang*, black pepper, jasmine, *ormenis flower, bergamot*, coriander, carnation, *tuberose*, cistus, pimento berry, lime, *cardamon, litsea cubeba*

Assisting

thyme linalol, *lavender, marjoram, jasmine, geranium*

Assuring

geranium, marjoram, patchouli, pine, *ginger, frankincense, cedarwood*

Astuteness

patchouli, *fennel, rosemary, eucalyptus citriodora, coriander*

Attentive

ormenis flower, *lemon, cypress, clove, litsea cubeba*

Attuned

grapefruit, *frankincense, sandalwood, juniper, neroli, chamomile roman*

Awakened

ylang ylang, *jasmine, juniper,*

black pepper

Awakening

basil, peppermint, *juniper, frankincense, petitgrain, rosemary, coriander, neroli, carnation*

Awareness (self)

grapefruit, lemon, jasmine, lavender, rosemary, helichrysum

Awareness (spiritual)

chamomile roman, *neroli, frankincense, juniper, rose otto*

Balanced

bergamot, cedarwood, clary sage, *cypress, mandarin, geranium, benzoin,* lavender, linden blossom, marjoram, orange, grapefruit, thyme linalol, *eucalyptus radiata*

Balanced (emotionally)

lavender, *lemon, rose otto, cedarwood, cardamon, orange, mandarin*

Balancing

petitgrain, sandalwood, *juniper,*

lavender, hyacinth, neroli   *sandalwood*

Benevolence

cinnamon, *benzoin, vetiver, patchouli, linden blossom, lavender*

Boosting

grapefruit, *orange, melissa, bergamot, pimento berry, myrtle*

Buffering

helichrysum, pine, *benzoin, vetiver, patchouli, sandalwood*

Calming (general)

hyacinth, lavender, melissa

Calmness

chamomile german, *chamomile roman, clary sage*, helichrysum, lemon, linden blossom, mandarin, *marjoram, neroli, ormenis flower*, ylang ylang

Calmness (spiritual)

vetiver, *benzoin, neroli, chamomile roman, rose otto, spikenard, frankincense*

Caring

helichrysum, lavender, rose otto, *chamomile roman,*

Centring

rosemary, tuberose, vetiver, *benzoin, myrrh, ginger*

Changeability

black pepper, *cinnamon, clove, hyacinth, bay, bergamot, geranium*

Changes (going through)

cypress, *eucalyptus radiata,* rosemary, *cedarwood, lemon*

Cheerful

melissa, grapefruit, orange, *mandarin*, basil, bergamot

Clarifying

basil, cardamon, peppermint, *rosemary, eucalyptus radiata,* petitgrain

Clarity

basil, cardamon, fennel, *grapefruit*, lavender, *lemon, rosemary*

Clarity (of thought)

lemon, rosemary, basil, pimento berry, clove, petitgrain

Cleansing

juniper, *cypress, pine, cedarwood, frankincense, neroli, lemon*

Clearing

fennel, *juniper, pine, cypress*

Comforting

black pepper, cedarwood, *chamomile roman*, cypress, eucalyptus citriodora, *frankincense, geranium*, marjoram, rose maroc, *rose otto*, lavender, *sandalwood, benzoin, melissa*

Communication

carnation, geranium, *chamomile german, grapefruit, peppermint, lemon, bay, linden blossom*

Compassionate

chamomile roman, lavender, rose otto, neroli, *nutmeg, pine, cypress, melissa*

Completeness

bergamot, neroli, rose otto, *cistus, chamomile roman*

Composed

ormenis flower, *frankincense,*

lavender, rose maroc, jasmine, cedarwood, eucalyptus radiata

Concentration

basil, bergamot, cardamon, peppermint, rosemary, cedarwood, eucalyptus citriodora, lemon, thyme linalol
Intellectual – *lemon, basil, lemongrass, litsea cubeba*, cardamon, bergamot, orange, cedarwood, *rosemary*, peppermint, *frankincense, eucalyptus radiata*
Spiritual – *frankincense*, neroli, *chamomile roman, rose otto*, narcissus, hyacinth

Confidence

bergamot, *cardamon*, cedarwood, clary sage, coriander, cypress, fennel, ginger, grapefruit, *jasmine*, ylang ylang, linden blossom, marjoram, pine, petitgrain, rose maroc, rosemary, tuberose, orange

Confusion

ginger, *rosemary, benzoin, cinnamon, clove, marjoram, lavender*

Connecting

rose otto, *neroli, petitgrain, fennel, coriander, jasmine*, sandalwood

Conscious

lemon, *rosemary, bergamot, basil, lavender*

Consoling

ormenis flower, *benzoin, chamomile roman, cypress,* linden blossom, *melissa, rose maroc, geranium*

Contentment

cypress, *rose otto, lavender,* neroli, *bergamot*, orange, sandalwood, patchouli, clove, ylang ylang, chamomile roman

Control (being in)

cypress, cedarwood, pine, vetiver, ginger, clove

Conviction

juniper, *vetiver, frankincense, thyme linalol, cedarwood*

Cooling

chamomile german, *peppermint, eucalyptus citriodora, eucalyptus radiata*

Co-operation

chamomile roman, grapefruit, *rose maroc, jasmine, ylang ylang*

Courage

cardamon, frankincense, ginger, hyacinth, marjoram, *cedarwood, benzoin,* fennel, orange, ormenis flower, thyme linalol

Creativity

carnation, coriander, eucalyptus citriodora, bergamot, cistus, lemon, narcissus, orange, rosemary, *frankincense*, geranium, *neroli*, rose maroc, jasmine, bay, clove, mimosa, litsea cubeba, sandalwood, cypress, *juniper*

Cushioning

carnation, geranium, *benzoin, rose otto, lavender, chamomile roman*

Decisiveness

basil, thyme linalol, *cedarwood, vetiver, patchouli, peppermint*

Devotion

rose otto, *chamomile roman, neroli*

Dignified

cedarwood, cypress, *frankincense, vetiver*

Direction

cardamon, cypress, *lemon*, pine

Directional

black pepper, *lemon*, *ginger*, *juniper*

Directness

pine, *cypress*, *cedarwood*, *clove*, *pimento berry*, cinnamon, marjoram

Discovery

narcissus, *grapefruit*, *black pepper*, *bay*

Dreams

helichrysum, *narcissus*, *mimosa*, *cedarwood*

Earthed

ormenis flower, *vetiver*, *ginger*

Elevating

frankincense, *rose otto*, *neroli*, *linden blossom*, geranium, *clary sage*, *spikenard*, *juniper*

Embracing

lavender, *benzoin*, *geranium*, *melissa*

Emotional clarity

lemon, *petitgrain*, *grapefruit*, *melissa*, *black pepper*

Emotionally invigorated

lemon, *grapefruit*, *rosemary*, *eucalyptus citriodora*

Emotionally purified

grapefruit, *frankincense*, *neroli*, *helichrysum*, *melissa*

Emotionally refreshed

peppermint, *helichrysum*, *lemon*, *grapefruit*

Emotionally stable

chamomile roman, frankincense, *vetiver*, *sandalwood*

Empathetic

ormenis flower, *melissa*, chamomile roman, lavender

Empathy

chamomile german, ginger, eucalyptus citriodora, *ormenis flower*

Empowering

narcissus, thyme linalol, *jasmine, cedarwood, frankincense*

Encompassing

carnation, *benzoin, hyacinth, rose maroc*

Encouraging

bergamot, cardamon, coriander, ginger, *cinnamon, clove,* eucalyptus citriodora, tuberose, *jasmine*

Endurance

black pepper, *ginger, rosemary, thyme linalol, nutmeg, pine*

Energizing

orange, *rosemary, peppermint, thyme linalol, basil, juniper, pine,* cinnamon, *eucalyptus globulus, grapefruit, helichrysum*

Energy

helichrysum, rosemary, *orange, peppermint*

Enlightening

fennel, frankincense, hyacinth, juniper, *neroli, rose otto, chamomile roman, cistus,*

yarrow, spikenard, sandalwood

Enlivening

coriander, *rosemary, peppermint, eucalyptus citriodora,* fennel, *petitgrain, litsea cubeba, melissa*

Enthusiasm

cardamon, *carnation, orange, jasmine, lemon, grapefruit,* tuberose, *bay,* ylang ylang, basil, coriander, *geranium,* eucalyptus citriodora, *melissa, pimento berry*

Equilibrium (restores)

clary sage, hyacinth, *cedarwood, vetiver, litsea cubeba, patchouli, sandalwood*

Euphoria

clary sage, jasmine, rose otto, *rose maroc, tuberose, narcissus,* ylang ylang

Exhilaration

pine, *cypress, juniper, mandarin, coriander*

Expansive

tuberose, *benzoin, clary sage, nutmeg, spikenard, geranium, lavender*

Expressiveness

coriander, eucalyptus citriodora, petitgrain, *neroli, cardamon, pimento berry,* sandalwood, tuberose, *jasmine, cistus, rose maroc*

Extroverted

tuberose, *jasmine, rose maroc, carnation, cinnamon, clove, bay*

Fair-minded

cinnamon, *cedarwood, cistus, cypress, pine, vetiver, lavender, marjoram*

Faith

hyacinth, *frankincense, spikenard, juniper, basil, coriander, chamomile roman, neroli, linden blossom*

Flexibility

geranium, *lavender, clary sage, lemon, myrtle, black pepper, ylang ylang*

Focus

cedarwood, marjoram, *thyme linalol, lemon,* fennel, bergamot, *basil, cypress,* juniper, lemongrass, *litsea cubeba,* ginger, cinnamon, clove,

ylang ylang, linden blossom, nutmeg, *rosemary*

Forceful

fennel, *peppermint, cinnamon, clove, clary sage*

Forgiving

hyacinth, pine, rose maroc, *rose otto, chamomile roman, neroli*

Fortitude

cardamon, cedarwood, fennel, frankincense, ginger, rosemary, thyme linalol

Fostering

melissa, *chamomile roman, benzoin, linden blossom, cardamon*

Frankness

tuberose, *jasmine, ylang ylang, cedarwood, black pepper, cypress*

Freedom

eucalyptus citriodora, rose maroc, *rose otto, neroli, petitgrain, sandalwood, cistus*

Friendliness

geranium, *mandarin, orange,
lavender, marjoram, clove,
cinnamon, bergamot*

Fulfilled

rose maroc, *benzoin, jasmine,
clary sage, geranium,
lavender, chamomile roman,
ormenis flower, ylang ylang*

Generosity

grapefruit, *benzoin, nutmeg,
cinnamon, sandalwood,
melissa, lavender, geranium*

Generosity (of spirit)

cypress, *frankincense, lavender, geranium, coriander,
chamomile roman, petitgrain,
rose otto, neroli, carnation*

Gentle

lavender, mandarin, melissa,
rose otto, hyacinth

Gentleness

chamomile roman, helichrysum, mandarin, melissa

Grounded

clary sage, patchouli, vetiver,
spikenard, ginger

Grounding

cedarwood, *vetiver,
black pepper, ginger*

Growth

vetiver, *coriander, fennel,
cardamon, orange, mimosa*

Guided

neroli, chamomile roman,
frankincense, juniper

Happiness

rose otto, *orange*, jasmine,
coriander, ginger, clove,
cinnamon, benzoin, carnation,
pimento berry, geranium,
melissa

Harmonizing

chamomile roman, clary sage,
lavender, eucalyptus citriodora,
geranium, helichrysum,
rose maroc, rose otto

Harmony

bergamot, jasmine, sandalwood, petitgrain, geranium,
ormenis flower

Healers

All essential oils are healing – the following have a healing character.

chamomile german, geranium, chamomile roman, lavender, frankincense

Honourable

vetiver, *spikenard, lavender, cedarwood, cypress, myrrh, frankincense*

Humility

pine, *chamomile roman, chamomile german, ormenis flower*, juniper, *melissa*, neroli

Humour

geranium, *orange*

Hypnotic

narcissus, *carnation, tuberose*

Idealism

helichrysum, *bay, petitgrain, coriander, chamomile roman, neroli*

Imagination

coriander, *ginger, orange, helichrysum, pimento berry, jasmine, carnation*

Incorruptibility

cypress, *cedarwood, vetiver, lavender, frankincense, lemon, bay*

Independence

carnation, *tuberose, geranium, clary sage, lemon, grapefruit, peppermint*

Inner child (for a positive)

helichrysum, *melissa, mandarin, lavender, chamomile roman*

Inner freedom

rose otto, *helichrysum, neroli*

Inner peace

chamomile roman, cypress, lavender, *rose otto*

Inner strength

helichrysum, *geranium, chamomile roman, melissa*

Inner vision

juniper, rose otto, *petitgrain, linden blossom, sandalwood, chamomile roman, sage*

Inner visionary

narcissus, *frankincense, juniper, sandalwood, basil, cypress, sage*

Inner vitality

rose maroc, *lemon, pine, juniper, litsea cubeba*

Insightfulness

sandalwood, *juniper, sage, clary sage, pine, lavender*

Inspiration

frankincense, *neroli, rose otto, bergamot, lemon, benzoin, hyacinth, carnation, jasmine, bay*

Inspiring

clary sage, grapefruit, jasmine, mandarin, narcissus

Integrity

basil, mandarin, marjoram, vetiver, *lavender, cedarwood*

Introspection

frankincense, *rose otto, pine, chamomile roman, neroli, nutmeg*

Intuitiveness

jasmine, *neroli, cistus*

Invigorating

thyme linalol, *peppermint, rosemary, eucalyptus radiata, petitgrain, pine, cedarwood, cypress,* cinnamon, *patchouli, eucalyptus citriodora*

Joy

bergamot, lemon, *neroli*, orange, rose otto, sandalwood, frankincense, petitgrain, ylang ylang, chamomile roman, linden blossom, *mimosa*, grapefruit, jasmine, helichrysum, pimento berry

Liberating

carnation, bergamot, *tuberose, grapefruit, geranium, lavender*

Lifting of sorrow

neroli, chamomile roman, *cypress*

Light-hearted

orange, grapefruit, *petitgrain*

Lightness

neroli, petitgrain, *lemon, linden blossom, lavender*

Liveliness

lemon, *grapefruit, rosemary, peppermint, eucalyptus radiata*

Love

rose otto, *rose maroc, jasmine, chamomile roman, melissa*

Loving

rose otto, neroli, *jasmine*

Lucidity

patchouli, *black pepper, cardamon, litsea cubeba, coriander, lemon, rosemary*

Meditative

frankincense, helichrysum, juniper, lavender, narcissus, ormenis flower, sandalwood, ylang ylang, *spikenard*

Memory (good)

coriander, lemon, *rosemary, eucalyptus citriodora, peppermint*

Mesmerizing

narcissus, *tuberose, rose maroc, jasmine, clary sage, cistus*

Mind-body connection

vetiver, *benzoin, lavender, geranium, helichrysum*

Mindful

ormenis flower, pine, *cypress, lavender, yarrow*

Mothering

geranium, *lavender, marjoram*

Motivated

fennel, rose maroc, rose otto

Motivating

coriander, *lavender, clove, rosemary, grapefruit, lemon, pine, cypress, bay*, bergamot, black pepper, cardamon, tuberose

Mystic

ormenis flower, *myrrh, galbanham, frankincense, vetiver, spikenard*

Nobility of spirit

This section could apply to all essential oils; this list is therefore extremely limited.

cedarwood, *neroli, frankincense, chamomile roman, basil*

Nurturing (feelings)

carnation, *lavender, geranium, mandarin, ormenis flower*

Openness

carnation, *petitgrain, ylang ylang, fennel, mimosa,* jasmine, sandalwood, *palma rosa, helichrysum*

Optimism

coriander, eucalyptus citriodora, jasmine, petitgrain

Organized

chamomile german, *cedar-wood, eucalyptus radiata, peppermint, lemon*

Originality

carnation, *tuberose, hyacinth, litsea cubeba, black pepper, clove*

Passionate

rose maroc, *jasmine, ylang ylang, tuberose, pimento berry, clove, bay*

Patience

chamomile german, cypress, pine, helichrysum, rose otto, linden blossom

Peace

Each individual person has essential oils they can attune to for peace; these are only a guide.

juniper, chamomile roman, neroli, frankincense, rose otto, melissa, angelica seed, spikenard, yarrow, jasmine, carnation

Peaceful

chamomile german, mandarin, chamomile roman, melissa, sandalwood, neroli

Penetrating

peppermint, thyme linalol, galbanham

Performance

bay, bergamot, cistus, eucalyptus citriodora, *frankincense, lemon*, lavender, *grapefruit, helichrysum*, rose maroc, jasmine, geranium, *cypress*, ormenis flower, tuberose

Perseverance

fennel, helichrysum, *hyacinth*, marjoram, *pine*

Persistence

cedarwood, patchouli, vetiver

Positivity

All essential oils used in aromatherapy can have a positive effect.

basil, bay, lemon, cedarwood, *grapefruit*, pine, vetiver, *patchouli*, juniper, melissa, myrrh, cypress, cardamon, orange, petitgrain, *geranium*, *frankincense*, rosemary, hyssop, pimento berry

Powerful (self)

cedarwood, *cypress*, *thyme linalol*, *sandalwood*, *patchouli*, *cinnamon*

Practicality

cinnamon, *pine*, *lemon*, *thyme linalol*, *black pepper*, *peppermint*, *rosemary*, *lavender*

Profoundness

jasmine, *narcissus*, *spikenard*, *frankincense*, juniper, *chamomile roman*

Progressiveness

melissa, *cistus*, *helichrysum*

Protected

vetiver, *myrrh*, *spikenard*, *yarrow*, *chamomile german*, *chamomile roman*,

frankincense, rose otto, sandalwood

Protective

cypress, frankincense, *cedarwood*, *chamomile roman*, *geranium*, *lavender*, rose otto, sandalwood

Purifying

juniper, lemon, *pine*, *sage*, *lavender*, *cypress*, rosemary

Purity of heart

cypress, *neroli*, *rose otto*, *chamomile roman*, *melissa*, *helichrysum*

Purpose

cardamon, *cinnamon*, *vetiver*, *patchouli*, *cedarwood*, *cypress*, *black pepper*, *ormenis flower*, *carnation*, *jasmine*

Purposefulness

basil, *cedarwood*, *peppermint*, *eucalyptus radiata*, *bay*, *pimento berry*

Radiating

carnation, *grapefruit*, *tuberose*, *jasmine*, *ylang ylang*, *rose maroc*, *rose otto*

Realistic

cinnamon, *lavender, peppermint, black pepper, marjoram,
pine*

Reasonable

patchouli, *lavender, peppermint, lemon, thyme linalol,
clary sage*

Reassuring

rose maroc, *benzoin,
chamomile roman, bay,
helichrysum, sandalwood*

Reconciled

lavender, *geranium, bergamot,
sandalwood, clary sage,
helichrysum*

Refreshing

mandarin, *lemon, bergamot,
lavender, lime, juniper,
eucalyptus citriodora*

Regenerating

clary sage, geranium, neroli,
orange, eucalyptus citriodora,
melissa, lavender, rose otto,
peppermint

Relaxed

chamomile german, chamomile
roman, clary sage, jasmine,
lavender, linden blossom,
melissa, ormenis flower, petitgrain

Releasing

carnation, *palma rosa,
hyacinth, rose maroc,
linden blossom, lavender*

Reliable

fennel, *vetiver, cedarwood,
frankincense, myrrh, pine*

Resolute

fennel, orange, *patchouli,
ginger, black pepper*

Resolution

frankincense, *myrrh, lavender,
cistus*

Restfulness

lavender, geranium,
rose maroc, clary sage,
*linden blossom, neroli,
marjoram*, petitgrain,
sandalwood, mimosa

Restorative

rosemary, *eucalyptus radiata,
peppermint, pine, cinnamon,
cardamon,* clary sage, petitgrain, *lavender*, cypress,
bergamot

Restored

marjoram, patchouli, *ginger, pine, lavender*

Revitalizing

mandarin, petitgrain, *orange, grapefruit, melissa, rosemary,* clary sage, *lavender, neroli, lemon*

Reviving

rose otto, *eucalyptus citriodora, lavender, rosemary, melissa, linden blossom,* rose maroc, *bergamot, geranium, mandarin, palma rosa*

Sacredness

juniper, *neroli, chamomile roman, sandalwood, basil,* frankincense, spikenard, sage

Sagacious

narcissus, frankincense

Secretiveness

carnation, *bay, hyacinth, rose otto, lavender*

Secular

chamomile roman, cinnamon

Secure

geranium, *lavender, benzoin, linden blossom, chamomile roman*

Security

black pepper, *frankincense, cedarwood, cinnamon, clove, clary sage,* linden blossom, *geranium, benzoin,* sandalwood

Self-awareness

clary sage, ylang ylang, cypress, geranium, pine, *sandalwood,* bay, ormenis flower, *jasmine,* clove, pimento berry, mandarin, coriander, angelica seed, *sage,* cistus, *myrtle,* rosemary

Self-esteem

hyacinth, sandalwood, vetiver, *ylang ylang,* rose maroc, *jasmine,* carnation, *bergamot,* geranium, ormenis flower, *cedarwood,* tuberose

Self-forgiveness

pine, chamomile roman, frankincense, geranium, lemon

Self-image

orange, lavender, melissa, neroli, chamomile roman, ylang ylang, rose maroc,

jasmine, sandalwood, cypress,
juniper, cedarwood, pine,
black pepper, frankincense,
mandarin, nutmeg, myrtle, bay

Self-worth

carnation, juniper, rose otto,
mandarin, orange, patchouli,
bay

Sensitivity

cypress, jasmine, *hyacinth*,
rose otto, *neroli*,
linden blossom, marjoram,
sandalwood, tuberose,
carnation, melissa

Sensuality

jasmine, rose otto, rose maroc,
sandalwood, ylang ylang,
tuberose

Sensuous

tuberose, ylang ylang

Serene

chamomile roman, sandalwood

Serenity

chamomile roman,
linden blossom

Sharing

pine, lavender, ormenis flower,
hyacinth

Shielding

geranium, lavender, marjoram,
bergamot, cedarwood, benzoin

Simplicity

pine, chamomile roman,
chamomile german,
ormenis flower

Sincere

marjoram, rosemary, cypress,
cedarwood

Sincerity

coriander, juniper,
chamomile roman, clary sage

Softly

cypress, *chamomile roman,*
mandarin, rose otto, melissa

Softness

chamomile roman, *mandarin,*
rose otto, melissa

Soothed

clary sage, geranium,
linden blossom, mandarin,
ylang ylang, *benzoin*

Soothing

chamomile german,
chamomile roman, hyacinth,
jasmine, marjoram,
ormenis flower, patchouli

Soundness

eucalyptus citriodora, petitgrain, black pepper, mimosa

Spontaneous

grapefruit, tuberose, lemon,
coriander, orange, neroli,
chamomile roman

Sprightly

mandarin, melissa, grapefruit

Stability

chamomile roman, geranium,
linden blossom, neroli, rosemary, cedarwood, cypress,
petitgrain

Stamina

black pepper, *cinnamon*

Steadfast

cinnamon, *vetiver, patchouli*

Steadiness

geranium, *lavender, pine,
fennel, cedarwood*

Stillness

carnation, chamomile roman,
cypress, narcissus

Stimulating

basil, cardamon, patchouli,
eucalyptus citriodora, *peppermint*, ylang ylang, *rosemary,*
eucalyptus radiata, lemon

Straightforwardness

*black pepper, peppermint,
frankincense, cedarwood, basil,*
cardamon, cypress

Strength

basil, bergamot, *cedarwood,
cinnamon*, clary sage, *cypress*,
juniper, lemon, melissa, petitgrain, *vetiver*

Strengthening

cedarwood, *ginger*, marjoram,
rosemary

Strong

chamomile german, orange

Structured

cypress, linden blossom, rosemary

Supportive

melissa, thyme linalol

Sympathetic

mandarin, orange, lavender, geranium

Tenacity

pine

Tenderness

carnation, *rose otto, mandarin, benzoin*

Tolerant

thyme linalol, *peppermint, frankincense, clary sage, lavender, marjoram*

Tranquil

geranium, mandarin, *clary sage, chamomile roman*

Transformation

tuberose, carnation, *patchouli, sandalwood*

Trust

basil, hyacinth, cypress, *lavender*

Trusting

hyacinth, *pine*, sandalwood, eucalyptus citriodora, *cypress*

Truthful

narcissus, *frankincense*

Understanding

chamomile german, *chamomile roman, cypress*, eucalyptus citriodora, helichrysum, *neroli, pine*

Unhurried

ormenis flower, *marjoram, vetiver*

Unifying

ylang ylang, carnation

Unity

sandalwood

Unruffled

patchouli

Uplifted

clary sage, *grapefruit*, jasmine, juniper, mandarin, orange, *petit-grain*, ylang ylang

Upliftment

eucalyptus citriodora, *rosemary, basil*, bergamot

Versatile

lemon, *lavender*

Vibrancy

peppermint

Vigorous

rosemary

Visionary

juniper, sage

Visualization (relaxing)

lavender, neroli, rose otto, chamomile roman, clary sage

Visualization (stimulating)

rosemary, ginger, black pepper, thyme linalol

Vitality

eucalyptus citriodora, juniper, *peppermint*

Warming

cinnamon, clary sage, ginger, helichrysum, marjoram, orange, thyme linalol

Warmth

ginger, ylang ylang, sandalwood

Welcoming

jasmine

Willpower

cypress, cedarwood

Wisdom

frankincense, juniper, rose otto, vetiver, cypress, cedarwood

Wise

cypress, sandalwood, cedarwood

Violet Leaf

Part Four

APPENDICES I–IV

Author's Note:

Valerie Ann Worwood is always grateful to receive feedback
and readers' comments, but regrets that she is unable to reply
personally to all letters. Please write to:

> PO Box 2256
> Romford
> Essex RM7 7BU
> England

Workshops in Aroma-Genera are conducted in Britain,
Australia, New Zealand, Canada and the United States of
America. For details please see *Suppliers*. For information
please send a large, stamped, self-addressed envelope.

APPENDIX I – SAFETY DATA

NOT ALL NATURAL PLANTS OR PLANT PRODUCTS ARE BENEFICIAL to health. Deadly Nightshade can be poisonous and stinging nettles sting. The following essential oils should NOT be used under any circumstances:

Bitter Almond	Rue
Boldo leaf	Sassafras
Calamus	Savin
Yellow Camphor	Southernwood
Horseradish	Tansy
Jaborandi leaf	Thuja
Mugwort	Wintergreen
Mustard	Wormseed
Pennyroyal	Wormwood

(List as recommended by the International Federation of Aromatherapists code of practice.)

Essential oils are highly concentrated plant essences and should not be taken orally unless under medical supervision.

People with sensitive skin or allergic reactions to aromatic materials should always do a skin test twenty-four hours before use.

Some essential oils have been documented as being photo-sensitive and should not be applied to the skin before exposure to the sun. Of those mentioned in this book, those that may fall into this category are among the citrus oils – especially bergamot, and also angelica.

PREGNANCY

In pregnancy, the usual quantities should be reduced by at least half volumes of essential oil. Certain essential oils should be avoided altogether during pregnancy or when breastfeeding. These are:

Basil	Cinnamon	Aniseed
Fennel	Juniper	Marjoram
Peppermint	Rosemary	Thyme
Clary sage	Oregano	Clove
Nutmeg	Bay	Pimento Berry
Cistus	Hops	Sage
Valerian	Spikenard	Black Pepper
Tarragon	Cedarwood	

APPENDIX II – THERAPEUTIC COMPONENTS OF ESSENTIAL OILS AND ABSOLUTES

Principal chemical components of essential oils relevant to
The Fragrant Mind

MOST SCIENTISTS AND RESEARCHERS HAVE ATTRIBUTED THE therapeutic action of essential oils on the brain/mind to several identified groups of naturally occurring botanical chemicals. It is evident that there are other components, albeit traces, which are as yet unidentifiable, but which might play a significant part in the action of essential oils on the brain.

Although the following identified components account for some of the therapeutic effects, it cannot be said that they account for all the properties ascribed to many of the essential oils. In fact in aromatherapy some essential oils that are used for emotional conditions contain no known compound that would explain their efficacy, Frankincense being among them (Lunny V N). Essential oils extracted by methods other than steam distillation, such as flower absolutes, contain other heavier compounds which cannot be obtained by steam distillation. Carbon dioxide (CO_2) extraction yields even more compounds which would have been lost using either of the other methods. Therefore the process by which essential oils are obtained defines which chemical compounds they may contain.

Many essential oils are known to have an adaptogenic

character – having either a stimulant or sedative action depending upon the physiological and pathological condition of the body/brain to which it is/are applied. Another level of complexity occurs when essential oils are combined in formulations; it is possible that they form new synergistic compounds that are unidentifiable by scientific procedures. New methods of analysis are also identifying components not previously known to be part of a particular essential oil's makeup and with the advance of technology, undoubtedly more will come to light. However, whether for home use or for use in a clinical setting, these essential oils have a long successful history of safe therapeutic use.

Several researchers including Louis-Claude Vincent, Jean Mar and most recently Pierre Franchomme and Daniel Pénoël, have shown that essential oils have positive and negative charges, which at present are attributed to the major chemical groups. For example, Phenols which are known to be warming and potentially strong have been attributed with a positive charge. Aldehydes are thought to be cooling and calming with a negative charge, and so on. However, only certain individual components have been tested, rather than complete essential oils, which may in their entire synergistic form give an entirely different picture, and one must suspect that overall the story is far more complex. (See Chapter 2.)

The chemical components listed are only some of those contained in essential oils, those which are particularly relevant to the subject material of *The Fragrant Mind*. The list is by no means conclusive, and has been included for those who need foundational evidence for the aromatherapeutic use of essential oils and absolutes.

Basically, chemicals affect receptors in the body by sedating or stimulating:

ACIDS	Stimulant	ALCOHOLS	Stimulant, Sedative
ALDEHYDES	Calming	COUMARINS	Sedative, Hypnotic
ETHERS	Calming, Analgesic	ESTERS	Sedative, Calming
HYDROCARBONS	Calming	TERPENES	Stimulant, Tonic
PHENOLS	Stimulant, Tonic		

ANTI-SPASMODIC	BALANCING
Ethers, Esters, Phenols, Sesquiterpenes	Ethers, Esters, Alcohols

CALMING	COOLING
Aldehydes, Coumarins, Ethers, Esters, Sesquiterpenes	Aldehydes, Esters

ENERGIZING	HYPNOTIC
Alcohols	Alderhydes, Coumarins

HYPOTENSIVES	TONIC GENERAL
Alcohols, Coumarins, Esters	Alcohols, Esters, Sesquiterpenols

TONING	RELAXING
Alcohols, Terpenes	Alderhydes, Coumarins, Ethers, Esters, Lactones, Sesquiterpenes

SEDATIVE	SOOTHING
Alderhydes, Coumarins, Esters	Alderhydes, Ethers, Esters

STIMULATING	WARMING
Alcohols, Ethers, Ketones, Mono-terpenes, Monoterpenols, Oxides, Phenols, Terpenes, Acids	Phenols, Oxides, Terpenes

APPENDIX III – SUPPLIERS

ESSENTIAL OILS

Britain

Valerie Ann Worwood Aromatherapy

Comprehensive aromatherapy list and other related items. For price list and other information please send a large, stamped, self-addressed envelope or, from overseas, an International Response Coupon. Valerie Ann Worwood Aromatherapy, PO Box 2256, Romford, Essex RM7 7BU, England

Aroma-Genera

Details of workshops in the UK can be obtained from PO Box 2256, Romford, Essex RM7 7BU. Please send a stamped, self-addressed envelope.

Earthway Aromatherapy

Mail order service for essential oils, aromatherapy products for the professional and non-professional. For catalogue please send a large, stamped, self-addressed envelope or, from overseas, an International Response Coupon. Earthway Aromatherapy, PO Box 5278, Westcliffe-on-Sea, Essex, SS0 7TT, England

North America

The Anahata Centre

Mail order service for essential oils and related products, including Aroma-Genera oils and workshops. Please enclose a stamped addressed envelope for price list. PO Box 149, 185-9040 Blundell Road, Richmond, V6Y 1K3, British Columbia, Canada

Australasia

Aroma-Genera Workshops New Zealand

Mail order service for essential oils and related products, including Aroma-Genera Workshops. PO Box 8083, New Plymouth, New Zealand (Tel: 06 758 5859 Fax: 06 758 1556)

APPENDIX IV – USEFUL ADDRESSES

Please send a large, stamped, self-addressed envelope to these addresses if you require a reply. Many of the organizations listed below have local groups; see the telephone directories.

AROMATHERAPY

Valerie Ann Worwood Study Systems

Aromatherapy study courses. P.O. Box 2256, Romford, Essex RM7 7BU, England.

The Aroma-Genera Association of North America

For information and list of professional Aroma-Generists. 1917 West 4th, Vancouver, British Columbia V6S 1M7, Canada

International Federation of Aromatherapists

Information on aromatherapy and list of registered aroma-therapists; information on professional courses and training. Stamford House, 2–4 Chiswick High Road, London W4 0TZ

International Society of Professional Aromatherapists
Hinckley and District Hospital and Health Centre, The
Annexe, Mount Road, Hinckley, Leicestershire LE10 1AG

Register of Qualified Aromatherapists
PO Box 6941, London W8 9HF

COUNSELLING, CARE AND HEALING

British Association for Counselling

37A Sheep Street, Rugby, Warwickshire CV21 2BX (01788
78328/9)

British Association of Psychotherapists

121 Hendon Lane, London N3 3PR (0171 346 1747)

British Psychological Society

Provides information on counselling services.
St Andrews House, 48 Princes Road East, Leicester LE1
7DR (0116 2549568)

Carers National Association

Information and advice for people acting as carers.
20–25 Glasshouse Yard, London EC1A 4JS (0171 490 8818)

Confederation of Healing Associations

Suite 3, The Red and White House, 113 High Street,
Berkhamsted, Herts HP4 2DJ (01442 870660)

Co-Counselling International

c/o Westerly, Prestwick Lane, Chiddingfold, Surrey GU8
4XW

The Maitreya School of Healing

Courses in mental colour therapy, spiritual healing.
11 Holland Road, Ampthill, Bedford MK45 2RR (01525 403345)

National Federation of Spiritual Healers

Old Manor Farm Studio, Church Street, Sunbury-on-Thames, Middlesex TW16 6RG (01932 783164)

Westminster Pastoral Foundation

Provides advice on counselling services.
23 Kensington Square, London W8 5HN (0171 937 6956)

Who Cares Trust

National network providing advice for young people and their carers.
Citybridge House, 235–245 Goswell Road, London EC1V 7JD (0171 833 9047)

OTHER THERAPIES

Association for Humanistic Psychology

26 Huddlestone Road, London E7 0AN

Behavioural Therapy

British Psychological Society, St Andrews House, 48 Princes Road East, Leicester LE1 7DR (0116 549568)

Bio-Dynamic Therapy and Bio-Energetics

The Gerda Boysen Centre, Acacia House, Centre Avenue, Acton Park, London W3 7SX

Bio-Energetic

G. C. Whitfield, Westmount House, 146A Eastern Road, Brighton, East Sussex BN2 2AE

British Society of Medical and Dental Hypnosis

For information on hypnotherapy.
151 Otley Old Road, Leeds LS16 6HN

Council for Complementary and Alternative Medicine

A register of qualified practitioners of complementary
therapies and medicine.
Park House, 206–208 Latimer Road, London W10 6RE
(0181 968 3862)

Gestalt Therapy

Gestalt Centre, 64 Warwick Road, St Albans, Herts AL1 4DL
(01727 864806)

Humanistic Psychology

Personal and professional development.
7 Earlham Road, Norwich NR2 3RD

Institute of Psycho-Synthesis

The Barn, Nan Clark's Lane, London NW7 4HH (0181 202
4525)

The Open Centre

Encounter groups and self-awareness therapy.
118 Old Street, London EC1 9BP (0171 251 1504)

Positive Health Centre

For list of autogenic training practitioners, usually professionally qualified health workers.
101 Harley Street, London W1N 1DF

Psychosynthesis and Education Trust

48 Guildford Road, Stockwell, London SW8 2BV (0171 403
2100)

ADVICE ON DRINK, DRUGS AND SMOKING

Action on Alcohol Abuse

Advice and help with alcohol abuse.
26 Craven Street, London WC2N 5NT (0171 839 7345)

ADFAM National

Support, information and helpline for families and friends of drug users.
Chapel House, 18 Hatton Place, London EC1N 8ND (0171 405 3923)

Al-Anon Family Groups UK and Eire

Support and advice for relatives and friends of alcoholics.
61 Great Dover Street, London SE1 4YE (0171 403 0888)

Alcoholics Anonymous

Encouragement, advice and support in overcoming alchoholism.
PO Box 1 Stonebow House, Stonebow, York YO1 2NJ.
(01904 644026)
General Service Office, 11 Redcliffe Gardens, London SW10 9BG
Helplines: England 0171 352 3001 Scotland 0141 221 9027 Wales 01646 695555 Northern Ireland 01232 681084

CITA – Council for Involuntary Tranquilliser Addiction

Support and information for sufferers of prescribed drug addiction and their families.
Cavendish House, Brighton Road, Waterloo, Liverpool L22 5NG (0151 949 0102)

Drinkline

Information and advice for people worried about their alcohol drinking.
13–14 West Smithfield, London EC1A 9DH (0171 332 0150)

Families Anonymous

Self-help group for those affected by drug abuse or related problems.
Unit 37, Doddington & Rollo Community Association
Charlotte Despard Avenue, London SW11 5JE (0171 498 4680)

Narcotics Anonymous

Help and advice on coming off drugs.
PO Box 1980, London N19 3LS (0171 272 9040, 0171 498 9005)

Quit

Help and advice to smokers wishing to quit.
102 Gloucester Place, London W1H 3DA (0171 487 2858)

The Standing Conference on Drug Abuse

Up-to-date local information for drug users and their family and friends.
1–4 Hatton Place, Hatton Gardens, London EC1 8ND (0171 430 2341)
Freephone: Dial 100 and ask for Freephone Drug Problems

Turning Point

Help for people with drink, drug and mental health problems.
101 Back Church Lane, London E1 1LU (0171 702 2300)

SPECIALIST ADVICE AND SUPPORT

Age Concern

Direct services to older people in the UK.
Astral House, 1268 London Road, London SW16 4ER (0181 679 8000)
Bernard Sunley House, 60 Pitcairn Road, Mitcham, Surrey CR4 3LL and 54A Fountainbridge, Edinburgh, EH3 9PT

Alzheimer's Disease Society

Advice and information for carers and families.
Gordon House, 10 Greencoat Place, London SW1P 1PH (0171 306 0606)

Alzheimer's Scotland

Advice and information for carers and families.
8 Hill Street, Edinburgh, EH2 3JZ (0131 225 1453)

Associations of Widows

54–57 Allison Street, Digbeth, Birmingham B5 5TH

British Association of Cancer United Patients

Information and emotional support for cancer patients and their families.
3 Bath Place, Rivington Street, London EC2A 3JR (0171 696 9003)

British Dyslexia Association

Support and information for all those with dyslexia.
98 London Road, Reading, Berkshire RG1 5AU (01734 668271)

Cancerlink

Emotional support and information to people affected with cancer and their families.
17 Britannia Street, London WC1X 9JN (0171 713 7867)
9 Castle Terrace, Edinburgh EH1 2DP (0131 228 5557)
Macline for teenagers 0800 591028, Asian line 0171 713 7867

Childline

Free national help line for troubled children.
2nd Floor, Royal Mail Building, Studd Street, London N1 OQW (0171 239 1000)

Child Watch

Counsels adults and children who have been abused.
206 Hessle Road, Hull, North Humberside HU3 3BE (01482
25552)

Citizens Advice Bureau

Drop-in or appointment system for anyone needing advice to
do with finance, housing, employment, law and many other
matters. Very wide scope, and practical help and involvement.
See telephone directory for local offices.

The Compassionate Friends

Support groups for bereaved parents.
53 North Street, Bristol BS3 1EN (0117 966 5202)

Cruse (Bereavement care)

Help and advice plus contact with other bereaved people.
Cruse House, 126 Sheen Road, Richmond, Surrey TW9 1UR
(0181 940 4818)

Cry-sis

Self-help and support for families with demanding children.
BM CRY-SIS, London WC1N 3XX (0171 404 5011)

Cult Information Centre

Information on cults.
BCM Cults, London WC1N 3XX (0181 651 3322)

Eating Disorders Association

Information and support for those suffering from bulimia or
anorexia, as well as for their families.
Sackville Place, 44 Magdalen Street, Norwich, Norfolk NR3
1JU (Helpline: 01603 621414)

Gamblers Anonymous

Self-help for gambling problems.
PO Box 88, London SW10 OEU (0171 384 3040)

Headway

Advice and information for people with head injuries.
7 King Edward Court, King Edward Street, Nottingham NG1
1EW (0115 924 0800)

Home Start UK

Support, friendship and help for young families under stress.
2 Salisbury Road, Leicester LE7 7QR (0116 255 4988)

Life Line

Support, advice and counselling for women with unplanned
pregnancies as well as post-abortion counselling.
Cae Bach, 4 Pant-y-Wennol, Bodafon, Llandudno, Gwynedd,
LL30 3DE (01492 543741)

ME Association

Advice and support to people affected with ME.
Stanhope House, High Street, Stanford-le-hope, Essex SS17
0HA (01375 642466)

Meet-a-Mum Association

Advice for post-natal depression, friendship and support for
mothers.
14 Willis Road, Croydon CRO 2XX (0181 665 0357)

MENCAP

Services, advice and support for people with learning diffi-
culties, their families and carers.
Mencap National Centre, 123 Golden Lane, London EC1Y
ORT (0171 454 0454)

MIND (National Association for Mental Health)

Over 230 local associations providing counselling and other
services for people with mental health problems; and produces
publications on a wide range of issues including drug withdrawal, bereavement, tranquillizer addiction, dementia and
depression.

22 Harley Street, London W1 (0171 637 0741)
Granta House, 15–19 Broadway, Stratford, London E15 4BQ
(0181 519 2122)

Miscarriage Association

Support and advice for those who have been through mis-
carriage.
Head office c/o Clayton Hospital, Northgate, Wakefield, West
Yorkshire WF1 3JS (01924 200799)

Missing Persons Bureau

Help and support for families of missing persons.
Roebuck House, 284–286, Upper Richmond Road West, East
Sheen, London SW14 7JE (0181 392 2000)

National AIDS Helpline

Twenty-four hour, free and confidential phoneline, with advice
on any aspect of HIV and AIDS.
PO Box 1577, London NW1 3DE (0800 567123)

National Council for One Parent Families

Advice on issues relating to lone parenthood.
255 Kentish Town Road, London NW5 2XL (0171 267 1361)

National Debtline

Expert telephone advice on financial difficulties.
318 Summer Lane, Birmingham B19 3RL (0121 359 3562)

National Stepfamily Association

Advice, support and information for step-parenting families.
72 Willesden Lane, London NW6 7TA (0171 372 0844)

NCH Action for Children

Projects supporting children, throughout the UK.
85 Highbury Park, London N5 1UD (0171 226 2033)

Norcap – National Organization for Counselling Adoptees and their Parents

Guidance and support for adoptees, adoptive and birth parents.
3 New High Street, Headington, Oxford OX3 7AJ (01865 750554)

NSF

Support charity for schizophrenia.
28 Castle Street, Kingston upon Thames, Surrey KT1 1SS (0181 547 3937; Advice Line: 0181 837 6436)

Parents Against Injustice (Pain)

Support and advice for parents mistakenly accused of abuse.
3 Riverside Business Park, Stansted, Essex CM24 8PL (01279 647171)

Parent Line

Support for parents under stress.
Westbury House, 57 Hart Road, Thundersley, Essex SS7 3PP (01268 757077)

Phobic Action

Practical help and support and advice for people suffering phobias.
Claygrounds Groups, Manor Road, Woodford Green, Essex IG8 8PR (0181 559 2459)

Phobics Society

Support and advice for people suffering phobias.
(0161 881 1937)

Positively Women

Confidential advice for women with HIV or AIDS.
5 Sebastian Street, London EC1V OHE (0171 490 5515 Helpline: 0171 490 2327)

Refuge

Emergency accommodation and advice for women.
(0181 995 4430 Crisisline: 0181 995 4430)

Relate – National Marriage Guidance

Counselling agency for relationship difficulties. Offices all over UK, see local phone book. Herbert Gray College, Little Church Street, Rugby, Warwickshire CV21 3AP (01788 573241)

Release

National helpline for drug and legal advice.
388 Old Street, London EC1V 9LT (0171 729 9904/0171 603 8654)

Samaritans

Confidential support for people feeling low and even suicidal: national number (Link Line) 0345 909090 and see local telephone directories.
Head Office: 10 The Grove, Slough SL1 1QP (01753 532713)

Saneline

Confidential support and information for anyone with mental illness.
199–205 Old Marylebone Road, London NW1 5QP (0171 724 8000)

Schizophrenic Association of Great Britain

Advice and support to schizophrenics and their families.
Bryn Hyfryd, The Crescent, Bangor LL57 2AG (01248 354048)

Scottish Association for Mental Health

Information on mental health issues.
Atlantic House, 38 Gardner's Crescent, Edinburgh EH3 8DQ (0131 229 9687)

Stillbirth and Neonatal Death Society

Support for those who have suffered stillbirth or neonatal death.
28 Portland Place, London W1N 4DE

Survivors of Sexual Abuse

Counselling advice and self-help groups.
Feltham Open Door Project, The Debrome Building, Boundaries Road, Feltham TW13 SDT (0181 890 4732)

Terrence Higgins Trust

Advice, counselling, and services for people with HIV and AIDS.
52–54 Gray's Inn Road, London WC1X 8JU (0171 831 0330; Helpline: 0171 242 1010; Legal line 0171 405 2381)

The National Autistic Society

Advice, information and schools and centres for people with autism.
276 Willesden Lane, London NW2 5RB (0181 451 1114)

Women Against Rape

Counselling, support and advice regarding rape.
Kings Cross Women's Centre, 71 Tonbridge Street, London WC1H 9DZ (0171 837 7509)

Women's Aid Federation England

Emergency and temporary accommodation and advice for abused women.
PO Box 391, Bristol BS99 7WS (0117 963 3542)

Women's Aid Scotland

Information and support for women and children.
12 Torphichen Street, Edinburgh EH3 8JQ (0131 221 0401)

Young Minds

Provides information and advice on issues relating to the mental health of children and young people.
22A Boston Place, London NW1 6ER (0171 724 7262)

NOTES TO CHAPTERS 1–14

Notes to Chapter 1

[1]Varro E. Tyler, *Natural Products and Medicines*, in *Herbalgram*, 1993, **28**

[2]Peter Gorman, *Making Magic, Omni*, July 1993, p 86

[3]*Ibid*, p 86

[4]Richard Evans Schultes and Albert Hofmann, *Plants of The Gods*, Rochester, Healing Arts Press, 1992, p 173

[5]*Ibid*

Notes to Chapter 2

[1]Richard Thompson, *The Brain, A Neuroscience Primer*, New York, W. H. Freeman and Company, 1993, p4

[2]*Ibid*, p5

[3]*Ibid*, p3

[4]Peter Tompkins and Christopher Bird, *Secrets of The Soil*, London, Penguin/Arkana, 1992, p126

[5]Pierre Franchomme and Daniel Pénoël, *L'Aromathérapie Exactement*, Limoges, Rogor Jollois, 1990

[6]Peter Tompkins and Christopher Bird, *Secrets of The Soil*, London, Penguin/Arkana, 1992

[7]Craig Warren and Stephen Warrenburg, 'Mood Benefits of Fragrance', *The International Journal of Aromatherapy*, Summer 1993, **5**, 2

[8]W. Jager G. Buchbauer, L. Jirovetz, M. Fritzer, 'Percutaneous Absorption of Lavender Oil from a Massage Oil', *J. Soc. Cosmet. Chem.*, **43**, p49–54

[9]Richard Thompson, *The Brain*, p121

[10]*Ibid*, p151

[11]*Ibid*, p150

[12]*Ibid*, p175

[13]*Ibid*, p159

[14]Rob McCaleb, *Herbalgram*, Vol 29, 1993, p20

[15]Buchbauer, *International Journal of Aromatherapy*, Spring 1993, p13

[16]*Ibid*, p12

[17]Peter Tompkins and Christopher Bird, *Secrets of The Soil*, London, Penguin/Arkana, 1992, p103

[18]*After Dark,* Channel 4 TV, Open Media Productions

[19]Tompkins and Bird, *Secrets of The Soil*, London, Penguin/Arkana, 1992, p101

[20]Christopher Bird, *The Persecution and Trial of Gaston Naessens – The True Story of The Effort to Suppress an Alternative Treatment for Cancer, AIDS, and Other Immunologically Based Diseases*, Tiburon, California, H. J. Kramer Inc, 1991, p15

[21]*Ibid*, pp300–301

[22]*Ibid*, p304

[23]Michael Talbot, *The Holographic Universe*, New York, HarperCollins, 1991

[24]Johnson and Goldfinger, *Health Letter Book*, p418

[25]'Prozac' (fluoxetine hydrochloride) Data Sheet IFDO2MAR93, Dista Products Ltd, Basingstoke, Hants RG21 2XA

[26]*Chemical Marketing Reporter*, 4 June, 1990

[27]Brendan O'Regan, 'Healing, Remission, and Miracle Cures', *Institute of Noetic Sciences Special Report*, May 1987, p3

[28]*Ibid*, p3

[29]Thomas J. Hurley III, 'Placebo Effects: Unmapped Territory of Mind/Body Interactions', *Investigations* 1985, **2**, p9

[30]*A Prescription for Improvement*, Audit Commission, London, HMSO, March 1994, p18

[31]*Ibid*, p23

Notes to Chapter 3

[1]Jane Butterworth, 'The Day I Went Insane . . .', *Practical Health*, p82

[2]William Lowther, 'Beaming up . . . a human computer', *Mail on Sunday*, 13 February 1994

[3]Bill Moyers, *Healing and The Mind*, London, Thorson, HarperCollins, 1993, p182

[4]Jeanne Achterberg, 'Mind and Medicine: The Role of Imagery in Healing', *ASPR Newsletter* 14, June 1988, **3**, p20

[5]Michael Talbot, *The Holographic Universe*, New York, HarperCollins, 1991, p105

[6]*Ibid*, p105

[7]*The British Medical Association Complete Family Health Encyclopedia*, London, Dorling Kindersley, 1990

[8]*A Prescription for Improvement*, Audit Commission Report, 1994, HMSO Publications, p 21

[9]Russell Murray, Donna Hurle and Anthony Grant, *Tranquillizers, The MIND Guide to Where to Get Help*, MIND/Bradford University, 1991, (available from MIND, Granta House, 15–19 Broadway, Stratford, London E15)

[10]Bill Moyers, *Healing and The Mind*, Thorson, 1993, p97

[11]P. Goldberg, *The Intuitive Edge*, Turnstone Press, Wellingborough, 1985

Notes to Chapter 4

[1]James A. Duke, PhD, 'Father Nature's Farmacy', *HerbalGram*, Spring 1987, **12**, p6

[2]Erin P. Reed, 'Environmental Fragrancing Technology Makes Dollars & Scents', *The Aroma-Chology Review*, September 1993, p6

[3]Valerie Ann Worwood, *The Fragrant Pharmacy*, London, Bantam Books, 1990

[4]Erin P. Reed, op. cit., p5

[5]Quoted in *Crains Chicago Business*, 2–8 December, 1991, p1

[6]See *V. A. W. Aromatherapy* in Appendix III, p558

[7]*Daily Express*, 12 February 1994

[8]Georgia Persinos, PhD, *Herbalgram*, 1992, **26**, p14

[9]*Washington Insight*, 15 June, 1989 and 15 September 1991

[10]A. R. Hirsch, P. M. Piecinski and K. M. Rankin, 'Trichloro-ethylene Exposure and Headache', *Headache*, p275

Notes to Chapter 5

[1]Valerie Ann Worwood, *The Fragrant Pharmacy*, London, Bantam Books, 1990, pp17–21

Notes to Chapter 7

[1]Valerie Ann Worwood, *Fragrant Sensuality*, London, Bantam Books, 1993

[2]Dr Seymour Epstein, *Sunday Express*, 10 January 1993, p34

Notes to Chapter 8

[1]Debbie Taylor, 'Women: An Analysis', *Women: A World Report*, New Internationalist/Methuen, London, 1985, p65

[2]J. Kleijnen and P. Knipschild, 'Ginkgo biloba', *The Lancet*, 1992, 340(7): 1136–9, see also Kleijnen and Knipschild 'Ginkgo biloba for cerebral insufficiency', *British Journal of Clinical Pharmacology*, 1992, **34**, 352–8

[3]Glyn Jones, 'A Shrinking of The Spirit', *Guardian*, 8 March 1994, p21

[4]I am grateful to *Herbalgram* for this information: No 14, *Fall* 1987, p3, referring to a report in *Planta Medica* **53** (1) pp5–8

[5]'Femail', *Daily Mail*, 1 March 1993

[6]*Los Angeles Times*, 1 October 1991

[7] *A Prescription for Improvement*, Audit Commission, HMSO, 1994, p23

[8]Tony Buzan, *The Mind-Map Book*, London, BBC Books, 1993

[9]NSF Information Sheet *What is Schizophrenia?*, NSF, Kingston upon Thames, Surrey

Notes to Chapter 9

[1]See *Positive Health Centre* listing in addresses for list of practitioners

Notes to Chapter 10

[1]*Carers National Association*, 20–25 Glasshouse Yard, London EC14 4JS (0171 490 8818)

[2]*Westminster Pastoral Foundation*, 23 Kensington Square, London W8 5HN (0171 376 2404)

[3]*Psychological Society*, St Andrews House, 48 Princes Road East, Leicester LE1 7DR

[4]Dr Roger J. Woolger, *Other Lives, Other Selves*, New York, Doubleday, 1987

Notes to Chapter 12

[1]Roger Woolger, *Other Lives, Other Selves*, Wellingborough, Crucible, 1990, p16

[2]Truddi Chase, *When Rabbit Howls*, New York, EP Dutton, 1987

[3]Dr Ronald Livingston, 'Natrum muriaticum', *Health and Homeopathy*, Summer 1992, London, The Hahnemann Society of Great Britain

BIBLIOGRAPHY

Adams, R. B., Victor, M., *Principles of Neurology*, New York, McGraw-Hill, 1991, p 307

Aikman, Lonnelle, 'Nature's Gifts to Medicine', *National Geographic*, September 1974

Alexander, F. M., *The Use of Self*, New York, Dutton, 1932

Anholt, R. R. H., 'Primary Events in Olfactory Reception', *Trends Biochem Sci*, 1987 **12**, p 58

Anholt, R. R. H. 'Odor recognition and olfactory transduction', *Chem. Senses*, 1991 **16**, p 421

Argyle, M., *The Psychology of Interpersonal Behaviour*, London, 1967

Atanassova-Shopova, S., Roussinov, K., 'Effects of Salvia sclarea essential oil on the central nervous system', *Bulletin of the Institute of Physiology*, Bulgarian Academy of Sciences, 1970, **13**, pp 89–95

Badia, P., Wesensten, N., Lammers, W., Culpepper, J., and Harsh, J. 'Responsiveness to Olfactory Stimuli Presented in Sleep', *Physiology & Behaviour*, 1990 **48**, pp 87–90

Badia, P., 'Olfaction Sensitivity in Sleep: The Effects of Fragrance on the Quality of Sleep', *Perfumer and Flavorist*, 1991, **16**, pp 33–4

Baerheim Svendsen A., and Scheffer J. J. C. (ed), *Essential*

Oils and Aromatic Plants, Nederlands, Dr W. Junk Publications, 1984

Balz R., *Les Huiles Essentielles; et comment les utiliser*, Crest, Balz Publications, 1986

Bardeau, F., *La Medicine Aromatique*, Paris, Robert Laffont, 1976

Baron, R. A. 'Environmentally-induced positive effect: Its impact on self-efficacy, task performance, negotiation, and conflict', *J Appl Soc Psycho*, 1990, **20**, pp 368–84

Baron, R., Byrne, D., *Social psychology; Understanding Human Interaction*, 5th edn, Allyn and Bacon inc, 1974

Beck, A. T., *Cognitive Therapy and the Emotional Disorders*, New York, Penguin, 1991

Benson, D. F., 'Treatable dementias' in: Benson, D. F., Blumer, D. (eds), *Psychiatric Aspects of Neurologic Disease*, **11**, New York, Grune & Stratton, 1992, p 139

Bernadet, M., *La Phyto-aromatherapie practique*, Paris, Editions Dangles, 1983

Blakeslee, T., *The Right Brain; A new understanding of the unconscious mind and its powers,* London, Macmillan

Bromberg, J. J., *Fasting Girls*, Massachusetts, Harvard University Press, 1988

Brown, G. W., Harris, T., *Social Origins of Depression; A study of psychiatric disorders in women*, London, Tavistock, 1978

Buchbauer, G., Jirovetz, I., Jager, W., Dietrich, H., Plack, C., 'Aromatherapy: evidence for sedative effects of the essential oil of lavender after inhalation', Zeitschrift fur Naturforschung, Section C, *Journal of Biosciences*, Nov-Dec 1991, **46**, pp 11–12, pp 1067–72

Buchbauer, G., 'Biological effects of Fragrance and Essential oils', *Perfumer & Flavorist*, 1993, **18**, pp 19–23

Buchbauer, G., Jirovetz, I., Jager, W., 'Aromatherapy: Evidence for Sedative Effects of the Essential Oil of Lavender after Inhalation', Institute of Pharmaceutical Chemistry, University of Vienna, 1991

Buchbauer, G., Jirovetz, I., Jager, W., 'Kurzmitteilungen: Passiflora and Lime Blossoms: Motility Effects after Inhalation of the Essential oils and of some of the Main

Constituents in Animal Experiment', *Aech. Pharm. (Weinheim)*, 1992, **325**, pp 247–8

Budlong, Ware T., *Performing Plants*, New York, Simon & Schuster, 1969

Burbank, L., *The Training of the Human Plant*, New York, Century Co, 1907

Burbank, L., *How Plants are Trained to Work for Man*, New York, P. F. Collier & Son, 1921

Capeland, I., Gurnsey, J., *Managing Stress*, London, Constable & Company Ltd, 1987

Chase, T., *When Rabbits Howl*, London, Pan Books, 1987

Chopra, Deepak, *Perfect Health*, London, Bantam Books, 1990

Cousins, N., *Anatomy of an Illness as Perceived by the Patient: Reflections on healing and regeneration*, London/New York, Bantam, 1981

Dally, P., Watkins, M. J., *Psychology and Psychiatry*, Sevenoaks, Hodder & Stoughton, 1986

Dimoff, T., Carper, S., *How to tell if your kids are on drugs*, New York, Facts and File Inc, 1992

Dossetor, D. R., Couryer, S. and Nicol, A. R., 'Massage for severe self-injurious behaviour in a girl with Cornelia de Lange syndrome', *Developmental Medicine & Child Neurology*, July 1991, **33(7)**, pp 636–40

Doty, R., Reyes, P., Gregor, T., 'Presence of both odor identification and detection in Alzheimer's Disease', *Brain Res Bull*, 1987, **18**, p 598

Dowden, A. O., T*he Secret Life of Flowers*, New York, Odyssey Press, 1964

Dryden, W., *Rational Emotive Counselling in Action*, London, Sage Publications 1990

Duraffourd, P., *The Best of Health: Thanks to Essential Oils*, Perigny, La Vie Clair, 1984

Dywer, J., *The Body at War*, London, Unwin Hyman, 1988

Ehrlichman, H., Bastone, L., 'Odor experience as an affective state: Effects of odor pleasantness on cognition', *Perfumer & Flavorist*, 1991, **16**, pp 11–12

Ehrlichman, H., Bastone, L., 'Olfaction and Emotion' in: Serby, M. J., Chobor, K. L. (eds) *Science of Olfaction*, 1992,

Springer-Verlag, New York, pp 410–17

Ehrlichman, H., Halpern, J. N., 'Affect and Memory: Effects of Pleasant and Unpleasant Odors on Retrieval of Happy and Unhappy Memories', *Journal of Personality and Social Psychology*, 1988, **55**, pp 769–79

England, Marjorie A., Wakely, Jennifer, *A Colour Atlas of the Brain and Spinal Cord*, London, Wolfe Publishing, 1991

Fakouri, C., Joners, P., 'Relaxation RX: slow stroke back rub', *Journal of Gerontological Nursing*, Feb 1987, **13(2)**; pp 32–5

Field, T. *et al.*, 'Massage reduces anxiety in child and adolescent psychiatric patients', *J Am Acad Child Adolesc Psychiatry*, 1992, **31(1)**, pp 125–31

Forward, S., *Toxic Parents*, London, Bantam Press, 1990

Franchomme, P., Pénoël, D., *L'aromatherapie Exactement*, Limoges, Roger Jollois Editeur, 1990

Fraser, J., Kerr, J. R., 'Psychophysiological effects of back massage on elderly institutionalized patients', *Journal of Advanced Nursing*, 1993, **18(2)**, pp 238–45

Fredrickson, R., *Repressed Memories*, New York, Fireside Publications, 1992

Gardner, H., *The Shattered Mind*, London, Routledge & Kegan Paul, 1977

Gattefosse, R. M., *Aromatherapy*, Saffron Walden, C. W. Daniel, 1993

Gatti, G., 'L'azione delle essenze sul sistema nervosa', Cayola, *Rivista Italiana Essenza e Perfumi*, 1923, **5(12)**

Giannitrapani, D., *The Electrophysiology of Intellectual Functions*, Basel, Karger, 1985

Gilling, D., Brightwell, R., *The Human Brain*, London, Orbis Publishing Ltd, 1982

Graham, H., *Time Energy and Psychology of Healing*, London, Jessica Kingly, 1990

Grieve, M., *A Modern Herbal*, London, Jonathan Cape, 1979

Grof, Stanislav, M.D., *The Holotropic Mind*, Harper, San Francisco, 1990

Grof, Stanislav, M.D., *The Adventure of Self-Discovery*, New York, State University Press, 1988

Guenther, E., *The Essential Oils*, 4 vols, 1948–52

Guillemain, J., Rousseau, A., Delaveau, P., 'Neurodepressive effects of the essential oil of Lavendula angustifolia Mill', *Annales Pharmaceutiques Francaises*, 1989, **6**, pp 337–43

Hall, M. P., *The Mystical and Medical Philosophy of Paracelsus*, Philosophical Research Society, Los Angeles, 1969

Harris, B., Lewis, R., 'Psychophysiological effects of odour', Part 1–2, *International Journal of Alternative & Complementary Medicine*, Jan/March, 1994

Hassett, J., White, K. M., *Psychology in Perspective*, New York, Harper & Row, 1989

Hernandez-Peon, R., Lavin, A., Alcocer-Cuaro, C., Marcelin, J. P., 'Electrical activity of the olfactory bulb during wakefulness and sleep', *EEG Clinical Neurophysiology*, 1960, **12**, pp 41–58

Hirsch, A. R., Trannel, T. J., *Depression and Chemosensory Dysfunction*, Chicago, Smell & Taste Treatment and Research Foundation Ltd

Hirsch, A. R., 'Olfaction and Psychiatry', 144th Annual Meeting, American Psychiatric Association, New Orleans, LA, 16 May 1991

Hirsch, A. R., 'Nostalgia, the odors of childhood and society', *The Psychiatric Times: Medicine and behaviour*, August 1992, p 29

Hirsch, A. R., 'Olfaction and Anxiety', *Clinical Psychiatry*, 1993, **16**, p 4

Hirsch, A. R., Gay, S. E., 'Effect of Ambient Olfactory Stimuli on the Evaluation of a Common Consumer Product', *Chem. Senses*, 1991, **5**, p 535

Hope, M., *The Psychology of Healing*, London, Element Books, 1989

Hopkins, S. J., *Principle Drugs*, London, Faber & Faber, 1988

Jacobsen, C. F., 'Electrical measurements of neuromuscular states during mental activities: imagination involving skeletal muscle', *American Journal of Physiology*, **91**, pp 597–608

Jager, W., Buchbauer, G., Jirovetz L., Fritzer, M., 'Percutaneous Absorption of Lavender Oil from a Massage Oil', *J Soc Cosmet*, 1992, **43**, pp 49–54

Jones, P. F., Hanson, A. J., Grey, E. F., 'Startle as a paradigm of malposture'

Jori, A., Bianchetti, Prestini, P. E., 'Effects of Essential Oils on Drug Metabolism', *Biochemical Pharmacology,* 1969, **18**, pp 2081–5

Kaada B., Torsteinbo O., 'Increase of plasma beta-endorphins in connective tissue', *General Pharmacology*, 1989, **20(4)**, pp 487–9

Keeny, B. P., *Aesthetics of Change*, London, Guildford Press 1983

Kirk-Smith, M. D., Van Toller, S., Dodd, G. H., 'Unconscious odour conditioning in human subjects', *Biol Psychol*, 1983, **17**: pp 221–31

Klemm, W. R., Lutes, S. D., Hendrix D. V., Warrenburg S., 'Topographical EEG maps of human responses to odors', *Chemical Senses,* 1992, **17**, 3, pp 347–61

Kline, N., Rausch, J., 'Olfactory precipitants of Flashbacks in Post Traumatic Stress Disorders: Case Reports', *Journal of Clinical Psychiatry,* 1985, **46**, pp 383–4

Knasko, S. C., 'Ambient odor and shopping behaviour', *A Chem*, S-XI, 1989

Knasko, S. C., 'Ambient Odor's effect on creativity, mood and perceived health', *Chemical Senses* 1992, **17**, 1, pp 27–35

Knasko, S. C., Gilbert, A. N., Sabini, J., 'Emotional State, Physical Well-Being, and Performance in the Presence of Feined Ambient Odor', *Journal of Applied Social Psychology*, 1990, **20**, pp 1345–57

Kobal, G., Hummal, T., 'Olfactory evoked potentials' in: Getchell, T. V. *et al.* (eds), *Smell and Taste in Health and Disease*, New York, Raven Press, pp 255–75

Koob, G. F., 'Neuropeptides and Memory' in: Iversen, I. I., Iversen, S. D., Snyder, S. H. (eds). *Handbook of Psychopharmacology*, Plenum Press, New York, 1987, p. 532

Kreig, M. B., *Green Medicine*, London, George Harrap, 1964 (New York, Rand McNally, 1964)

Kuipeis, L., Bebbington, P., *Living with Mental Illness*, London, Souvenir Press Ltd, 1987

Landis, C., Hunt, A. W., *The Startle Pattern*, New York, Farrar & Rinehart, 1939

Landis, C., Hunt, A.W., *Perceptual and Motor Skills,* 1964, 19, pp 21–2

Langland, R. M., Panicucci, E., 'Effects of touch on communication with elderly confused patients', *Journal of Gerontology and Nursing*, 1982, **8(3)**, pp 152–5

Lautie, R., Passebecq, A., *Aromatherapy*, Wellingborough, Thorson, 1979

Lavabre, M., *Aromatherapy Workbook*, Rochester, Healing Arts Press, 1990

Lawrence, B., *Essential Oils*, 3 vols, 1976–87

Lee, C., *Safety Guide on the Use of Essential Oils*, London, Nature by Nature Ltd, 1993

Lele, R., *Ayurveda and Modern Science*, Bombay, Brharatiya Vida Bhavan, 1986

Lewis, D., *Fight Your Phobia and Win*, London, Sheldon Press, 1984

Linskens, H. F., Jackson, J. F, (ed) *Essential Oils and Waxes*, Vol 2, New York, Springer Verlag, 1991

Lis-Balchin, Dr M., *Aroma Science, The Chemistry and Bioactivity of Essential Oils,* East Horsley, Amberwood Publishing Ltd, 1995

Loehr, Franklin, *The Powers of Prayer on Plants*, New York, Signet Books, 1969

Long, T. S., Huffman, E., Demartino, A. B., Demarco, J., 'EEG and Behavioural Responses to Low-level Galaxolide Administration', *Assoc. Chemoreception Sci. Ann. Meet.*, 1989, Sarasota, Fla, USA

Lorenzetti, B. B., Souza, G. E., Sarti, S. J., Santos, Filho, D., Ferreira, S.H., 'Myrcene mimics the peripheral analgesic activity of Lemongrass tea', *Journal of Enthnopharmacology*, 1991, **34(1)**: pp 43–8

Lorig, T. S., Schwartch, G. E., Brain and odor 11: 'EEG alpha activity during administration of perceptually similar odors', *Psychophysiology*, 1987, **24**, p 599

Lowen, A., *Bioenergetics*, London, Penguin Books, 1976

Ludvigson, H. W., Rottman, T. R., 'Effects of Ambient Odors of Lavender and Cloves on Cognition, Memory, Affect and Mood', *Chem. Senses*, 1989, **14**, pp 525–36

Luscher, Max, *Luscher/Colour Test* (trans. Ian Scott), London,

Pan Books, 1971

McCaffery, M., Wolff, M., 'Pain relief using cutaneous modalities, positioning, and movement', *Hospice Journal*, 1992, **8(1–2)**, pp 121–53

McKechnie, A. A., Wilson, F., Watson, N., Scott, D., 'Anxiety states; a preliminary report on the value of connective tissue massage', *Journal of Psychosomatic Research*, 1983, **27(2)**, pp 125–9

MacLean, P. D., 'The Limbic system (Visceral Brain) incidence of interdependent and emotional processes', *Psychosomatic Medicine*, **42**

Mair, R. G., Harrison, L. M., 'Influence of Drugs on Smell Function' in: Laing, D. G., Doty, R. L., Preipohl, W. (eds), *Human Sense of Smell*, 1991, Springer-Verlag, Berlin

Manley, C. H., 'Psychophysiological Effect of Odor', *Critical Reviews in Food and Sciences and Nutrition*, 1993, **33(1)**, pp 57–62

Maslow, A., *Towards a Psychology of Being*, New York, Van Nostrand Reinhold, 1966

Maury, M., *The Secret of Life and Youth*, London, Macdonald & Co, 1964

Meek, S. S., 'Effects of slow stroke back massage on relaxation in hospice patients', *Image – The Journal of Nursing Scholarship*, 1993 **25(1)**, pp 17–21

Melody, P., Miller, A. W., Miller, J. K., *Facing Codependence*, San Francisco, Perennial Library, Harpers & Row, 1989

Melville, A., Johnson, C., *Cured to Death*, London, Secker & Warburg Ltd, 1982

Melzig, M., Teucsher, E., 'Investigations of the influence of essential oils and their main components on the adenosine uptake by cultivated endothelial cells', *Planta Med*, Feb 1991, **57(1)**, pp 41–2

Milne, I., Milne, M., *The Nature of Plants*, Philadelphia, B. Lippincott, 1971

Morton, I., Hall, J., Halliday, J., *Tranquillizers*, London, Bloomsbury, 1991

Moyers, Bill, *Healing and the Mind*, London, Thorsons, 1993

Naranjo, Claudio, *Ennea-Type Structures*, Nevada City, Gateways/IDHHB, 1990

Nwaiwu J. L., Akah, P. A., 'Anticonvulsant activity of the volatile oil from the fruit of Tetrapleura tetraptera', *Journal of Ethnopharmacology*, 1986, **18(2)**, pp 103–7

Oldfield, Harry, Coghill, Roger, *The Dark Side of the Brain*, Shaftesbury, Element Books, 1988

Ornstien, R., Sobel D., *The Healing Brain*, London, Macmillan, 1988

Ortiz de Urbina, A. V., Martin, M. L. Montero, M. J., Moran, A., San Roman L., 'Sedating and antipyretic activity of the essential oil of Calamintha sylvatica subsp. ascendens', *Journal of Ethnopharmacology*, 1989, **25(2)**, pp 165–71

Pelletier, K., *Mind as Slayer, Mind as Healer*, London, Allen & Unwin, 1987

Penoel, D., Penoel, R., *Pratique Aromatique Familiale*, Aouste-sur-sye, Osmobiose, 1992

Perls, F. S., *The Gestalt Approach and Eye Witness to Therapy*, London, Bantam, 1976

Pustjarvi, K., Airaksinen, O., Pontinen, P. J., 'The effects of massage in patients with chronic tension headache', *Acupuncture & Electro-Therapeutics Research*, 1990, **15(2)**, pp 159–62

Ratsch, C., *Sacred and Magical Plants*, A. Hofmann, Trans. Dorset, Prism Press, 1992

Redd, W. H., Mann, S. L., *Fragrance Administration to Reduce Patient Anxiety During Magnet Resonance Imaging in Cancer Diagnosis Work-Up*, Memorial Sloane-Kettering Cancer Center, New York

Reed, B. V., Held, J. M., 'Effects of sequential connective tissue massage on autonomic nervous system of middle aged and elderly adults', *Physical Therapy*, 1988, **68 (8)**, pp 1231–4

Reese, A. J. M., *The Principles of Pathology*, London, Boston, Wright PSG, 1987

Rhoades, Robert E., 'The World's Food Supply at Risk', *National Geographic*, April 1991

Ridley, H. N., *Spices*, London, Macmillan & Co, 1983

Riordan, J., Whitmore, B., *Living with Dementia*, New York, Manchester University Press, 1990

Riso, Don Richard, *The Practical Guide to Personality Types*,

London, Aquarian/HarperCollins, 1991

Riso, Don Richard, *Personality Types*, London, Aquarian/HarperCollins, 1987

Roberts, A., 'Alzheimer's disease may begin in the nose and may be caused by Aluminosilicates', *Neuro-biol Aging*, 1986, **7**, pp 561–67

Rovesti, P., *In Search of Perfumes Lost*, Venice, 1980

Royal, D., *The Human Side to Plants*, New York, Frederick A. Stokes Co, 1914

Royal, D. and Fitch, F. E., *Personality of Plants*, New York, Bouilon-Biggs, 1923

Russell, P., *The Brain Book*, London, Routledge & Kegan Paul, 1990

Sacks, O., *Migraine*, London, Faber & Faber, 1991

Schaef, Anne Wilson, *Beyond Therapy, Beyond Science*, San Francisco, Harper

Schilcher, H., 'Effects and side-effects of Essential Oils', Baerheim Svenden and Scheffer (eds), *Essential Oils and Aromatic Plants*, The Netherlands, Dr Junk Publishers, 1985

Schultes, Richard Evans, Hofmann, Albert, *Plants of the Gods*, Rochester, Healing Arts Press, 1992

Schwing, G., *A Way to the Souls of the Mentally Ill*, New York, International Press, 1954

Selgman, M. E. P., *Helplessness*, San Francisco, Freeman & Company, 1975.

Serby, M., Corwin, J., Novatt, A., Conrad, P., Rotrosen, J., 'Olfaction in dementia', *Journal Neurol-neurosurg Psychiatry*, 1985, **48**, p 849

Sharma, Pandit Shiv (ed), *Realms of Ayurveda*, New Delhi, Arnold-Heinemann, 1979

Sheldrake, R. A., *A New Lease of Life*, London, Granada, 1988

Siegel, B. S., *Love, Medicine and Miracles*, London, Rider, 1986

Silverman, A. F., Pressman M. E., Bartel, H. W., 'Self-esteem and tactile communication', *Journal of Humanistic Psychology*, 1973, **13**, pp 73–7

Springer, S. P., Deusch, G., *Left Brain, Right Brain*, New York, 1989

Stanford, T. L., *Strong at the Broken Places*, London, Virago Press Ltd, 1991

Stern, J. A., Brown, M., Ulet, G. H., Stellen, I., 'A Comparison of Hypnosis, Acupuncture, Morphine, Valium, Aspirin and Placebo in the Management of Expression of Experimentally Induced Pain', Annals of New York Academy of Science, 1987, **296**, pp 175–93

Stoddart, D. Michael, *The Scented Ape*, Cambridge University Press, 1990

Stone, H., Winkelman, S., *Embracing Ourselves: The voice dialogue manual*, San Rafael, California, New World Library, 1989

Sugano, H., 'Effects of Odors on Mental Function (Abstract)', JASTS, XX11, 1988, p 8

Synge, Patrick, *Plants with Personality*, London, Lindsay Drummond Ltd, 1939

Talbot, Michael, *The Holographic Universe*, New York, HarperCollins, 1991

Taylor, J. E., *The Sagacity and Morality of Plants*, London, Chatto & Windus, 1884

Tecces, J. J., Scheff, N. M., 'Attention reduction and suppressed direct-current potentials in the human brain', *Science*, 1969, **164**, p 331

Thompson, Richard F., *The Brain*, New York, W. H. Freeman and Co, 1993

Tisserand, R., *Aromatherapy for Everyone*, London, Arkana, 1988

Tisserand, R., *The Safety Data Manual*, Brighton Association of Tisserand Aromatherapists, 1985

Torri, S., Fukuda, H., Kanemoto, H., Miyanchi, R., Hamauzu, Y., Kawasaki, M., 'Contingent Negative Variation (CNV) and the Psychological Effects of Odour' in: Van Toller, S., Dodd, G. H., (eds), *Perfumery: Psychology and Biology of Fragrance*, Chapman and Hall, New York, pp 107–120

Turner, P., Richens, A., Routledge, P., *Clinical Pharmacology*, London, Churchill Livingstone, 1986

Uphof, J. C., *Dictionary of Economic Plants*, New York, Verlag, Von J. Cramer 1968

Valnet, J., Duraffourd, C., Lapraz, J. C., *Phytotherapy &*

Aromatherapy, Paris Presse de la Renaissance, 1978

Valnet, J., *The Practice of Aromatherapy*, Saffron Walden, C. W. Daniel Company Ltd, 1982

Van Toller, S., 'Odours, emotion and psychophysiology', *International Journal of Cosmetic Science*, **10**, pp 171–97

Van Toller, S., Dodd, G. H., *Perfumery: The psychology and biology of fragrance*, London, Chapman and Hall, 1988

Van Toller, S., Dodd, G. H., *Fragrance: The Psychology and Biology of Perfume*, London, Elsevier Science Publishers, 1992

Viaud, H., Dufour, D., *Huiles essentielles-hydrolats; Distillation qualite controle de la purete indications majeures*, Sisteron, Editions Presence, 1983

Walker, J. T., 'The Anxious Patient', *Journal of Family Practitioners*, 1981, **12**, pp 733–8

Walker, M., *Dirty Medicine*, London, Slingshot Publications, 1993

Warm, J. S., Dember, W. N., Parasuraman, R., 'Effect of Olfactory Stimulation on performance and stress in a visual sustained attention task', *Journal of Cosmetic Chem.*, 1991, **42**, pp 199–210

Watson, Lyall, *Supernature*, London, Coronet/Hodder Paperbacks, 1974

Watt, M., *Plant Aromatics Data and Reference Manual*, Essex, Watt, 1991

Weinrich, S. P., Weinrich, M. C., 'The effect of massage on pain in cancer patients', *Applied Nursing Research*, 1990, **3(4)**, pp 140–5

Weisskopf-Joelsov E., *Father I have kept my promise*, Purdue Research Foundation, 1988

West, M., 'Meditation', *British Journal of Psychiatry*, 1979, **135**, pp 457–69

Wilson, Glen, *Your Personality and Potential*, Topsfield, MA, Salem House Publishers, 1989

Wilson, M., *Crossing the Boundaries*, London, Virago Press, 1993

Woolger, Roger J., *Other Lives, Other Selves*, New York, Dolphin/Doubleday, 1987

Worwood, V. A., *Fragrant Sensuality*, London, Bantam

Books, 1996 (previously published as *Aromantics*, 1987)

Worwood, V. A., *The Fragrant Pharmacy*, London, Bantam Books, 1990

Wren, R. C., revised Williamson, E. M., Evans F. J., *Potters New Cyclopaedia of Botanical Drugs and Preparations*, Saffron Walden, C. W. Daniel Company Ltd, 1989

Youngken, H. W., *Pharmaceutical Botany*, Dehra, R. P. Singh, 1986

INDEX

NOTE: Page numbers in bold refer to illustrations

Valerie Ann Worwood is internationally acknowledged as one of the world's leading aromatherapists. Awarded a Doctorate in 1990, she has served on the executive councils of the International Federation of Aromatherapists and The Aromatherapy Organisations Council, and has initiated research projects into the clinical use of essential oils.